Nursing
NONPRESCRIPTION
DRUG
HANDBOOK

Nursing NONPRESCRIPTION DRUG HANDBOOK

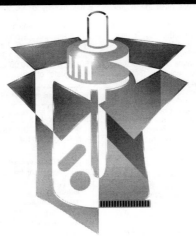

Springhouse Corporation
Springhouse, Pennsylvania

Staff

Editorial Director
William J. Kelly

Clinical Director
Marguerite S. Ambrose, RN, MSN, CS

Creative Director
Jake Smith

Art Director
Elaine Kasmer

Senior Associate Editor
Ann E. Houska

Clinical Project Editor
Eileen Cassin Gallen, RN, BSN

Drug Information Editor
Melissa M. Devlin, PharmD

Editors
Rita M. Doyle, Catherine E. Harold,
Audrey S. Hughes

Clinical Editors
Christine M. Damico, RN, MSN, CPNP;
Nancy LaPlante, RN, BSN;
Pamela S. Messer, RN, MSN;
Kimberly A. Zalewski, RN, MSN

Copy Editor
Leslie Dworkin

Designers
Arlene Putterman (associate art director),
Joseph John Clark, Jan Greenberg,
Donald G. Knauss

Manufacturing
Pat Dorshaw (manager), Beth Janae Orr

Electronic Production Services
Joy Rossi Biletz, Diane Paluba (manager)

Editorial Assistants
Carol A. Caputo, Arlene Claffee,
Danielle Jan Barsky

Indexer
Deborah K. Tourtlotte

Visit our Web site at NDHnow.com.

NNPDH- D N O S A J J M A M
04 03   10 9 8 7 6 5 4 3 2
ISBN 1-58255-101-4

Library of Congress Cataloging-in-Publication Data
Nursing nonprescription drug handbook.
    p.; cm.
    Includes index.
    1. Drugs, Nonprescription – Handbooks, manuals,
etc. 2. Nursing – Handbooks, manuals, etc.
I. Lippincott Williams & Wilkins. Springhouse
Division.
    [DNLM: 1. Drugs, Non-Prescription – Handbooks.
2. Drugs, Non-Prescription – Nurses' Instruction.
QV 735 N974 2001]
RM671.A1 N87 2001
615'.1—dc21   2001045721
ISBN 1-58255-101-4 (casebound)

Contents

Drug updates and news   NDHnow.com

Contributors and consultants

Tricia M. Berry, RPh, PharmD
Assistant Professor of Pharmacy
　Practice
St. Louis College of Pharmacy
St. Louis

Cheryl L. Brady, RN, MSN
Instructor
Kent State University
East Liverpool, Ohio

Michael Briggs, RPh, PharmD
Pharmacist, Co-owner
Lionville Natural Pharmacy
Exton, Pa.

Darlene Nebel Cantu, RNC, MSN
Director
Baptist Health System School of
　Professional Nursing
San Antonio, Tex.

Lawrence Carey, PharmD
Clinical Pharmacist Supervisor
Jefferson Home Infusion Service
Philadelphia

Elizabeth Chester, PharmD
Clinical Pharmacy Specialist,
　Primary Care
Kaiser Permanente, Colorado
Aurora, Colo.

Linda M. Eugenio Clark,
RPh, PharmD
Assistant Professor of Clinical
　Pharmacy
Massachusetts College of
　Pharmacy and Health Sciences
Boston

Jason C. Cooper, PharmD
Pharmacist
Bon Secours St. Francis Hospital
Charleston, S.C.

Ami Dansby, RPh
Pharmacist, Natural Medicine
　Consultant
Bruce's Pharmacy
Charlottesville, Va.

Tatyana Gurvich, PharmD
Clinical Pharmacologist
Glendale Adventist Family
　Practice Program
Glendale, Calif.

Nancy Hutton Haynes,
RN, MN, CCRN
Assistant Professor of Nursing
Saint Luke's College
Kansas City, Mo.

Jennifer H. Justice, PharmD
Clinical Assistant Professor of
　Pharmacy Practice
West Virginia University
Charleston, W.Va.

Julia N. Kleckner, PharmD
Pharmacy Manager
Option Care
Upper Darby, Pa.

Nancy L. Gindele Kranzley,
RN, MS
Pulmonary Clinical Nurse
　Specialist
The Christ Hospital
Cincinnati

Kristi L. Lenz, PharmD
Oncology Clinical Specialist and
　Assistant Professor
Medical University of South
　Carolina
Charleston, S.C.

John S. Markowitz, PharmD, BCPP
Assistant Professor, Department of
  Pharmaceutical Services
Medical University of South
  Carolina
Charleston, S.C.

Dawna Martich, RN, MSN
Clinical Trainer and Recruiter
American Healthways
Pittsburgh

Pamela Messer, RN, MSN
Drug Safety Surveillance Manager
AstraZeneca
Wilmington

Jolynne Myers, RNCS, MSN,
MSEd, ARNP
Adult Nurse Practitioner
Consultants in Gastroenterology
Independence, Mo.

Steven G. Ottariano,
RPh, BS Pharm
Clinical Staff Pharmacist
Veterans Affairs Medical Center
Manchester, N.H.

Robert Lee Page II, PharmD
Assistant Professor of Pharmacy
University of Colorado Health
  Sciences Center, School of
  Pharmacy
Denver

Susan Markel Poole, RN, BSN, MS,
CRNI, CNSN
Senior Director, Professional
  Services
Option Care, Inc.
Bannockburn, Ill.

Lorraine Flint Rother,
RN, MS, CNS
Clinical Specialist, Psychiatry
Department of Veterans Affairs,
  Palo Alto Health Care System
San Jose, Calif.

Cynthia A. Ruiz, PharmD
Assistant Professor of Pharmacy
  Practice
St. Louis College of Pharmacy
St. Louis

Marcia Silkroski, RD, CNSD
Owner, Clinical Director
Nutrition Advantage
Chester Springs, Pa.

Gary Smith, PharmD
Manager, Clinical Pharmacy
  Services
Fairview Physician Associates
Edina, Minn.

Kathleen M. Speer, RN, PhD, CPNP
Pediatric Nurse Practitioner
Children's Medical Center
Dallas

Barbara Strande, RN, MSN
Assistant Professor
Western Kentucky University,
  Department of Nursing
Bowling Green, Ky.

Allison J. Terry, RN, MSN
Staff Nurse
Central Alabama Veterans Health
  Care System
Montgomery, Ala.

Laurie Willhite, RPh, PharmD
Clinical Pharmacy Specialist,
  Clinical Assistant Professor
Fairview University Medical
  Center
Minneapolis

How to use this book

Nursing Nonprescription Drug Handbook, created by many of the same pharmacists and nurses who create *Nursing Drug Handbook*, provides information about the OTC drugs your patients are using. You'll learn about the therapeutic uses of OTC drugs, the interactions between OTC drug ingredients and prescription drugs, and more. The consistent format and helpful features of the book make the content readily accessible and easy to use.

Features

This handbook contains many features to enhance nursing knowledge and skills:
• Tables that show the route, onset, peak, and duration of each drug
• *Alert* logos that provide cautionary tips for avoiding common medication errors and draw your attention to drug names that sound alike or look alike
• An Interactions section that points out interactions between the OTC drug and other drugs, herbs, foods, and lifestyle behaviors
• Appendices that include ingredients found in combination OTC drugs, patient-teaching aids, sugar-free OTC drugs,

sunblocks, OTC multivitamin comparisons, oral rehydration solution components, OTC drug resources, and more
• Comprehensive index featuring generic names, trade names, therapeutic uses, indications, and combination products
• Drug updates and news on NDHnow.com

Introductory chapters

Chapter 1 explains what an OTC drug is and how important it is to find out which OTC drugs your patient is taking. It also discusses who uses OTC drugs and offers consumer safety information from the Food and Drug Administration (FDA) to pass on to your patients. The chapter also covers drug tampering and label requirements. Chapter 2 defines generic drugs and reviews FDA standards for approval of the three generic drug divisions—prescription, prescription-to-OTC, and OTC. It also lists the various categories and applications of generic OTC drugs.

Body system chapters

Chapters 3 through 8 classify all drugs according to the body system they affect. Each of these body system chapters includes an introductory section, a drug monograph section, and a combination drug table.

The introductory section provides general information on the normal anatomy of the body system. You'll also find information on common conditions affecting the body system, including the pathophysiology, signs and symptoms, possible serious conditions, complications if the symptoms go untreated, nursing considerations, and patient teaching information.

Alphabetized drug monographs follow the introductory section. Each monograph includes brand names; pregnancy risk category; how the drug is supplied; drug action with route, onset, peak, and duration; indications and dosages; adverse reactions; interactions with other drugs and with herbs, foods, and lifestyle behaviors; contraindications for taking the drug; overdose and treatment instructions; nursing considerations, including *Alert* warnings when applicable; and patient teaching tips.

Following the drug monographs is a table that reviews combination OTC drugs that include one or more of the drugs covered in the chapter—along with other ingredients. Combination drug tables include brand name and active ingredients, indications and dosages, and nursing considerations for these products.

Nutrition and miscellaneous drugs

Chapter 9 covers OTC products that affect nutrition, such as vitamins and other dietary supplements. Chapter 10 includes OTC products (such as insulin) that don't fit easily into any one body system chapter. These chapters contain introductory sections and drug monographs only.

Drug monographs

The drug monographs in each chapter are alphabetized by generic name. Following each generic name is a list of brand names, if applicable.

Brand names that are specifically Canadian are designated with a dagger (†); those that are specifically Australian are followed by a double dagger (‡); and those that are specifically British are followed by a section mark (§). A brand name with no symbol is available in the United States, Canada, and possibly Australia and the United Kingdom (U.K.). The mention of a brand name in no way implies endorsement of that product or guarantees its legality.

Some liquid OTC drugs contain alcohol. Although the slight sedative effect that alcohol produces isn't harmful for most patients, alcohol ingestion can be undesirable and even dangerous for some patients. Oral drugs that contain alcohol should be taken cautiously, if at all, by children and patients such as these:

• patients who take potent CNS depressants such as barbiturates

• patients who take drugs that may produce a disulfiram-type reaction (such as chlopropamide or metronidazole)

• patients who take disulfiram as part of a treatment program for alcoholism. Such patients, upon ingestion of alcohol, will develop severe signs or symptoms that may include blurred vision, confusion, dyspnea, flushing, sweating, and tachycardia.

To help prevent inadvertent alcohol consumption, the text signals alcohol content with a single asterisk (*) after each brand name of a liquid drug that contains it. In many of these drugs, the alcohol content is small. Nevertheless, these drugs should be avoided by patients susceptible to adverse effects after exposure to alcohol.

Each systemically absorbed drug has been assigned a pregnancy risk category based on available clinical and preclinical information. (See *Pregnancy risk categories,* page xii.) Although drugs are best avoided during pregnancy, this rating system lets you rapidly assess the risk-to-benefit ratio of a particular drug. Drugs in category A are generally considered safe to use in pregnancy; drugs in category X are contraindicated.

How supplied

This section lists the forms available for each drug (for example, tablets, capsules), specifying available dosage forms and strengths. Strengths specifically available in Canada are designated with a dagger (†), those available in Australia with a double dagger (‡), and those in the U.K. with a section mark (§).

Action

This section succinctly describes the mechanism of action—that is, how the drug provides its therapeutic effect. For example, although all antihypertensives lower blood pressure, they don't all do so by the same pharmacologic process.

Pregnancy risk categories

The Food and Drug Administration assigns the following categories to reflect a drug's potential to cause birth defects.

- A: Adequate studies in pregnant women have failed to show a risk to the fetus.
- B: Animal studies have not shown a risk to the fetus, but controlled studies have not been conducted in pregnant women; or animal studies have shown an adverse effect on the fetus, but adequate studies in pregnant women have not shown a risk to the fetus.
- C: Animal studies have shown an adverse effect on the fetus, but adequate studies have not been conducted in humans. The benefits from use in pregnant women may be acceptable despite potential risks.
- D: The drug may cause risk to the human fetus, but the potential benefits of use in pregnant women may be acceptable despite the risks (such as in a life-threatening situation or a serious disease for which safer drugs can't be used or are ineffective).
- X: Studies in animals or humans show fetal abnormalities, or adverse reaction reports indicate evidence of fetal risk. The risks involved clearly outweigh potential benefits.
- NR: Not rated.

Also included in table form is the route, onset, peak (described in terms of effect or peak blood level), and duration of drug action, if data are available or applicable. Values listed are for patients with normal renal function, unless otherwise specified.

Indications & dosages

This section lists general dosage information for adults, children, and special patient populations, as applicable. Dosage directions reflect the therapeutic directions on OTC package inserts and standard clinical references, but they shouldn't be considered as absolute recommendations.

Adverse reactions

This section lists adverse reactions to each drug by body system. The most common adverse reactions are in *italic* type; reactions that are less common are in roman type. Life-threatening adverse reactions are in ***bold italic*** type; and reactions that are common *and* life-threatening are in **BOLD CAPITAL LETTERS**.

Interactions

This section lists each drug's clinically significant interactions with other drugs, herbs, foods, and lifestyle behaviors, detailing additive, potentiated, and antagonistic effects, as applicable. Drug interactions are listed under the drug that is adversely affected. To check on the possible effects of using two or more drugs at the same time, refer to the interaction entry for each of the drugs in question.

Contraindications

This section lists any conditions, especially diseases, for which the use of the drug is undesirable, unwarranted, or dangerous.

Overdose & treatment

This section explains the signs and symptoms a patient experiences when he takes an overdose of the drug, followed by the treatment needed to counteract the overdose.

Nursing considerations

This section lists recommendations for cautious use of the drug, along with other useful information about the drug, such as suggestions for preventing and treating adverse reactions.

An *Alert* logo signals cautionary tips to help you and your patients avoid medication errors.

Patient teaching

This section focuses on teaching your patient how to use the drug safely and effectively. It includes steps for preparing the drug, adverse reactions to watch for, developments that should be reported to a doctor, and more.

Photoguide to tablets and capsules

This full-color photoguide includes the most commonly used OTC tablets and capsules in the United States, to make drug identification easier for nurses and to enhance patient safety. The drugs are arranged alphabetically by brand name for quick reference, and the most common dosage strengths are shown.

Guide to abbreviations

ACE	angiotensin-converting enzyme	FDA	Food and Drug Administration
ACTH	adrenocorticotropic hormone	g	gram
		G	gauge
ADH	antidiuretic hormone	GFR	glomerular filtration rate
AIDS	acquired immuno-deficiency syndrome	GGT	gamma-glutamyltransferase
ALT	alanine transaminase		
AST	aspartate transaminase	GI	gastrointestinal
AV	atrioventricular	gtt	drops
b.i.d.	twice daily	GU	genitourinary
BPH	benign prostatic hypertrophy	G6PD	glucose-6-phosphate dehydrogenase
BSA	body surface area	H_1	histamine$_1$
BUN	blood urea nitrogen	H_2	histamine$_2$
cAMP	cyclic adenosine monophosphate	HbA_{1c}	glycosylated hemoglo-bin
CBC	complete blood count	HIV	human immuno-deficiency virus
CK	creatine kinase		
CMV	cytomegalovirus	HNKC	hyperosmolar non-ketotic coma
CNS	central nervous system		
COPD	chronic obstructive pul-monary disease	h.s.	at bedtime
		I.D.	intradermal
CSF	cerebrospinal fluid	I.M.	intramuscular
CV	cardiovascular	INR	international normal-ized ratio
CVA	cerebrovascular accident		
		IPPB	intermittent positive-pressure breathing
D_5W	dextrose 5% in water		
DIC	disseminated intravas-cular coagulopathy	IU	international unit
		I.V.	intravenous
DKA	diabetic ketoacidosis	kg	kilogram
dl	deciliter	l	liter
DNA	deoxyribonucleic acid	LD	lactate dehydrogenase
ECG	electrocardiogram	M	molar
EEG	electroencephalogram	m^2	square meter
EENT	eyes, ears, nose, throat	MAO	monoamine oxidase

mcg	microgram	SIADH	syndrome of inappro-priate antidiuretic hormone
mEq	milliequivalent		
mg	milligram		
MI	myocardial infarction	S.L.	sublingual
ml	milliliter	sp.	species
mm³	cubic millimeter	T_3	triiodothyronine
Na	sodium	T_4	thyroxine
NaCl	sodium chloride	t.i.d.	three times daily
ng	nanogram	U	units
NG	nasogastric	USP	United States Pharmacopeia
NSAID	nonsteroidal anti-inflammatory drug		
OTC	over-the-counter	UV	ultraviolet
PABA	para-aminobenzoic acid	WBC	white blood cell
PCA	patient-controlled anal-gesia		
P.O.	by mouth		
P.R.	by rectum		
p.r.n.	as needed		
PT	prothrombin time		
PTT	partial thromboplastin time		
PVC	premature ventricular contraction		
q	every		
q.d.	every day; once daily		
q.i.d.	four times daily		
RBC	red blood cell		
RDA	recommended daily allowance		
REM	rapid eye movement		
RNA	ribonucleic acid		
RSV	respiratory syncytial virus		
SA	sinoatrial		
S.C.	subcutaneous		

1

Introduction to nonprescription drugs

The sheer number of nonprescription or over-the-counter (OTC) drugs available today is staggering. Consider that your patients can choose from among more than 100,000 such drugs without consulting a health care professional.

Of course, this freedom of choice can be beneficial in many ways, including financially and therapeutically. But it also can impede therapy and lead to confusion. And more often than not, when a patient turns to a health care professional for answers, he turns to a nurse. This introductory chapter, which covers fundamental questions, definitions, and techniques, will help you give the right answers.

What is an OTC drug?

Deciding what qualifies as an OTC drug and what doesn't isn't always simple. Although some drugs, such as aspirin, are easy to identify as OTC drugs, lines can blur between OTC drugs and food products, OTC drugs and cosmetics, OTC drugs and herbal therapies, OTC drugs and diet supplements, OTC drugs and

home remedies, and a number of other crossover categories. Caffeine, capsaicin, and oatmeal have therapeutic applications but are also unremarkable food products. Hand cream, body lotion, and makeup may contain several active ingredients, or none.

The definition of *over-the-counter* has never been precise, but in the past it was somewhat firmer than it is now. The term once referred to all types of products and merchandise sold without regulatory restriction. The acronym "OTC" has been popular for decades, roughly referring to a wide range of remedies and personal hygiene preparations.

In the 1990s, the pharmaceutical industry and regulatory authorities assigned a formal definition to "over-the-counter." The impetus was their need to distinguish between prescription drugs and drugs approved by the Food and Drug Administration (FDA) for conversion from prescription to OTC status. The broad definition of OTC drugs still encompasses all nonprescription drugs, plus many products popularly viewed as safe for general use. The formal FDA definition applies to *specific drugs that have been thoroughly screened and approved as safe and effective for use without a prescription.*

The FDA is in the process of reviewing the significant active ingredients of many of the drugs in the broad OTC category and producing an authoritative monograph about each one. The review of the 800 active ingredients, divided into 80 therapeutic categories, is designed to move steadily through a benefit-risk evaluation, which would be prohibitively time consuming if attempted for individual drugs in the dynamic OTC drug market.

Why people use OTC drugs

The benefits of health care management have prompted many nurses and doctors to encourage appropriate OTC drug use. A busy practice can effectively manage a larger number of patients who are well informed and confident about using OTC drugs. Plus, changes in state and federal regulation, health care delivery systems, third-party payer involvement, retail merchandising, and consumer education all contribute to the growing popularity of self-treatment.

Independent and cash-conscious consumers see OTC drugs as emancipating. The lowered economic barrier improves access to effective treatment for a large segment of the population. Busy schedules can more easily accommodate a quick stop to pick up an OTC drug than a visit to a clinic or doctor's office followed by another stop at the pharmacy.

Over-the-counter drugs provide a sense of taking positive action during that uncertain period between symptom onset and the decision to seek medical attention. Given the choice between seeking professional medical care and self-treatment of conditions they consider personal, insignificant, or embarrassing, many consumers choose self-treatment.

Self-determination is a strong force. This is true in all age groups but has the longest and most deeply ingrained history in the elderly population. Self-treatment helps preserve an independent self-image and delays or avoids the label "patient." The conservation of effort is another benefit to the elderly age group.

Prescription drugs are relative newcomers in the health care arena. Home remedies, folk medicine, and patent medicines hold a long, colorful, and deeply entrenched position in our culture. This strong cultural climate is not lost on manufacturers. An advertising campaign that featured "Doctor Mom" administering an OTC cough and cold remedy is an example of the direct-to-consumer messages that treatment begins at home, not in a doctor's office or health care facility. The overriding message in today's health care environment promotes OTC drugs as first-line intervention.

In 1999, Americans spent nearly $19 billion on OTC drugs. Cough and cold remedies led the pack with $3.5 billion in sales, followed by pain remedies at more than $3 billion. Laxatives, in sixth place, brought in $870 million. (See *OTC drugs: Top 10 categories.*)

Consumers are used to receiving mixed messages concerning health care recommendations in the media and from the health care industry. Cautionary warnings about the dangers of delaying professional treatment are counterbalanced by mandatory third-party preapproval procedures, restricted access to doctors, and anticipated rebukes from busy health care professionals for using valuable time for mi-

---

OTC drugs: Top 10 categories

This ranking of therapeutic categories is based on dollars spent in 1999.
 1. Cough and cold
 2. Pain relief
 3. Mouth care
 4. Antiperspirants
 5. Antacids
 6. Laxatives
 7. Eye care
 8. Feminine hygiene
 9. First aid
10. Foot care

---

nor complaints. Using an OTC drug doesn't remove the option of professional intervention.

Approving OTC drugs

Consumer safety is the FDA's first concern in approving a drug; in short, benefits *must* outweigh risks. The law gives the prescriber responsibility to monitor and manage the risks and benefits of prescription drug use and to adjust doses as needed to maintain a positive benefit-to-risk balance.

Drugs approved for OTC use must meet FDA requirements for safety and efficacy without a doctor's prescription. The patient is now responsible for monitoring the benefit-to-risk balance. Consumer education and new labeling standards are intended to help maintain a positive benefit-to-risk balance in OTC drug use. Consumers must be aware that using an OTC drug carries the risk of interactions, adverse effects, and unexpected harmful events. Allergic reactions and product sensitivity can develop even after the patient has used the same product for a year or longer. Certain patients may have increased sensitivities to some OTC drugs and must avoid unintentional exposure to potentially harmful active ingredients. Pregnant and breast-feeding women are generally advised to avoid all drugs not specifically approved by their doctor—and that includes OTC drugs. (See *Using OTC drugs safely.*)

Product tampering is of special concern to the FDA. Consumers are advised to carefully inspect OTC packaging before purchase and to exercise extreme caution if any of the tamper-resistant features have been compromised. (See *Protection from product tampering,* page 6.)

The FDA has two approval processes for OTC drugs. The OTC Drug Review Program is an ongoing review of the safety and efficacy of products that are already on the market without prior approval. The program to switch from prescription to OTC regulates the transition of a prescription drug to OTC status.

OTC Drug Review Program

The goal of the OTC Drug Review Program is to establish drug monographs for each of the 80 classes (therapeutic categories) of OTC drugs that predate regulation. The therapeutic class monographs provide detailed information concerning acceptable ingredients, doses, formulations, and labeling. The continual updating of monographs provides current information about additional ingredients and labeling requirements.

Any drug company, doctor, consumer, or citizen's group can submit data for a drug monograph. Anyone can request that the FDA amend an existing drug monograph or submit an opinion regarding a drug monograph by submitting a citizen petition or correspondence to an established monograph docket.

Drugs that conform to the therapeutic-class monograph can be marketed without fur-

Using OTC drugs safely

The following safety tips are based on the Food and Drug Administration's recommendations to consumers.

Read the label
Just as a patient wouldn't ignore his doctor's instructions for using a prescription drug, he shouldn't ignore the label when taking an OTC drug. Here's what to tell your patient to look for on the package:
- a description of tamper-resistant features to check before buying the product
- product name
- ingredients
- recent significant product changes
- indications—what the product is used for
- usual dosage—directions for use
- warnings
  - when to stop taking the drug
  - when to see the doctor
  - possible side effects
- expiration date—when to throw the drug away

Special considerations
Tell your patient to follow these instructions:
- When you read the label, always wear your glasses or contact lenses if you need them.
- Read with enough light; it usually takes three times more light to read the same line at age 60 than at age 30.
- More is not better; never take the drug longer or in higher doses than the label recommends.
- Persistent symptoms are a clear signal that it's time to see the doctor.
- If you still have questions after you read the label, talk to the doctor, nurse, or pharmacist.

ther FDA approval; those that don't must be submitted for review and approval through the New Drug Application (NDA) process. As new ingredients are introduced to the OTC market, they must go through the NDA process.

Prescription-to-OTC switch
The goal of the FDA program to switch from prescription to

<table>
<tr><td>

Protection from product tampering

To help your patient protect himself from product tampering, give him this advice from the Food and Drug Administration:

- If anything looks suspicious, be suspicious.
- Don't buy an OTC product if the packaging is damaged.
- Be alert to the tamper-resistant features on the package before you open it. These features are described on the label.
- When you get home, inspect the drug inside the package.
- Don't use any drug that is discolored or different in any way. If it is, contact the store where you bought the product and take it back.
- Never take drugs in the dark.

</td></tr>
</table>

OTC is to help consumers take a more active role in their health care. Switch candidates are drugs that were previously approved for prescription use via the NDA process. These drugs must be resubmitted for NDA review before being marketed as OTC drugs. Safety and efficacy are the dual requirements for FDA approval of any drug, prescription or nonprescription. Approval for release of an OTC drug requires evidence that a typical patient can use it safely without medical supervision.

More than 600 of the FDA-defined OTC drugs were available only by prescription 20 years ago. Of course, this represents a very small portion of the 100,000 OTC drugs available today.

Access to information

At one time, a phone call to the doctor's office was a quick and easy way of getting a doctor's or nurse's advice or reassurance regarding self-treatment. Patients had the alternative of making an appointment if the signs and symptoms warranted further professional evaluation; the doctor was aware of the patient's ongoing health concerns and could monitor progress, as needed. Few professional practices can still offer this option.

When OTC drugs were sold predominantly in drug stores, the pharmacist was available to provide answers and guidance for selecting an OTC drug. Today, patients can purchase OTC drugs in grocery stores, department stores, specialty shops, gas stations, on the Internet, and in various other retail outlets.

News stories provide incomplete and sometimes distorted

health care information. Web site sources can be risky. Consumers seeking sound advice about selecting an OTC drug must find answers to their questions elsewhere.

Direct-to-consumer advertising is one of the largest resources immediately available to all consumers. Advertising, by intent, presents a bias in favor of the product. Even with its limitations, advertising does provide guidance on the appropriate use of an OTC drug. Information on the package is the next immediate source of information.

Manufacturers' Web sites can be an excellent source of product-specific information and often provide answers to frequently asked consumer questions. Web site addresses are routinely included in broadcast and print ads, as well as on the product label. Some of these sites include links to the Web sites of credible organizations and groups dealing with the conditions for which the OTC drug is indicated. The FDA Web site (www.fda.gov) is another good source of general consumer information. The focus, however, isn't on medical conditions, and the FDA doesn't recommend drugs.

Labeling requirements

Over-the-counter drug labeling is changing for the better. Current labeling is inconsistent in almost every way and can be very difficult to read. Current labeling is designed to conform to the package size and shape. The print size can be so small that it becomes meaningless. Regardless of its quality, the information on the label seldom reaches the consumer. Terms and language can be confusing and difficult to understand.

According to the FDA, "The safety and effectiveness of OTC drugs depend not only on the ingredients but also on clear and truthful labeling that can be understood by consumers." New labeling will clearly show the drug's ingredients, dose, and warnings.

The FDA's OTC drug–labeling regulation, "Drug Facts," is meant to improve the way consumers choose and use OTC drugs, just as the "Nutrition Facts" regulation has helped consumers make informed food choices. The regulation applies to all OTC drugs, and its goal is to help consumers understand the benefits and risks of each drug and the correct way to use it. Manufacturers will be required to use a standardized format, plain language, approved type sizes (with a minimum allowable size limit), and graphic features designed to help consumers.

Nursing considerations

Your patient assessment includes finding out about your patient's OTC drug history and use, occult OTC drug use, and any allergies, sensitivities, or adverse effects he has experienced through OTC drug use. Other considerations may include drug recalls, labeling changes, and drug tampering.

Drug history and use profile

As a nurse, you discuss your patient's OTC drug use as part of a broader interview to identify medical concerns. You may also advise parents in well-baby clinics or counsel senior citizens at monthly blood pressure clinics. Whatever the setting and whatever the patient's state of health, you can be fairly certain he uses OTC drugs.

When serious health care issues arise, you must obtain a good history of signs, symptoms, and OTC remedies. Although obtaining an accurate prescription drug history may be difficult, you can usually construct it from the patient's medicine containers or from the records on file with the prescribers and pharmacy. But there's no paper trail for OTC drug use, and the container trail is often cluttered and unclear.

To obtain a complete history, explain to the patient that by including all remedies (home, herbal, prescription, and OTC), he is helping the health care team make the best choices in planning care and treatment. Phrase questions to include examples of OTC drug use and ask about daily routines that might involve self-treatment. "Do you have any trouble sleeping?" may be answered "No." But "Do you take anything to help you get to sleep?" may be answered "Yes" and be followed by an accurate accounting of the sleep aids the patient uses.

Communication barriers

To enhance your ability to get an accurate and complete drug history and use profile from your patient, you'll need to be aware of two important communication barriers: familiarity and effectiveness.

Familiarity

Familiarity creates a mental blind spot that prevents the patient from identifying OTC drugs as treatment drugs. Sheer volume and availability blend OTC drugs into the background of daily life, even for people who rarely use them.

Consumers are comfortable with OTC drugs. They purchase them along with their groceries and routinely keep them close at hand: in cupboards, desk drawers, purses, briefcases, diaper bags, glove compartments, and medicine cabinets. These are "safe and familiar" items, not attracting any special attention or warranting any extra consideration. (See *OTC drugs: Common misconceptions.*)

Effectiveness

Over-the-counter drugs work. They frequently succeed as therapeutic agents, and they're easy to use. Whether the signs and symptoms are episodic or chronic, most patients continue to use what they perceive to be successful remedies, even when other, apparently unrelated, health care concerns arise.

Over-the-counter drugs prevent minor conditions from worsening and allow people to continue the activities of daily living. Sunburn prevention and treatment products enable many people to enjoy outdoor activities. The muscle-aching "weekend warrior" can still

---

OTC drugs: Common misconceptions

- The expiration date can be ignored; drugs can't go bad.
- Smaller doses of adult OTC drugs are safe for children.
- Expensive drugs work better than inexpensive drugs.
- Higher-than-recommended doses are safe because the dose on the label is deliberately low for safety.
- If it can be treated with an OTC drug, it can't be serious.

---

show up ready to work on Monday.

For the self-employed, productivity is critical. OTC drugs keep minor accidents, upper respiratory tract infections, and headaches from causing major disruptions to workflow.

A patient who discusses concerns about blood pressure medications or cholesterol levels with you may not mention his favorite antacid or nighttime cold preparation. The patient with concerns about vision changes may not realize that her routine use of vitamin A, taken to prevent dry skin, is a piece of valuable information.

The success of OTC drugs lets a patient dismiss the ailment and the OTC drug use. The ailment is no longer a concern, and the patient may believe that the drug isn't important enough to mention to you.

Occult use of OTC drugs

Be aware that self-treatment is not easily abandoned and that it can silently continue along with prescribed therapies, complicating treatment and possibly endangering the patient.

A patient who is told to avoid caffeine may not comply because caffeine relieves his headaches. Your skillful interview may reveal that headaches have been relieved, and you might even find out which OTC drug was used, but you may have difficulty learning the size and frequency of doses or whether headaches continue to occur.

Allergy, sensitivity, adverse effects

Allergic reactions and drug sensitivity can arise when your patient takes an OTC drug, just as they can when he takes a prescription drug. Both are adverse effects and may or may not be labeled as such. As discussed earlier, the benefits of the OTC drug must exceed the risks, to obtain approval from the FDA. Known adverse effects included in labeling are considered by the FDA to be acceptable risks when measured against the drug's health benefits.

Not every patient experiences adverse effects, but many do. The particular term used to describe the event is less important than a clear description of signs and symptoms and of the sequence of events. Ask the patient to describe the adverse effect, including specific symptoms and when they occurred. Keep in mind that labeled adverse effects can be serious. Don't dismiss them just because they are predictable.

Additional considerations

Be aware that the drugs taken off the market may remain in many homes. Patients will rely on personal supplies of OTC drugs they have found to be effective. Stay informed about drug recalls and drugs taken off the market and help the patient identify any of these drugs in their supply.

Drug labeling changes must be approved by the FDA and are a part of the NDA or monograph review process. Patients relying on memory may be unaware of current dose and duration limits. They also might not be aware of the addition of active ingredients or changes of dose strength.

Drug tampering gained national attention when a number of people died after taking deliberately poisoned OTC drugs. The murderer placed the products back on the retail shelf for random purchase and didn't know the victims. The pharmaceutical industry instituted tamper-resistance measures to reduce the potential for ingestion of poisoned drugs. Tampering still occurs and is still a concern; however, tamper-resistant features make it more difficult to conceal tampering. If the package or any portion of the tamper-resistant device is damaged, the shopper should immediately turn it over to store personnel. If the OTC drug is in any way unusual, the consumer should return it to the store.

Patient teaching

• Advise patients to carefully read the labels of all OTC drugs every time they start using them and every time they buy a new container.

• Advise patients to closely follow recommendations for contacting a doctor if they are not seeing results or if adverse events occur.

• Caution patients never to take medicine in the dark.

• Warn patients that many OTC drug manufacturers produce a range of drugs with similar names and different active ingredients.

• Advise a pregnant patient to check with her doctor before taking any drugs, including OTC drugs.

• Advise a patient who is breast-feeding that the baby may be exposed via breast milk to any drugs she is taking orally. Tell her she should completely remove any topical preparation from the breast before breast-feeding, to prevent its accidental ingestion by the baby.

• Advise parents that child-*resistant* caps are not child-*proof*. Containers should be kept where children can't see them or reach them. Provide parents with the phone number of the local poison control center.

• Advise parents that children's doses must be exact and should never be estimates. Encourage them to use a measuring spoon or, better still, a pediatric medicine device, rather than an eating utensil to give their child's dose.

• Advise parents to always check with a pharmacist, doctor, or nurse practitioner before giving a child two medicines at the same time.

• Warn the patient about potential interactions involving OTC drugs. Tell him to avoid drinking alcohol when taking antihistamines, cold and cough drugs containing detromethorphan, or sleep aids. Tell the patient he shouldn't use OTC sleep aids when taking prescription sedatives or tranquilizers.

• If your patient is taking an anticoagulant or has diabetes or gout, tell him to consult his doctor before taking aspirin or any OTC drug that contains aspirin.

2

Generic drugs

Generic drugs save consumers an estimated $8 to $10 billion a year in retail drug purchases. Additional savings are estimated to be in the billions of dollars for hospitals. Yet the reliability of generic drugs has generated much discussion and debate over the years. We are familiar with the differences among nondrug generic products, and we know that product quality can vary widely, even when the label lists the same ingredients. Even though the Food and Drug Administration (FDA) must approve all drugs marketed in the United States, many patients and health care professionals have their doubts about the quality of a generic drug that may cost surprisingly less than the brand name version. Justified questions arise:
• Can it really be as good?
• Did they leave something out or substitute some inferior ingredient?
• Has the brand name drug simply been overpriced all these years?

Patients will be asking you their questions as they seek an explanation of the differences between generic and brand name drugs. In many ways, there are no significant differences, but there are some minor ones. Knowing the facts can help you answer your patient's questions.

Approval standards

Patients commonly think of generic drugs as less expensive clones of brand name drugs, but there are actually three categories of generic drugs:
• *Prescription drugs*. The FDA allows some minor differences, but the generic drug must meet the same requirements as the specific brand name drug already on the market.
• *Prescription-to-OTC drugs*. These drugs have made the transition from prescription to over-the-counter (OTC) drug status. The FDA holds these drugs to the same product-specific standards as it does generic prescription drugs.
• *OTC drugs*. Because these drugs must meet the standards of an active ingredient monograph, all OTC drugs can be considered generic drugs.

Prescription drugs

Generic prescription drugs were created to provide consumers with an inexpensive alternative to expensive brand name prescription drugs. In 1984, the Drug Price Competition and Patent Term Restoration Act (Waxman-Hatch Act) became law. The Act establishes standards, protects drug developers, and has sparked a proliferation of generic drugs.

Manufacturing a clone of an established brand name prescription drug avoids the cost of research and development. The savings in production costs is passed on to the consumer, making inexpensive generic drugs available to consumers without compromising safety.

A drug manufacturer seeking approval to market a generic drug in the United States must submit a generic drug application (abbreviated New Drug Application) to the FDA. The first requirement is the existence of a model, pioneer (reference) drug, approved by the FDA and no longer under exclusivity protection. New brand name prescription drugs are developed and approved under patent protection. As with any product, the patent provides a period of protected exclusive

marketing. This allows the manufacturer of the pioneer drug to recover research and development costs and other expenses of bringing the drug to market. The cost of drug research and development, including clinical trials, is extremely high, and it takes years of expense-intensive activity to bring a new drug onto the market. As long as a drug is under patent, no generic version can be marketed. By the time market exclusivity has expired, the drug is an established brand name and the manufacturer has usually recovered the initial investment and realized some profit. Therapeutic performance is already accepted by the health care community, as well as by consumers, and demand has been established; the market is ready for competition. Once the patent has expired, drug manufacturers are free to submit generic drug applications to the FDA. (See *Generic drug requirements*.)

Producing a generic drug is much less expensive than developing a new drug. All required clinical trials were satisfactorily completed by the New Drug Application (NDA) holder before the brand name drug was approved. The FDA accepts as valid the safety, efficacy, and positive benefit-to-risk balance established for the reference drug. Once the generic drug application is approved, the manufacturer can begin marketing the generic drug with minimal promotion.

Generic drugs must be *true copies* of the originals. A generic drug *must* have the same active ingredients in the same strengths in the same dosage form and with the same route of administration as the pioneer drug. (See *Myths and facts about generic drugs,* page 16.)

Identical drug performance is the next requirement. Bioequivalence must be shown to be identical to that of the brand name product. The active ingredients of the generic product must be delivered to the patient's bloodstream at the same rate and the same level as the reference drug.

Scientific evidence of bioequivalence is submitted with the NDA and can be measured in a number of ways. The following is one method that the FDA finds acceptable:
• Measure the time it takes for the generic drug to reach the bloodstream in 24 to 36 healthy volunteers.
• Compare the rates of absorption (also known as bioavail-

Generic drug requirements

The list below summarizes the requirements set by the Food and Drug Administration (FDA) for generic drugs.
• Pioneer drug already approved by the FDA
• Demonstrated bioequivalence to the pioneer drug
• Approval of active and inactive ingredients
• Proof of adherence to good manufacturing practices
• Review of generic drug testing
• Review of generic drug labeling
• Reporting of all adverse reactions and serious adverse health effects
• FDA approval for major manufacturing changes or drug reformulation
• Periodic inspection of manufacturing plants
• FDA quality control monitoring.

---

ability) of the generic and reference drugs.
• If the rates match, the generic drug passes the bioequivalence test.

Labeling contents must be identical. The label of a generic drug is required to contain the same information as that of the brand name drug—indications,

Myths and facts about generic drugs

- *Myth:* Generic drugs aren't as safe as brand name drugs.
  Fact: Generic and pioneer drugs have the same demonstrated risk-to-benefit balance.
- *Myth:* Generic drugs are made in inferior facilities.
  Fact: Brand name companies produce 50% of generic drugs.
  Fact: All facilities are subject to the same regulations and inspections.
- *Myth:* Side effects are more likely with generic drugs.
  Fact: The rates of side effects reported to the FDA are the same.
- *Myth:* Generic drugs have delayed therapeutic effect or lower potency.
  Fact: The generic and brand name versions must have the same quality, strength, purity, and stability; the generic version must deliver the same amount of active ingredient at the same rate.

Production standards must be identical. Raw materials and the product must meet the same *United States Pharmacopeia (USP)* specifications.

A generic drug on the market in the United States must be proven to be stable under extremes of heat and humidity. The manufacturer must demonstrate that the container and its closure system don't interact with the drug. Other standards the applicant must meet include strict sterility assurance and microbiologic integrity standards, when applicable.

The abbreviated NDA must include a detailed description of the facilities used to manufacture, process, test, package, label, and control the drug and a certification of compliance with federal regulations of current good manufacturing practices (GMPs).

Finally, the FDA conducts an inspection. After approval, the manufacturer must maintain the same standards, and periodic FDA inspections for quality assurance must continue.

Allowable variations

Generic drugs are allowed some variations from the brand name drug. The FDA considers that the allowed variations are insignificant and don't compro-

dose range recommendations, duration, contraindications, interactions, cautions, adverse effects, and all other FDA-mandated information.

mise drug safety, efficacy, or benefit-to-risk ratio. Permitted variations include:
• inactive ingredients
• shape, color, and size of a tablet or capsule
• dyes used in enteric coatings (See *Patient safety: Generic drug cautions*.)

Prescription-to-OTC drugs
The FDA encourages brand name drug manufacturers to submit supplemental applications for *prescription-to-OTC drug* approval of current prescription drugs. This transition usually involves a reduction in strength or some other product adjustment.

It's the responsibility of the manufacturer, without prescriber supervision, to provide clinical research that demonstrates safety and efficacy; this creates considerable additional expense. When the supplemental application for the switch is approved, a new period of exclusivity goes into effect, allowing the manufacturer to recover prescription-to-OTC drug expenses. As with prescription drugs, when the period of exclusivity has expired, the door is open for generic drug manufacturers.

Patient safety: Generic drug cautions

Alert your patient to the possibility that generic drugs may look different or contain additives to which he may be sensitive.

Drug identification
Safety often depends on visual cues. In the past, the patient could look at the drug and recognize it. If it didn't look right, the patient would know not to take it. Today, each refill can look different and still be the same drug. Or it could be the wrong drug. Encourage the patient, when in doubt, to ask the pharmacist to verify the drug's identity.

Sensitivities
Dyes and lactose contained as inactive ingredients in some generic drugs can cause adverse symptoms. Patients who aren't sensitive to the drug may be sensitive to these ingredients.

OTC drugs
Active ingredients, rather than individual drugs, are subjected to a review and approval process. For active ingredients introduced after May 1992, the

potential manufacturer must submit an NDA or supplemental application.

Active ingredients that were on the market before May 1992 undergo safety and effectiveness reviews by an Advisory Review Panel. An OTC drug monograph is developed for each Category I active ingredient. The monograph sets standards specifying ingredients, dosage, indications for use, and labeling. All products that meet the requirements of the OTC drug monograph are eligible for marketing. Those that do not are classified as Category II or III and are removed from the market.

Active ingredient groups

Indications and examples for each group of active ingredients are presented here.

Anesthetics
• Indications: sore throat, hemorrhoid pain, sunburn, insect bites, poison ivy dermatitis
• Examples: benzocaine, phenol, benzyl alcohol, tetracaine, pramoxine, dibucaine

Antipruritics
• Indications: pruritus
• Examples: antihistamines (to block histamine [H_1] receptor);

counterirritants; hydrocortisone, menthol, phenol, camphor

Antiseptics
• Indications: topical, oral, ophthalmic, anorectal conditions
• Examples: alcohols (ethyl and isopropyl), iodine, chlorhexidine, thimerosal, hydrogen peroxide, phenol, hexylresorcinol

Astringents
• Indications: poison ivy dermatitis, hemorrhoids, acne
• Examples: witch hazel, aluminum acetate, boric acid, calamine

Keratolytics
• Indications: hemorrhoids; dandruff; seborrhea; desquamation, débridement, or sloughing of epidermal cells
• Examples: resorcinol, aluminum chlorhydroxy allantoinate (for hemorrhoids); salicylic acid, sulfur (for dandruff or seborrhea)

Lubricants
• Indications: dry eyes, vaginal dryness
• Examples: artificial tears (for dry eyes); water-soluble lubricants (for vaginal dryness)

Protectants
• Indications: unprotected injured skin
• Examples: calamine lotion, aluminum hydroxide, bismuth subgallate

Vasoconstrictors
• Indications: hemorrhoids, allergy symptoms
• Examples: ephedrine, epinephrine, phenylephrine (to shrink hemorrhoids and treat allergy symptoms [ophthalmic and otic preparations])

3

Central nervous system

The central nervous system (CNS) consists of the brain and spinal cord. It controls the entire body by transmitting complex electrical and chemical impulses in response to internal and external stimuli. The CNS is the body system most protected from external trauma. The bony rigid box of the cranium houses the brain, and the vertebral column protects the spinal cord. Three layers of connective tissue provide additional protection.

CNS symptoms for which patients may take over-the-counter (OTC) drugs include sleep disturbances, pain and headache, appetite and weight control, low energy, fever, and nicotine addiction.

Anatomy

Briefly review the anatomy of the brain and spinal cord.

Brain

The brain controls basic functions such as breathing, heart rate, temperature regulation, thirst, hunger, sleep, sexual drive, and muscle movement. It also controls higher functions such as cognitive skills, thought process, judgment, and creativity. Serotonin, dopamine, norepinephrine, epinephrine, acetylcholine, and gamma aminobutyric acid are primary neurochemicals involved in neurotransmission. The pituitary and pineal glands also lie within the brain.

The brain has three anatomically and functionally distinct parts—the cerebrum, cerebellum, and brain stem.

Cerebrum

The cerebrum is the upper portion of the brain, divided into right and left hemispheres, each of which is further divided into four lobes: frontal, parietal, occipital, and temporal. At the center of the cerebrum is the diencephalon, which consists of the thalamus, hypothalamus, and epithalamus. The thalamus relays nerve impulses. The hypothalamus registers temperature, water metabolism, appetite, thirst, emotional expression, and part of the sleep-wake cycle. The epithalamus regulates the endocrine system.

Cerebellum

The cerebellum, located behind and below the cerebrum, controls and coordinates muscle movement and equilibrium.

Brain stem

The brain stem, at the base of the brain, controls the basic functions of respiration and heart rate; it consists of the midbrain, the pons, and the medulla oblongata.

Spinal cord

The spinal cord is the column of communication pathways between the brain stem and the peripheral nervous system. Damage to the spinal cord disrupts neurotransmission and can deprive areas of the body from registering sensation and receiving response commands. CNS malfunctions can range from minor to life threatening.

Sleep disturbances

Sleep disturbances, such as insomnia or daytime drowsiness, are a cause for concern. The brain controls the sleep-wake cycle. The average person needs about 8 hours of sleep per night, but this can range from 4 to 12 hours. Disturbed sleep can result from narcolepsy, sleep apnea, and depression. The patient who purchases OTC sleep aids may be neglecting a serious medical condition.

Signs and symptoms

Identifying the underlying cause of a sleep disorder requires a precise identification of signs and symptoms. Insomnia is classified as initial, middle, or early. *Initial insomnia* is difficulty falling asleep. *Middle insomnia* is difficulty staying asleep. *Early insomnia* is early morning awakening. Daytime drowsiness or sedation can be a sign of lack of sleep, inefficient sleep, or some other health condition, or it may be a side effect of medication. Other signs and symptoms to assess are snoring and breathing pauses during sleep; these can signal sleep apnea.

When recording signs and symptoms, specify the time, frequency, and length of episodes of sleep disruption; number of nights without sleep; baseline sleep pattern (normal bedtime, normal time to arise, and routine daytime napping); and current sleep pattern. Include the total number of hours of sleep per 24-hour period.

Serious conditions

Disturbed sleep can result from dietary indiscretion (including caffeine use), situational anxiety, medical disorders (including chronic pain), depression, manic-depressive illness, anxiety disorder, narcolepsy, sleep apnea, or posttraumatic stress disorder. If the underlying cause and the exact nature of the sleep disturbance aren't ascertained, treatment is unlikely to be successful.

Complications

Left untreated, sleep disturbances can predispose a person to accidents, physical problems, and even psychosis caused by sleep deprivation. A weakened immune system caused by lack of sleep reduces resistance to infection. Diminished mental acuity compromises judgment and response times. Drowsiness while operating equipment, driving a vehicle, or performing other potentially hazardous activities can lead to injury and death.

The frustration of sleep disturbance can lead to a self-defeating, self-medication cycle of drugs to promote sleep and then drugs to enhance wakefulness, culminating in reduced mental acuity and physical reserve.

Nursing considerations

• Assess the patient's sleep pattern: hours slept per night, frequency and pattern of interruptions, baseline sleep pattern, length of time the sleep problem has persisted, snoring, and breathing pauses.

• Find out if the patient ever experiences a good night's sleep and, if so, the circumstances under which this occurs.

• Assess the patient's perception of environmental barriers to sleep (noise, light level, aromas, temperature control, and bed comfort).

• Assess dietary habits (patterns of meals and caffeine and alcohol intake).

• Determine patterns of physical activity, job-related issues (traveling, shift rotation, demanding schedule), and situation concerns (domestic, social, financial).

• Identify nocturnal physical signs and symptoms such as back pain, aching legs, upper respiratory congestion, gastrointestinal (GI) disorders, or abnormal urinary patterns.

• Assess the patient for depression, mood swings, or irritability.

• Ask about past or recent traumas, such as combat or assault, and about nightmares.

• When appropriate, advise the patient to seek help from a mental health or sleep therapy professional.

Patient teaching

• Teach the patient about proper sleep hygiene, which includes establishing routine hours of sleep, decreasing or eliminating caffeine intake, promoting a quiet environment, avoiding alcohol, and keeping a sleep and dream record.
• Teach the patient the signs and symptoms of depression, which include sad mood or irritability, low energy or fatigue, a change in appetite, diminished ability to concentrate, and feelings of hopelessness.
• Explain the hazards of mixing alcohol or street drugs with OTC sleep aids.

Pain and headache

Pain is a mechanism for signaling that something is wrong and a corrective action is needed to avoid damage. The sensation of pain is relayed from the source of irritation via the peripheral nervous system and spinal cord to the brain. Pain response impulses signal the body system to attempt corrective action, such as muscle contraction, to remove the body from an external stimulus. When the pain is internal, response signals may initiate changes of activity or posture to minimize stress on the affected organ or body system. Pain medications can inhibit or change conduction of pain messages or perception and response to pain. Some medications that relieve pain also treat the underlying cause.

Signs and symptoms

The patient must fully describe the pain so that the doctor can make an accurate diagnosis and determine if use of an OTC medication is appropriate. Pain is considered the fifth vital sign in many health care systems today. Description should include location, intensity, duration, and consistency. Pain threshold and perception are unique to each individual and can vary widely from person to person. Pain descriptions should be recorded first in the patient's own words, and then quantitative and qualitative descriptors should be offered for the patient to choose from (sharp, throbbing, burning, dull, sudden onset, slow onset). A scale of intensity ranging from 1 to 10, with 10 representing the most severe pain, is a useful subjective tool.

Serious conditions

Headaches can indicate such serious problems as a cerebral aneurysm, CVA, or brain tumor. Pain with loss of sensation or tingling can signal nerve compression, irritation, or damage; a herniated disc; or a vertebral fracture. Chest pain, particularly when accompanied by pain radiating down either arm, suggests an MI. Sharp abdominal pain may reflect a medical emergency, such as appendicitis, perforated ulcer, or ectopic pregnancy.

Pain can be referred to an area unassociated with the actual source of the pain. For example, the pain associated with an MI can be felt as GI pain. Chronic pain, which may be caused by any one of many underlying conditions, is also a serious medical problem, often inadequately treated.

Complications

Treating pain with OTC pain medications can mask a serious underlying condition and might delay appropriate medical intervention. Pain resulting from sudden episodes of physical activity like exercise, sports, or yard work can often be treated successfully with an OTC product if the patient recognizes that masking the pain doesn't remove or reduce the damage. However, while the patient is using an OTC pain medication, additional activity stressing the same muscles or joints can cause unperceived damage, requiring a doctor's attention.

Long-term use or high doses of some OTC pain medications, such as aspirin and acetaminophen, can cause serious complications, including renal damage, bleeding disorders, and GI problems.

Nursing considerations

• Assess and document the patient's pain.
• Ask about the patient's nonpharmacologic management techniques for treating aches, pains, and headaches.
• Refer chronic pain patient to pain specialists.

Patient teaching

• Inform the patient that the need for prolonged use of OTC drugs might indicate a condition best managed by a doctor.
• Instruct the patient to read the labels of any OTC pain preparations, to carefully follow the directions, and to discontinue use if he experiences any adverse effects.
• Encourage the patient with chronic pain to seek medical attention.
• Encourage the patient to get a proper diagnosis.
• Encourage the patient to use relaxation techniques and diversionary activities to enhance the effectiveness of medication.

Appetite and weight control

Weight is in a continual state of fluctuation and is the result of a complex set of variables, including: genetic makeup, calorie intake, activity level, metabolism rate, hormonal levels, endocrine activity, fluid-electrolyte balance, environmental demands (arctic versus equator), resource availability, and general state of health.

Desired weight is a goal driven by many cultural and psychosocial objectives, as well as some health objectives. Height-weight ratio and body fat measures are used to clinically determine the ideal weight range for an individual. However, these are not the only factors to consider. Anorexia nervosa, bulimia, obesity, and morbid obesity are medical conditions and should be fully evaluated by a doctor for appropriate treatment.

Normal baseline appetite is driven by the requirement to fuel activities. Appetite is influenced by activity level, habit, psychosocial factors, sensory stimulation, and changes in health. Appetite disorder (increased or decreased) can be the result of many things, including medication side effects, head trauma, endocrine disorders, psychological disorders, and CNS disorders.

Signs and symptoms

Patients with appetite disorder may have an insatiable appetite, increased appetite, decreased appetite, or total loss of appetite. Weight is of concern when the patient is a large percentage over or under the normal range based on height. Sudden unexplained weight loss or weight gain should be fully evaluated by a doctor.

Serious conditions

Sudden or steady weight change can be the first indication of changes in thyroid hormone levels or other endocrine disorders. Undiagnosed pregnancy has prompted more than one woman to seek relief from unexplained weight gain. Weight gain accompanied by dyspnea, other respiratory problems, or peripheral edema may be an indication of heart failure.

Drastic unexplained weight loss should be evaluated immediately. It may be a sign of cancer, GI parasites, or other GI disorders.

Use of OTC weight control medication by a patient with normal or low weight suggests that the patient may have an eating disorder, such as anorexia nervosa, bulimia, or bulimia nervosa.

Complications
Prolonged obesity predisposes the patient to diabetes, hypertension, vascular problems, and joint strain. Acute or chronic starvation can be life threatening, causing death from dehydration and malnutrition. Bulimia has been known to cause esophageal bleeding and varices and even gastric rupture. Another result of excessive vomiting is hypokalemia, which can cause cardiac arrhythmias that are life threatening. Chronic starvation can cause permanent muscle tissue loss, renal damage caused by vitamin deficiency, and malnutrition.

Nursing considerations
• Evaluate the patient for eating disorders if he is of normal or low weight and using OTC appetite or weight control medications, especially for prolonged periods.
• Assess the patient's overall weight-loss program if he is using OTC appetite suppressants. The program should also include a proper diet and exercise routine.
• Ask if the patient experiences the "roller coaster" of weight loss and subsequent weight gain.
• Assess the patient's past attempts at weight control.
• Monitor the patient for adverse effects of OTC diet aids, such as irritability, jitteriness, or insomnia.

Patient teaching
• Instruct the patient to read carefully and follow the directions on the labels of all OTC diet aids.
• Inform the patient that slow steady weight loss is the most effective rate of reduction.
• Help the patient determine a healthy and realistic weight goal.
• Encourage regular daily exercise to improve general muscle tone and health, to stimulate appetite for those trying to gain weight, and to burn calories for those trying to lose weight.
• Encourage diversionary activities for patient with appetite control problems.
• Encourage water intake for those trying to lose weight, and encourage fruit juice intake for those trying to gain weight.

Low energy
A person's energy level is determined by diet, sleep pattern, age, exercise habits, and overall health. Energy level normally varies from person to

person and in the same person from day to day. The important measure is how the person's energy level compares with his norm. As a general rule, energy level diminishes with increasing age.

Signs and symptoms
Any report of loss of energy should be taken seriously. A marked increased need for sleep, lethargy, and difficulty getting up in the morning are serious signs and symptoms. Any disruption or discontinuation of employment, recreational activities, family and social interaction, or activities of daily living should be considered significant.

Serious conditions
Low energy can be indicative of chronic fatigue syndrome, anemia, depression, hypothyroidism, or cancer. A thorough physical, including a mental health assessment, is indicated if this is the patient's complaint.

Complications
Left undiagnosed, underlying causes of low energy can progress. Chronic fatigue syndrome can prevent a patient from working and severely limit his ability to meet family and social obligations. Depression can lead to chronic disability or to suicide. Anemia can become chronic. Hypothyroidism can become a medical emergency. Cancer left undetected and untreated can progress to an untreatable state.

Nursing considerations
• Assess the patient's signs and symptoms of fatigue.
• Determine the patient's baseline level of activity and when a change in routine pattern was noticed.
• Find out what OTC drugs the patient is using to treat his fatigue.

Patient teaching
• Assess the patient for adequate sleep, nutrition, and exercise.
• Instruct the patient to read and follow the instructions on any OTC drug used to treat fatigue.
• Encourage the patient to contact a doctor if fatigue is prolonged or disrupts normal activities.
• Encourage the patient to have a thorough medical evaluation if signs and symptoms persist and are unexplained.
• Assess the patient for signs and symptoms of depression; when appropriate, refer the patient to a doctor for evaluation.

Fever

Body temperature is controlled by the CNS. Temperature regulation allows for adaptation to differing climates and environmental conditions. Heat produced by metabolism and during exertion is released or retained through the skin, respiratory system, and products of elimination. Body heat regulation can fail in response to extreme environmental conditions (sunstroke, heat exhaustion, and hypothermia) or to CNS disorders. Body temperature rises naturally in the presence of pathogens, making fever one of the ways the immune system protects the body from bacteria and viruses.

Signs and symptoms

Normal body temperature falls within a narrow range around 98.6° F (37° C), and slight fluctuations are normal. In the presence of an invasive pathogen, the temperature rises; the patient may experience chills caused by peripheral vasoconstriction, as the body initiates a shivering response to produce adequate heat. Prolonged elevations to 100° to 102° F (38° to 39° C) can occur, with accompanying dehydration and malaise. Malfunctions of body temperature regulation, as well as defensive response to patho-gen invasion, can create dangerously high fevers, placing the brain at risk. Temperatures higher than 104° F (40° C) are considered excessive.

Because elderly patients can have a decreased response to infectious organisms, infection may be harder to recognize in them than in younger people. Therefore, a slight fever in an elderly patient should be taken seriously.

Serious conditions

Pituitary tumors can cause hyperthermia, resulting in death. Medications affecting dopamine, most often antipsychotic drugs, can cause neuroleptic malignant syndrome, a potentially fatal adverse reaction leading to autonomic dysregulation; elevated temperature is a hallmark symptom. Other possible causes of temperature elevation include dehydration and respiratory compromise.

Complications

Seizures, delirium, dehydration, coma, or neurologic damage are common with body temperatures exceeding 106° F (41° C). It is vital to determine the cause of the fever and render proper treatment, rather than mask this important indicator. Otherwise, a chronic infection, such as subacute bacterial endocarditis, can be missed.

Nursing considerations

• Use a consistent and reliable method to check the patient's temperature.
• Determine the duration of the fever. Prolonged low-grade fever may reflect undiagnosed infection.
• Discuss the patient's use of pharmacologic and nonpharmacologic methods for fever reduction.
• A sudden elevated temperature in the absence of signs and symptoms of infection can indicate autonomic dysregulation or pituitary tumor.
• Suspect neuroleptic malignant syndrome if temperature rises in a patient taking a neuroleptic drug, such as a phenothiazine.
• Make sure the patient stays adequately hydrated.
• Monitor fluid and electrolyte status.

Patient teaching

• Instruct the patient to read and follow directions on any OTC medications taken to control fever.
• Instruct the patient to report to a doctor any prolonged or excessive temperature elevation.

• When needed, teach the patient to accurately take temperatures.
• Instruct the patient to increase fluid intake and to immediately report any signs or symptoms of infection.
• Advise the patient not to use an alcohol sponge bath to reduce fever; this may result in alcohol poisoning because of excessive inhalation or cutaneous absorption.

Nicotine addiction

Tobacco use begins as a learned behavior that often progresses to physical and psychological dependence because of the highly addictive component, nicotine. The body develops a tolerance for nicotine, requiring increased exposure to meet the craving.

Signs and symptoms

Nicotine addiction should be suspected in a person who can't stop using tobacco products after repeated attempts to quit or who excessively and compulsively uses tobacco products. Withdrawal signs and symptoms include shakiness, irritability, fatigue, anxiety, and impaired concentration.

Serious conditions

The use of tobacco products presents serious threats to

health, and the use of OTC products to reduce nicotine exposure is unlikely to mask serious conditions. Cigarette smoking has been deemed the single most avoidable cause of death in the United States. Patients trying to reduce nicotine exposure because they have dyspnea, excessive coughing, chest pain, or intermittent claudication should have a full medical evaluation.

Complications
Exposure to nicotine and tar contributes to the development of CV disease, certain forms of cancer, emphysema, and other lung disorders.

Nursing considerations
• Ask every patient during initial assessment about the use of tobacco products.
• If the patient is trying to quit smoking by using an OTC drug, evaluate other strategies used in conjunction with smoking cessation medication to enhance the success of this attempt.
• Smoking cessation can benefit the patient, no matter how long he has smoked.

Patient teaching
• Inform the patient that a comprehensive smoking cessation program enhances the success rate of using OTC nicotine replacement products.
• Encourage the patient to use diversionary techniques.
• Advise the patient to read and follow OTC instructions and to report any signs and symptoms of respiratory and CV disorders.
• Warn the patient not to smoke while using nicotine replacement products.
• Advise the patient who is successful at quitting smoking to notify a doctor, especially if the patient currently takes theophylline. The dose of theophylline will need to be reduced to avoid possible toxicity.

acetaminophen
aspirin
aspirin, buffered
caffeine
capsaicin
choline salicylate
diphenhydramine
　hydrochloride
doxylamine succinate
ibuprofen
ketoprofen
magnesium salicylate
　tetrahydrate
naproxen sodium
nicotine polacrilex
nicotine transdermal
　system

---

acetaminophen (APAP, paracetamol)
Abenol†; Aceta Elixir*; Acetaminophen Uniserts; Aceta Tablets; Actamin; Actamin Extra; Actimol†; Aminofen; Aminofen Max; Anacin-3; Anacin-3 Extra Strength; Apacet Capsules; Apacet Elixir*; Apacet Extra Strength Caplets; Apacet Extra Strength Tablets; Apacet, Infants'; Apacet Regular Strength Tablets; Apo-Acetaminophen†; Arthritis Pain Formula Aspirin Free; Atasol Caplets†; Atasol Drops†; Atasol Forte Caplets†; Atasol Forte Tablets†; Atasol Tablets†; Banesin; Dapa; Dapa X-S; Datril Extra-Strength; Dymadon‡; Dymadon P‡; Exdol†; Exdol Strong†; Feverall, Children's; Feverall, Junior Strength; Feverall Sprinkle Caps, Children's; Feverall Sprinkle Caps Junior Strength; Genapap Children's Elixir; Genapap Children's Tablets; Genapap Extra Strength Caplets; Genapap Extra Strength Tablets; Genapap, Infants'; Genapap Regular Strength Tablets; Genebs Extra Strength Caplets; Genebs Regular Strength Tablets; Genebs X-Tra Halenol Children's*; Liquiprin Infants' Drops; Mapap, Children's*; Mapap Infant Drops; Meda Cap; Neopap; Oraphen-PD; Panadol; Panadol, Children's; Panadol Extra Strength; Panadol, Infants'; Panadol Junior Strength Caplets; Panadol Maximum Strength Caplets; Panadol Maximum Strength Tablets; Panamax‡; Paralgin‡; Redutemp; Robigesic†; Rounox†; Snaplets-FR; St. Joseph Aspirin-Free Fever Reducer for Children; Suppap-120; Suppap-325; Suppap-650; Tapanol Extra Strength Caplets; Tapanol Extra Strength Tablets; Tempra; Tempra Caplets; Tempra Chewable Tablets; Tempra

---

Drops; Tempra D.S.; Tempra, Infants'; Tempra Syrup; Tylenol Arthritis; Tylenol Caplets; Tylenol Children's Chewable Tablets; Tylenol Children's Elixir; Tylenol Children's Tablets; Tylenol Drops; Tylenol Elixir*; Tylenol Extended Relief; Tylenol Extra Strength Adult Liquid Pain Reliever; Tylenol Extra Strength Caplets; Tylenol Extra Strength Gelcaps; Tylenol Extra Strength Tablets; Tylenol, Infant's Drops; Tylenol Infants' Suspension Drops; Tylenol Junior Strength Caplets; Tylenol Junior Strength Chewable Tablets; Tylenol Regular Strength Caplets; Tylenol Regular Strength Tablets; Tylenol Tablets; Valorin; Valorin Extra

Pregnancy Risk Category B

HOW SUPPLIED
Tablets: 160 mg, 325 mg, 500 mg, 650 mg
Tablets (chewable): 80 mg, 160 mg
Caplets: 160 mg, 500 mg
Caplets (extended-release): 650 mg
Capsules: 325 mg, 500 mg
Gelcaps: 500 mg
Geltabs: 500 mg
Oral drops: 80 mg/0.8 ml

Oral liquid: 160 mg/5 ml, 500 mg/15 ml
Oral solution: 48 mg/ml, 100 mg/ml
Oral suspension: 80 mg/ml, 120 mg/5 ml‡, 160 mg/5 ml
Oral syrup: 16 mg/ml
Elixir: 80 mg/5 ml, 120 mg/5 ml, 160 mg/5 ml*, 325 mg/5 ml*
Sprinkles: 80 mg/capsule, 160 mg/capsule
Suppositories: 80 mg, 120 mg, 125 mg, 300 mg, 325 mg, 650 mg

ACTION
Unknown. Thought to produce analgesia by blocking generation of pain impulses, probably by inhibiting prostaglandin synthesis in the CNS or the synthesis or action of other substances that sensitize pain receptors to mechanical or chemical stimulation. Thought to relieve fever by central action in the hypothalamic heat-regulating center.

Route	Onset	Peak	Duration
P.O., P.R.	Unknown	0.5-2 hr	3-4 hr

INDICATIONS & DOSAGES
Mild pain or fever—
Adults: 325 to 650 mg P.O. q 4 to 6 hours p.r.n.; or 1 g P.O. t.i.d. or q.i.d., p.r.n. Or, two extended-release caplets P.O. q 8 hours p.r.n. Or, 650 mg P.R. q 4 to 6 hours, p.r.n. Maximum

dose shouldn't exceed 4 g daily. Dose for long-term therapy shouldn't exceed 2.6 g daily.
Children older than age 14: 650 mg P.O. q 4 to 6 hours p.r.n.
Children ages 12 to 14: 640 mg P.O. q 4 to 6 hours p.r.n.
Children age 11: 480 mg P.O. q 4 to 6 hours p.r.n.
Children ages 9 to 10: 400 mg P.O. q 4 to 6 hours p.r.n.
Children ages 6 to 8: 320 mg P.O. q 4 to 6 hours p.r.n.
Children ages 4 to 5: 240 mg P.O. q 4 to 6 hours p.r.n.
Children ages 2 to 3: 160 mg P.O. q 4 to 6 hours p.r.n.
Children ages 12 to 23 months: 120 mg P.O. q 4 to 6 hours p.r.n.
Children ages 4 to 11 months: 80 mg P.O. q 4 to 6 hours p.r.n.
Children up to age 3 months: 40 mg P.O. q 4 to 6 hours p.r.n.
Children ages 6 to 12: 325 mg P.R. q 4 to 6 hours p.r.n.
Children ages 3 to 6: 120 to 125 mg P.R. q 4 to 6 hours p.r.n.
Children ages 1 to 3: 80 mg P.R. q 4 to 6 hours p.r.n.
Children ages 3 to 11 months: 80 mg P.R. q 6 hours p.r.n.

ADVERSE REACTIONS
Hematologic: hemolytic anemia, *neutropenia, leukopenia, pancytopenia.*
Hepatic: *severe liver damage,* jaundice.

Metabolic: hypoglycemia.
Skin: rash, urticaria.

INTERACTIONS
Drug-drug
Barbiturates, carbamazepine, hydantoins, rifampin, sulfinpyrazone: high doses or long-term use of these drugs may reduce therapeutic effects and enhance hepatotoxic effects of acetaminophen. Advise patient to avoid using together.
Warfarin: anticoagulant effects may increase during long-term use with high doses of acetaminophen. Monitor patient closely.
Zidovudine: may increase incidence of bone marrow suppression. Monitor patient closely.

Drug-herb
Watercress: may inhibit oxidative metabolism of acetaminophen. Advise patient to avoid using together.

Drug-food
Caffeine: may enhance analgesic effects of acetaminophen. Monitor patient for effect.

Drug-lifestyle
Alcohol use: increases risk of hepatic damage. Advise patient to avoid using together.

Reactions may be *common*, uncommon, *life-threatening*, or COMMON AND LIFE-THREATENING.

CONTRAINDICATIONS
Contraindicated in patients who are hypersensitive to the drug.

OVERDOSE & TREATMENT
In acute overdose, hepatotoxicity causes plasma levels of 300 mcg/ml 4 hours after ingestion or 50 mcg/ml 12 hours after ingestion. Signs and symptoms of overdose include cyanosis, anemia, jaundice, skin eruptions, fever, emesis, CNS stimulation, delirium, methemoglobinemia progressing to depression, coma, vascular collapse, seizures, and death.

Acetaminophen poisoning develops in stages:
- *Stage 1:* 12 to 24 hours after ingestion; nausea, vomiting, diaphoresis, anorexia.
- *Stage 2:* 24 to 48 hours after ingestion; clinically improved but elevated liver function tests.
- *Stage 3:* 72 to 96 hours after ingestion; peak hepatotoxicity.
- *Stage 4:* 7 to 8 days after ingestion; recovery.

To treat toxic overdose of acetaminophen, empty the patient's stomach immediately by inducing emesis with ipecac syrup if patient is conscious or by gastric lavage. Administer activated charcoal via NG tube. Oral acetylcysteine (Mucomyst) is a specific antidote for acetaminophen poisoning and is most effective if started within 10 to 12 hours after ingestion, but it can help if started within 24 hours after ingestion. Administer a loading dose of 140 mg/kg P.O., followed by maintenance doses of 70 mg/kg P.O. q 4 hours for an additional 17 doses. Doses vomited within 1 hour of administration must be repeated. Remove charcoal before giving acetylcysteine because it may interfere with absorption of this antidote.

Acetylcysteine minimizes hepatic injury by supplying sulfydryl groups that bind with acetaminophen metabolites. Hemodialysis may help remove acetaminophen from the body. Monitor laboratory values and vital signs closely. Provide symptomatic and supportive measures (respiratory support, correction of fluid and electrolyte imbalances). Determine plasma acetaminophen levels at least 4 hours after overdose. If plasma acetaminophen levels indicate hepatotoxicity, perform liver function tests every 24 hours for at least 96 hours.

NURSING CONSIDERATIONS
- Use cautiously in patient with history of chronic alcohol use; hepatotoxicity has occurred after therapeutic doses.
- Many other OTC and prescription drugs contain acetamino-

phen; be aware of this when calculating total daily dose.

• Use liquid form for children and patients who have difficulty swallowing.

• Acetaminophen may cause false-positive decreases in blood glucose levels in home monitoring systems.

• Alcoholics must not exceed a daily dose of 2 g.

• Less than 1% of the dose of acetaminophen appears in breast milk. Drug may be used safely if therapy is short-term and doesn't exceed recommended dosages.

PATIENT TEACHING

• Tell parents to consult doctor before giving drug to children younger than age 2.

• Advise patient that the daily maximum dose is 4 g and shouldn't be exceeded.

• Advise patient that many OTC and prescription products contain acetaminophen. These should be accounted for when calculating total daily dose.

• Tell patient that drug is only for short-term use and to consult doctor if giving to children for longer than 5 days or adults for longer than 10 days.

• Tell patient not to use for self-medication of marked fever (over 103.1° F [39.5° C]), fever persisting longer than 3 days, or recurrent fever unless directed by a doctor.

• **Alert:** Warn patient that high doses or unsupervised long-term use can cause hepatic damage. Excessive ingestion of alcohol may increase the risk of hepatotoxicity.

• Tell breast-feeding patient that acetaminophen may be used safely if therapy is short-term and doesn't exceed recommended dosages.

aspirin (acetylsalicylic acid)

Artria S.R., ASA, Aspergum, Aspirin Regimen Bayer, Aspirin Regimen Children's, Aspro‡, Bayer Aspirin, Coryphen†, Easprin, Ecotrin, Empirin, Entrophen†, Extra Strength Bayer Arthritis Regimen, Halfprin, Norwich Extra Strength, Novasen†, ZORprin

aspirin, buffered (acetylsalicylic acid)

Adprin-B, Arthritis Pain Ascriptin, Bayer Buffered Aspirin, Bufferin, Extra Strength Adprin-B, Extra Strength Bayer Plus, Extra Strength Bufferin, Maximum Strength Ascriptin, Regular Strength Ascriptin, Tri-Buffered Bufferin

Pregnancy Risk Category D

HOW SUPPLIED
aspirin
Tablets: 325 mg, 500 mg
Tablets (chewable): 81 mg
Tablets (enteric-coated): 81
mg, 165 mg, 325 mg, 500 mg,
650 mg, 975 mg
Tablets (controlled-release):
800 mg
Tablets (timed-release): 81 mg,
650 mg, 800 mg
Gelcaps: 500 mg
Chewing gum: 227.5 mg
Suppositories: 120 mg, 200 mg,
300 mg, 600 mg

aspirin, buffered
Tablets: 325 mg, 500 mg

ACTION
Produces analgesia by blocking
peripheral prostaglandin synthesis. Pain threshold becomes
lower when prostaglandins sensitize pain receptors to mechanical and chemical stimulation;
aspirin and other salicylates
may prevent that effect. Exerts
anti-inflammatory effect by inhibiting prostaglandin synthesis; also may inhibit synthesis
or action of other mediators of
the inflammatory response. Relieves fever by acting on hypothalamic heat-regulating center
to cause peripheral vasodilation, thus increasing peripheral
blood supply and promoting
sweating; clinical effect is heat
loss and cooling by evapora-

tion. In low doses, appears to
impede clotting by blocking
prostaglandin synthesis, which
prevents formation of the
platelet-aggregating substance
thromboxane A.

Route	Onset	Peak	Duration
P.O.			
tablet	5-30 min	25-40 min	1-4 hr
buffered	5-30 min	1-2 hr	1-4 hr
extended	5-30 min	1-4 hr	1-4 hr
enteric-coated	5-30 min	Variable	1-4 hr
solution	5-30 min	15-40 min	1-4 hr
P.R.	Unknown	3-4 hr	Unknown

INDICATIONS & DOSAGES
*Rheumatoid arthritis, osteo-
arthritis, or other polyarthritic
or inflammatory conditions—*
Adults: initially, 2.4 to 3.6 g
P.O. daily in divided doses.
Maintenance dosage is 3.2 to
6 g P.O. daily in divided doses.

Juvenile rheumatoid arthritis—
Children: 60 to 110 mg/kg/day
P.O. in divided doses q 6 to 8
hours.

Mild pain or fever—
**Adults and children older
than age 11:** 325 to 650 mg
P.O. or P.R. q 4 hours, p.r.n.
Children ages 2 to 11: 10 to 15
mg/kg per dose P.O. or P.R. q 4
hours up to 80 mg/kg/day.

*Liquid contains alcohol.   **May contain tartrazine.   †Canada   ‡Australia   §U.K.

Prevention of thrombosis (transient ischemic attack)—
Adults: 1.3 g P.O. daily in two to four divided doses.

Reduction of risk of heart attack in patients with previous MI or unstable angina—
Adults: 160 to 325 mg P.O. daily.

Acute rheumatic fever—
Adults: 5 to 8 g P.O. daily.
Children: 100 mg/kg/day P.O. for 2 weeks; then 75 mg/kg/day P.O. for 4 to 6 weeks.

ADVERSE REACTIONS
EENT: tinnitus, hearing loss.
GI: nausea, GI distress, occult bleeding, dyspepsia, *GI bleeding.*
Hematologic: *leukopenia, thrombocytopenia*, prolonged bleeding time.
Hepatic: abnormal liver function tests, *hepatitis.*
Skin: rash, bruising, urticaria.
Other: *angioedema, hypersensitivity reactions* (*anaphylaxis*, asthma), *Reye's syndrome.*

INTERACTIONS
Drug-drug
ACE inhibitors: may decrease antihypertensive effects. Monitor blood pressure closely.
Activated charcoal: decreases aspirin absorption (dose and frequency related). Give aspirin between activated charcoal doses.
Antacids, urinary alkalinizers: decreases serum salicylate levels. Monitor patient for decreased therapeutic salicylate effect.
Anticoagulants: increases risk of bleeding. Advise patient to avoid using together.
Beta blockers: decreases antihypertensive effect. Advise patient to avoid long-term aspirin use if he's taking antihypertensives.
Carbonic anhydrase inhibitors: causes salicylate intoxication. Monitor patient closely.
Corticosteroids: enhances salicylate elimination. Monitor patient for decreased salicylate effect.
Exogenous insulin and sulfonylureas: may increase risk of hypoglycemia. Monitor patient closely. Assess for dose adjustment.
Loop diuretics (in patient with renal dysfunction, or cirrhosis with ascites): may decrease therapeutic effect of diuretic. Monitor patient closely. Assess for dose adjustment.
Methotrexate: increases risk of methotrexate toxicity. Advise patient to avoid using together.
Nitroglycerin: increases potential for hypotension. Adjust nitroglycerin levels, as needed.

Nizatidine: may increase risk of salicylate toxicity in patient receiving high doses of aspirin. Monitor patient closely.

NSAIDs, including diflunisal, fenoprofen, ibuprofen, indomethacin, meclofenamate, naproxen, piroxicam: decreases NSAID serum levels, resulting in decreased NSAID therapeutic effect. Advise patient to avoid using together.

Oral antidiabetics: increases hypoglycemic effect. Monitor patient closely; assess for dose adjustment.

Probenecid, sulfinpyrazone: decreases uricosuric effect. Advise patient to avoid using together.

Urine acidifiers (ascorbic acid, methionine): increases salicylate blood levels. Monitor patient for aspirin toxicity.

Valproic acid: increases valproic acid therapeutic effect. Advise patient to avoid using together.

Drug-herb
Horse chestnut, kelpware, red clover: increases risk of bleeding. Discourage patient from using together.

Drug-food
Caffeine: may increase absorption of aspirin. Monitor patient for increased aspirin effects.

Drug-lifestyle
Alcohol use: increases risk of GI ulceration and prolonged bleeding time. Advise patient to avoid using together.

CONTRAINDICATIONS
Contraindicated in patients who are hypersensitive to drug and in those with NSAID-induced sensitivity reactions; G6PD deficiency; or bleeding disorders, such as hemophilia, von Willebrand's disease, or telangiectasia.

OVERDOSE & TREATMENT
Signs and symptoms of overdose include GI discomfort, oliguria, acute renal failure, hyperthermia, electroencephalogram (EEG) abnormalities, and restlessness. Patients also may have metabolic acidosis with respiratory alkalosis, hyperpnea, and tachypnea caused by increased carbon dioxide production and direct stimulation of the respiratory center.

To treat aspirin overdose, empty the patient's stomach immediately by inducing emesis with ipecac syrup if patient is conscious or by gastric lavage. Administer activated charcoal via NG tube. Provide symptomatic and supportive measures (respiratory support and correction of fluid and electrolyte imbalances). Closely monitor laboratory values and vital signs. Enhance renal excretion by giving sodium bicarbonate to alkalinize urine. Use cooling blanket or sponging if patient's rectal temperature is higher than 104° F (40° C).

Hemodialysis is effective in removing aspirin but is only used in severely poisoned individuals or those at risk for pulmonary edema.

NURSING CONSIDERATIONS

• Use cautiously in patient with GI lesions, impaired renal function, hypoprothrombinemia, vitamin K deficiency, thrombocytopenia, thrombotic thrombocytopenic purpura, or severe hepatic impairment.

• *Alert:* Because of possible link to Reye's syndrome, the Centers for Disease Control and Prevention recommends not giving salicylates to children or teenagers with chickenpox or flulike illness.

• For inflammatory conditions, rheumatic fever, and thrombosis, give aspirin on a schedule, rather than as needed.

• Enteric-coated and sustained-release tablets are slowly absorbed and therefore aren't suitable for rapid relief from acute pain, fever, or inflammation. They do cause less GI bleeding and may be better suited for long-term therapy, such as treatment of arthritis.

• Aspirin irreversibly inhibits platelet aggregation. It should be discontinued 5 to 7 days before elective surgery, as ordered, to allow time for the production and release of new platelets.

• During prolonged therapy, hematocrit, hemoglobin level, PT, INR, and renal function should be assessed periodically, as ordered.

• For patient with swallowing difficulties, crush non–enteric-coated aspirin and dissolve in soft food or liquid. Administer liquid immediately after mixing because drug will break down rapidly.

• Buffered aspirins may include calcium carbonate, magnesium oxide, magnesium carbonate, or alumina-magnesia.

• Pregnant patients should avoid aspirin, especially during last trimester of pregnancy, unless directed by a doctor.

• Salicylates are excreted in breast milk in low concentrations.

• Febrile, dehydrated children can develop toxicity rapidly.

• Monitor elderly patient closely because he may be more susceptible to aspirin's toxic effects.

Reactions may be *common*, uncommon, *life-threatening*, or COMMON AND LIFE-THREATENING.

PATIENT TEACHING

• Instruct patient with history of tartrazine dye (F&D 6) allergy to avoid aspirin.

• Advise patient on sodium-restricted diet that 1 tablet of buffered aspirin contains 553 mg of sodium.

• Advise patient to take aspirin with food, milk, antacid, or large glass of water to reduce adverse GI reactions.

• Tell patient that sustained-release or enteric-coated preparations shouldn't be crushed or chewed but should be swallowed whole.

• Instruct patient to discard aspirin tablets that have a strong vinegar-like odor.

• Tell patient to consult doctor before giving drug to a child for longer than 5 days or to an adult for longer than 10 days.

• Advise patient receiving prolonged treatment with large doses of aspirin to watch for petechiae, bleeding gums, and signs of GI bleeding, and to maintain adequate fluid intake. Encourage use of a soft-bristled toothbrush.

• Because of many possible drug interactions involving aspirin, warn patient taking prescription drugs to check with doctor or pharmacist before taking aspirin or OTC products containing aspirin.

• Instruct pregnant patient to avoid aspirin, especially during last trimester of pregnancy, unless directed by a doctor.

• Caution parents to keep aspirin out of reach of children because aspirin is a leading cause of poisoning in children. Encourage use of child-resistant containers.

caffeine

Caffedrine, Enerjets, Keep Alert, NoDoz, Quick Pep, Vivarin

Pregnancy Risk Category C

HOW SUPPLIED

Tablets: 100 mg, 150 mg, 200 mg
Tablets (timed-release): 200 mg
Caplets: 200 mg
Capsules (timed-release): 200 mg
Lozenges: 75 mg

ACTION

Inhibits phosphodiesterase, the enzyme that degrades cyclic adenosine monophosphate (cAMP). Caffeine stimulates all levels of the CNS; improves level of arousal and psychomotor coordination.

Route	Onset	Peak	Duration
P.O.	Unknown	50-75 min	Unknown

INDICATIONS & DOSAGES
Mental or physical fatigue or drowsiness—
Adults: 100 to 200 mg anhydrous caffeine P.O. q 3 to 4 hours, p.r.n.

ADVERSE REACTIONS
CNS: insomnia, restlessness, nervousness, headache, excitement, agitation, muscle tremor, twitching.
CV: tachycardia, palpitations, extrasystoles.
EENT: tinnitus.
GI: nausea, vomiting, diarrhea, stomach pain.
GU: diuresis.
Other: irritability after abrupt withdrawal.

INTERACTIONS
Drug-drug
Beta agonists, cimetidine, fluoroquinolones, oral contraceptives, theophylline: excessive CNS stimulation. Advise patient to avoid using together.

Drug-food
Beverages containing caffeine: excessive CNS stimulation. Advise patient to use with caution.

CONTRAINDICATIONS
Contraindicated in patients who are hypersensitive to caffeine.

OVERDOSE & TREATMENT
Signs and symptoms of overdose in adults may include insomnia, dyspnea, altered states of consciousness, muscle twitching, seizures, diuresis, arrhythmias, and fever. In infants, symptoms may include alternating hypotonicity and hypertonicity, opisthotonoid posture, tremors, bradycardia, hypotension, and severe acidosis.

Treat overdose symptomatically and supportively; gastric lavage and charcoal may help. Carefully monitor vital signs, ECG, and fluid and electrolyte balance. Seizures may be treated with diazepam or phenobarbital; diazepam can exacerbate respiratory depression.

NURSING CONSIDERATIONS
• Patient with a history of peptic ulcer, symptomatic arrhythmias, or palpitations should use drug with caution.
• Caffeine doesn't reverse alcohol intoxication or CNS depressant effects of alcohol. Overly vigorous therapy with caffeine may aggravate depression in an already depressed patient.
• Caffeine content of 8 fluid ounces of coffee ranges from 70 to 250 mg; content can be as high as 47.5 mg per 8 fluid ounces in carbonated beverages (depending on brand); and content in tea can range from 35 to

128 mg per fluid ounce. Unsweetened baking chocolate contains 35 to 60 mg per ounce.
• **Alert:** A single dose shouldn't exceed 1 g.
• Watch for signs and symptoms of overdose, such as GI pain, mild delirium, insomnia, diuresis, dehydration, and fever. Treat with short-acting barbiturates, gastric emesis, or lavage, as ordered.
• Monitor patient for excessive use. Use for longer than 5 to 7 days should be medically evaluated.
• Sudden discontinuation of caffeine may cause headache and irritability.

PATIENT TEACHING
• Advise patient that OTC caffeine is for occasional use only.
• Stress importance of not exceeding recommended dosage.
• Instruct patient to stop taking caffeine if increased or abnormal heart rate, dizziness, or palpitations occur.
• Advise patient that caffeine shouldn't be used as a substitute for sleep.
• Advise patient to minimize use of medications, food, or beverages that contain caffeine while taking OTC caffeine.
• Tell patient to take drug at least 6 hours before bedtime to avoid sleep interference.

• Warn patient with a seizure disorder that drug may decrease seizure threshold. Instruct him to notify doctor if a seizure occurs.

capsaicin
Axsain, Benejoint, Capzasin-HP, Capzasin-P, Dolorac, No Pain-HP, Pain-X, R-Gel, Zostrix, Zostrix-HP

Pregnancy Risk Category NR

HOW SUPPLIED
Cream: 0.025% (Benejoint, Zostrix), 0.075% (Axsain, Capzasin-HP, Zostrix-HP), 0.25% (Dolorac)
Roll-on gel: 0.025%, 0.05%, 0.075%

ACTION
Unknown. May increase release of substance P, a principal neurotransmitter for pain, from peripheral type C sensory fibers to central neurons.

Route	Onset	Peak	Duration
Topical	Unknown	Unknown	Unknown

INDICATIONS & DOSAGES
Temporary relief from pain after herpes zoster infections; neuralgias, such as postoperative pain and painful diabetic neuropathy; pain associated

*with osteoarthritis or rheuma-
toid arthritis—*
**Adults and children older
than age 2:** apply to affected
areas not more than q.i.d.

*Temporary relief from arthritis
pain—*
(Dolorac)
**Adults and children ages 12
and older:** apply thin film to
affected area b.i.d.
(Capzasin-HP)
Adults: apply to affected area
t.i.d. or q.i.d.

*Temporary relief from aches
and pains associated with
arthritis—*
(Zostrix, Zostrix-HP)
**Adults and children ages 2
and older:** apply a thin film to
affected area t.i.d. or q.i.d.

ADVERSE REACTIONS
Respiratory: cough, irritation.
Skin: redness, stinging, or
burning on application.

INTERACTIONS
None significant.

CONTRAINDICATIONS
Contraindicated in patients who
are hypersensitive to drug.

OVERDOSE & TREATMENT
No information available.

NURSING CONSIDERATIONS
• Drug is for external use only.
• Burning or stinging may occur
initially but decreases with cautious use.

PATIENT TEACHING
• Warn patient to avoid getting
drug in eyes or on broken skin.
• Advise patient not to bandage
area tightly after applying drug.
• Tell patient to wash hands
with oil-cutting soap or detergent after applying drug.
• Inform patient that transient
burning or stinging is usually
evident at initial therapy but decreases with cautious use. This
effect persists in patients who
use drug less often than t.i.d. If
burning is severe, tell patient to
discontinue use of drug.
• Tell patient not to expose
treated area to heat or direct
sunlight.
• Caution patient against using
capsaicin oil (food additive) as
a topical treatment because of
the potential for severe skin reaction.
• Tell patient who is treating
himself with capsaicin to contact doctor if symptoms persist
longer than 2 to 4 weeks or resolve and shortly reappear.

choline salicylate
Arthropan

Pregnancy Risk Category C

HOW SUPPLIED
Liquid: 870 mg/5 ml

ACTION
Produces analgesia by affecting the hypothalamus (central action) and by blocking pain impulses (peripheral action). The peripheral action may involve inhibition of prostaglandin synthesis. Anti-inflammatory effect is produced by inhibiting synthesis of prostaglandins and perhaps inhibiting synthesis or action of other inflammation mediators. Relieves fever by acting on the hypothalamic heat-regulating center to produce peripheral vasodilation, which promotes sweating. Clinical result is cooling by evaporation. These drugs don't affect platelet aggregation and shouldn't be used to prevent thrombosis.

Route	Onset	Peak	Duration
P.O.	Variable	1-2 hr	4-6 hr

INDICATIONS & DOSAGES
Analgesia and antipyresis—
Adults and children ages 12 and older: 870 mg P.O. q 3 to 4 hours, p.r.n., not to exceed 6 doses per day.

Rheumatoid arthritis, osteoarthritis, and other inflammatory conditions—
Adults: 4.8 to 7.2 g (28 to 41 ml) P.O. daily in divided doses.
Children: 107 to 134 mg (0.6 to 0.8 ml) per kg daily in divided doses.

ADVERSE REACTIONS
EENT: tinnitus, hearing loss.
GI: GI bleeding, GI distress, nausea, vomiting.
GU: *acute tubular necrosis with renal failure.*
Skin: rash.
Other: elevated free T_4 levels, *hypersensitivity reactions (anaphylaxis), Reye's syndrome.*

INTERACTIONS
Drug-drug
Ammonium chloride and other urine acidifiers: increases choline salicylate blood levels. Monitor patient closely.
Antacids, urine alkalizers: delays and decreases absorption of choline salicylates. Monitor patient for decreased salicylate effect.
Corticosteroids: enhances salicylate elimination. Monitor patient for decreased effect.
GI-irritant drugs (such as antibiotics, other NSAIDs, steroids): increases GI irritation.

---

*Liquid contains alcohol.   **May contain tartrazine.   †Canada   ‡Australia   §U.K.

Advise patient to avoid using together.

Highly protein-bound (phenytoin, sulfonylureas, warfarin): may displace either drug. Monitor patient closely.

Lithium carbonate: increases serum lithium levels and risk of adverse effects. Monitor patient closely.

Methotrexate: may displace bound methotrexate and inhibit renal excretion. Monitor patient closely.

Sulfonylureas: enhances hypoglycemic effects. Monitor patient closely.

Warfarin: enhances anticoagulation effects. Advise patient to avoid using together.

Drug-food
Food: delays and decreases absorption of choline salicylate. Tell patient to take drug on an empty stomach.

CONTRAINDICATIONS
Contraindicated in patients who are hypersensitive to drug; with hemophilia, bleeding ulcers, or hemorrhagic states; who consume 3 or more alcoholic beverages per day; and in children or teenagers with chickenpox or flulike illness. Use cautiously in patient with impaired renal or hepatic function, peptic ulcer disease, or gastritis.

OVERDOSE & TREATMENT
Signs and symptoms of overdose include metabolic acidosis with respiratory alkalosis, hyperpnea, and tachypnea from increased carbon dioxide production and direct stimulation of the respiratory center.

To treat overdose of choline salicylate, empty stomach immediately by inducing emesis with ipecac syrup, if patient is conscious, or by gastric lavage. Give activated charcoal via NG tube. Provide symptomatic and supportive measures (respiratory support and correction of fluid and electrolyte imbalances). Monitor laboratory values and vital signs closely. Hemodialysis is effective in removing choline salicylate but is used only in severe poisoning. Forced diuresis with alkalinizing agent accelerates salicylate excretion.

NURSING CONSIDERATIONS
• Don't mix choline salicylate with antacids.
• Mix choline salicylate with fruit juice followed by a full 8-oz (240-ml) glass of water to ensure passage into stomach.
• Choline salicylate has fewer side effects than aspirin.
• Warn women to avoid use of choline salicylate in the third trimester of pregnancy.

PATIENT TEACHING
• Advise patient to avoid use of antacids while taking choline salicylate.
• Caution patient to carefully read the label and follow directions.
• Explain that choline salicylate should be mixed with fruit juice, a carbonated beverage, or water before administration.

---

diphenhydramine hydrochloride
Compoz Nighttime Sleep Aid Maximum Strength, Dormin, Maximum Strength Nytol, Midol PM, Miles Nervine, Nytol, Sleep-eze 3, Sleepinal, Sominex, Twilite, Unisom Sleepgels

Pregnancy Risk Category B

HOW SUPPLIED
Tablets: 25 mg, 50 mg
Capsules: 25 mg, 50 mg
Caplets: 25 mg, 50 mg
Softgels: 50 mg

ACTION
Competes with histamine for H_1-receptor sites on effector cells. Prevents, but doesn't reverse, histamine-mediated responses, particularly histamine's effects on the smooth muscle of the bronchial tubes, GI tract, uterus, and blood vessels. Structurally related to local anesthetics, diphenhydramine provides local anesthesia by preventing initiation and transmission of nerve impulses. Also suppresses cough reflex by a direct effect in the medulla of the brain.

Route	Onset	Peak	Duration
P.O.	15 min	1-4 hr	6-8 hr

INDICATIONS & DOSAGES
Nighttime sleep aid—
Adults: 25 to 50 mg P.O. h.s., if needed, or as directed by a doctor.

ADVERSE REACTIONS
CNS: drowsiness, confusion, insomnia, headache, vertigo, sedation, sleepiness, dizziness, incoordination, fatigue, restlessness, tremor, nervousness, *seizures.*
CV: palpitations, hypotension, tachycardia.
EENT: diplopia, blurred vision, nasal congestion, tinnitus.
GI: nausea, vomiting, diarrhea, dry mouth, constipation, epigastric distress, anorexia.
GU: dysuria, urine retention, urinary frequency.
Hematologic: hemolytic anemia, *thrombocytopenia, agranulocytosis.*
Respiratory: thickening of bronchial secretions.

Skin: urticaria, photosensitivity, rash.
Other: *anaphylactic shock.*

INTERACTIONS
Drug-drug
CNS depressants: increases sedation. Advise patient to use together cautiously.
MAO inhibitors: increases anticholinergic effects. Advise patient to avoid using together.

Drug-lifestyle
Alcohol use: increases CNS depression. Advise patient to use together cautiously.
Sun exposure: photosensitivity reactions may occur. Tell patient to avoid prolonged or unprotected sun exposure.

CONTRAINDICATIONS
Contraindicated in patients who are hypersensitive to drug; in those with angle-closure glaucoma, stenosing peptic ulcer, symptomatic prostatic hyperplasia, bladder neck obstruction, or pyloroduodenal obstruction; in newborns with ongoing acute asthmatic attacks; and in premature neonates or breast-feeding women. Avoid use in patient taking MAO inhibitors.

OVERDOSE & TREATMENT
Drowsiness is the usual symptom of overdose. Seizures, coma, and respiratory depression may follow profound overdose. Anticholinergic symptoms, such as dry mouth, flushed skin, fixed and dilated pupils, or GI symptoms, are common, especially in children.

In a conscious patient, treat overdose by inducing emesis with ipecac syrup followed by activated charcoal to reduce further drug absorption. If the patient is unconscious or ipecac fails, use gastric lavage. Treat hypotension with vasopressors, and control seizures with diazepam or phenytoin. Don't give stimulants.

NURSING CONSIDERATIONS
• Don't give drug to patient with breathing problems such as emphysema or chronic bronchitis, or with glaucoma or difficulty in urination caused by enlargement of the prostate gland, unless directed by a doctor.
• Evaluate environmental and physical factors contributing to insomnia.
• If insomnia persists for longer than 2 weeks, patient should consult a doctor.
• Pregnant patient should avoid taking drug.
• Breast-feeding patient should avoid drug because newborns are particularly sensitive to antihistamines.

• Children younger than age 12 should use only as directed by a doctor.

• Elderly patient is more sensitive to drug and should be monitored.

PATIENT TEACHING

• Advise patient not to exceed recommended dosage.

• Tell patient to take diphenhydramine with food or milk to reduce GI distress.

• Warn patient to avoid alcohol and driving or other hazardous activities that require alertness until drug's CNS effects are known.

• Tell patient that coffee or tea may reduce drowsiness and to use the drug cautiously if palpitations develop.

• Inform patient that sugarless gum, sugarless sour hard candy, or ice chips may relieve dry mouth.

• Tell patient to notify doctor if tolerance develops.

• Advise patient to consult doctor before using any other OTC products; many contain diphenhydramine.

• Warn patient of possible photosensitivity reactions; advise use of a sunblock.

• Teach patient the principles of good sleep hygiene such as following a regular sleep pattern, not exercising late in the evening, avoiding large meals or snacks before bedtime, eliminating daytime naps, and limiting caffeine intake.

• Tell pregnant or breast-feeding patient not to take diphenhydramine without the advice of a doctor.

---

doxylamine succinate
Unisom Nighttime Sleep-Aid

Pregnancy Risk Category NR

HOW SUPPLIED
Tablets: 25 mg

ACTION
Drug is an antihistamine, which acts on the CNS by producing prominent sedative effects.

Route	Onset	Peak	Duration
P.O.	Unknown	2-3 hr	Up to 10 hr

INDICATIONS & DOSAGES
Reduces difficulty in falling asleep—
Adults and children ages 12 years and older: 1 tablet (25 mg), P.O., 30 minutes before bedtime. Don't exceed one dose per day.

ADVERSE REACTIONS
CNS: anticholinergic effects (dry mouth, urinary retention, confusion, constipation, tachycardia), excessive sedation.

INTERACTIONS
Drug-drug
CNS depressant: increases sedation. Advise patient to use together cautiously.
MAO inhibitors: increases anticholinergic effects. Advise patient to avoid using together.

Drug-lifestyle
Alcohol: causes excessive sedation. Advise patient to avoid using together.

CONTRAINDICATIONS
Contraindicated in patients with breathing problems such as emphysema or chronic bronchitis; in those who have glaucoma or difficulty urinating caused by enlarged prostate gland; and in pregnant and breast-feeding patients.

OVERDOSE & TREATMENT
Effects include mild CNS depression, CV collapse, hypotension, respiratory depression, hallucinations, tremors, and convulsions which occur 30 minutes to 2 hours after ingestion and are usually a poor prognostic factor. Anticholinergic effects may also develop.

Treatment includes induction of emesis, and administration of a cathartic laxative and supportive measures.

NURSING CONSIDERATIONS
• Patient may experience mental status changes and confusion.
• Evaluate environmental and physical factors contributing to insomnia.
• Pregnant patient should avoid using drug.
• Breast-feeding patient should not take drug unless directed by a doctor.
• Elderly patient is more sensitive than younger adults to the anticholinergic effects of antihistamines.

PATIENT TEACHING
• Advise patient not to use this medication for longer than 2 weeks, unless directed by a doctor.
• Instruct patient to take drug 30 minutes before bedtime.
• Advise patient not to drive or operate machinery after taking this drug.
• Warn patient against using drug and alcohol together.
• Advise patient to consult doctor if drug is used for longer than 14 consecutive days.
• Teach patient the principles of good sleep hygiene such as following a regular sleep pattern, not exercising late in the evening, avoiding large meals or snacks before bedtime, eliminating daytime naps, and limiting caffeine intake.

Reactions may be *common,* uncommon, *life-threatening,* or COMMON AND LIFE-THREATENING.

• Instruct pregnant or breast-feeding patient not to take medication without consulting a doctor.

---

ibuprofen

Advil, Advil Liqui-Gels, Advil Migraine, Children's Advil, Children's Motrin, Ibu-Tab 200, Infant's Motrin, Junior Strength Advil, Junior Strength Motrin, Medipren, Midol Maximum Strength Cramp Formula, Motrin, Motrin IB, Motrin Migraine, Nuprin, Pediatric Advil Drops, Pediacare Fever, Profen

Pregnancy Risk Category B

HOW SUPPLIED
Tablets: 100 mg, 200 mg
Caplets and gelcaps: 200 mg
Tablets (chewable): 50 mg, 100 mg
Capsules: 200 mg
Oral suspension: 100 mg/2.5 ml, 100 mg/5 ml
Oral drops: 40 mg/ml

ACTION
Unknown. Produces analgesic, anti-inflammatory, and antipyretic effects, possibly by inhibiting prostaglandin synthesis.

Route	Onset	Peak	Duration
P.O.	Variable	1-2 hr	4-6 hr

INDICATIONS & DOSAGES
Rheumatoid arthritis, osteoarthritis, arthritis—
Adults: 300 to 800 mg P.O. t.i.d. or q.i.d. not to exceed 3.2 g daily.

Mild to moderate pain, dysmenorrhea—
Adults: 400 mg P.O. q 4 to 6 hours, p.r.n.

Minor aches, pains, and fever—
Adults: 200 to 400 mg P.O. q 4 to 6 hours. Don't exceed 1.2 g daily or give longer than 3 days.
Children ages 6 months to 12 years: fever below 102.5° F (39° C), 5 mg/kg P.O. q 6 to 8 hours; higher fevers, 10 mg/kg q 6 to 8 hours. Don't exceed 40 mg/kg daily.

Juvenile arthritis—
Children: 30 to 70 mg/kg/day P.O. in three or four divided doses.

ADVERSE REACTIONS
CNS: headache, dizziness, nervousness, *aseptic meningitis.*
CV: peripheral edema, fluid retention, edema.
EENT: tinnitus.
GI: epigastric distress, nausea, occult blood loss, peptic ulceration, diarrhea, constipation, dyspepsia, flatulence, heartburn, decreased appetite.

---

*Liquid contains alcohol.   **May contain tartrazine.   †Canada   ‡Australia   §U.K.

GU: *acute renal failure,* azotemia, cystitis, hematuria, increased BUN and creatinine levels.
Hematologic: prolonged bleeding time, anemia, *neutropenia, pancytopenia, thrombocytopenia, aplastic anemia, leukopenia, agranulocytosis.*
Hepatic: elevates liver enzyme levels.
Metabolic: hypoglycemia, hyperkalemia.
Respiratory: *bronchospasm.*
Skin: pruritus, rash, urticaria, *Stevens-Johnson syndrome.*
Other: decreases serum uric acid levels.

INTERACTIONS
Drug-drug
Antihypertensives, furosemide, thiazide diuretics: ibuprofen may decrease effectiveness of diuretics or antihypertensives. Monitor patient closely.
Aspirin: may decrease serum levels of ibuprofen. Advise patient to avoid using together.
Corticosteroids: increases risk of adverse GI reactions. Advise patient to avoid using together.
Cyclosporine: may increase nephrotoxicity of both drugs. Advise patient to avoid using together.
Digoxin, lithium, oral anticoagulants: ibuprofen may increase plasma levels or effects of these drugs. Monitor patient for toxicity.
Methotrexate: decreases methotrexate clearance and increases toxicity. Advise patient to use together cautiously.

Drug-herb
Dong quai, feverfew, garlic, ginger, horse chestnut, red clover: may increase risk of bleeding. Advise patient to avoid using together.
St. John's wort: increases photosensitivity. Advise patient to use sunscreen.

Drug-lifestyle
Alcohol use: increases risk of adverse GI reactions. Advise patient to avoid using together.
Sun exposure: may cause photosensitivity reactions. Advise patient to use sunscreen.

CONTRAINDICATIONS
Contraindicated in patients who are hypersensitive to drug or who have angioedema, syndrome of nasal polyps, or bronchospastic reaction to aspirin or other NSAIDs.

OVERDOSE & TREATMENT
Signs and symptoms of overdose include dizziness, drowsiness, paresthesia, vomiting, nausea, abdominal pain, headache, sweating, nystagmus, apnea, and cyanosis.

To treat drug overdose, empty stomach immediately by inducing emesis with ipecac syrup or by gastric lavage. Administer activated charcoal via NG tube. Provide symptomatic and supportive measures (respiratory support and correction of fluid and electrolyte imbalances). Monitor laboratory values and vital signs closely. Alkaline diuresis may enhance renal excretion. Dialysis is of minimal value because ibuprofen is strongly protein-bound.

NURSING CONSIDERATIONS

- Use cautiously in patient with GI disorders, history of peptic ulcer disease, hepatic or renal disease, cardiac decompensation, hypertension, or known intrinsic coagulation defects.
- Serious GI toxicity, including peptic ulceration and bleeding, can occur in patient taking NSAIDs, despite absence of GI symptoms.
- Use of drug in pregnant patient isn't recommended.
- Anti-inflammatory and antipyretic actions of NSAIDs may mask the signs and symptoms of infection.
- Blurred or diminished vision and changes in color vision have occurred.
- Full anti-inflammatory effects may take 1 to 2 weeks to occur.

- Only insignificant amounts of the drug appear in breast milk, but drug manufacturer recommends that patient should stop breast-feeding during therapy.
- Safety and efficacy in children younger than age 6 months haven't been established.
- Patient older than age 60 may be more susceptible to toxic effects of drug, especially adverse GI reactions. Advise patient to use lowest dose possible.
- Drug's effect on renal prostaglandins may cause fluid retention and edema. Elderly patient should avoid use.

PATIENT TEACHING

- Tell patient to take with meals or milk to reduce adverse GI reactions.
- **Alert:** Instruct patient not to take more than 1.2 g daily, not to give to children younger than age 12, and not to self-medicate for extended periods without consulting doctor.
- Caution patient that use with aspirin, alcohol, or corticosteroids may increase risk of adverse GI reactions.
- Teach patient signs and symptoms of GI bleeding, and tell him to notify doctor immediately if they occur.
- Instruct patient to carefully read and follow package instructions and not to take drug

for longer than 10 days for pain or 3 days for fever.
- Warn patient to avoid hazardous activities that require mental alertness until CNS effects are known.
- Advise patient to wear sunscreen to avoid photosensitivity reactions.

---

ketoprofen
Orudis KT

Pregnancy Risk Category B

HOW SUPPLIED
Tablets: 12.5 mg

ACTION
Unknown. Produces anti-inflammatory, analgesic, and antipyretic effects, possibly by inhibiting prostaglandin synthesis.

Route	Onset	Peak	Duration
P.O.	1-2 hr	0.5-2 hr	3-4 hr

INDICATIONS & DOSAGES
Minor aches and pain or fever—
Adults: 12.5 mg q 4 to 6 hours while symptoms are present. If pain or fever doesn't diminish, can take 1 more tablet (12.5 mg). Don't exceed 25 mg (2 tablets) in a 4- to 6-hour period or 75 mg (6 tablets) in 24 hours.

For elderly patient and patient with impaired renal function, reduce initial dose to between one-third and one-half of normal initial dose.

ADVERSE REACTIONS
CNS: headache, dizziness, CNS excitation or depression.
EENT: tinnitus, visual disturbances.
GI: nausea, abdominal pain, diarrhea, constipation, flatulence, *GI bleeding,* peptic ulceration, dyspepsia, anorexia, vomiting, stomatitis.
GU: *nephrotoxicity,* elevated BUN level.
Hematologic: prolonged bleeding time.
Hepatic: elevated liver enzyme levels.
Respiratory: dyspnea.
Skin: rash, photosensitivity.
Other: peripheral edema.

INTERACTIONS
Drug-drug
Aspirin, corticosteroids: increases risk of adverse GI reactions. Advise patient to avoid using together.
Aspirin, probenecid: increases plasma levels of ketoprofen. Advise patient to avoid using together.
Cyclosporine: increases nephrotoxicity. Advise patient to avoid using together.

Reactions may be *common*, uncommon, *life-threatening*, or COMMON AND LIFE-THREATENING.

Hydrochlorothiazide, other diuretics: decreases diuretic effectiveness. Monitor patient for lack of effect.
Lithium, methotrexate, phenytoin: increases levels of these drugs, leading to toxicity. Monitor patient closely.
Warfarin: increases risk of bleeding. Monitor patient closely.

Drug-herb
Dong quai, feverfew, garlic, ginger, horse chestnut, red clover: may increase risk of bleeding. Advise patient to avoid using together.
St. John's wort: increases photosensitivity. Advise patient to use sunscreen.

Drug-lifestyle
Alcohol use: increases risk of GI toxicity. Advise patient to avoid using together.
Sun exposure: may cause photosensitivity reactions. Advise patient to use sunscreen.

CONTRAINDICATIONS
Contraindicated in patients who are hypersensitive to drug or who have a history of aspirin- or NSAID-induced asthma, urticaria, or other allergy-type reactions.

OVERDOSE & TREATMENT
Signs and symptoms of overdose include nausea and drowsiness.

To treat, induce emesis with ipecac syrup or empty stomach via gastric lavage; give activated charcoal via NG tube. Provide symptomatic and supportive measures (respiratory support and correction of fluid and electrolyte imbalances). Monitor laboratory values and vital signs closely. Hemodialysis may be useful in removing ketoprofen and assisting in care of renal failure.

NURSING CONSIDERATIONS
• Use cautiously in patient with history of peptic ulcer disease, renal dysfunction, hypertension, heart failure, or fluid retention.
• Watch carefully for signs and symptoms of infection; the antipyretic and anti-inflammatory actions can mask these signs and symptoms.
• Monitor closely patient with preexisting renal failure, liver dysfunction, or heart failure.
• Serious GI toxicity, including peptic ulceration and bleeding, can occur in patient taking NSAIDs, despite absence of GI symptoms.
• Pregnant patient should avoid using drug during last trimester of pregnancy.

- Although most NSAIDs appear in breast milk, specific information about ketoprofen is unknown. Breast-feeding patient should avoid drug.
- NSAIDs impair synthesis of renal prostaglandins, which decreases renal blood flow and causes reversible renal impairment. Elderly patient is more sensitive to this and other toxic effects of the drug; monitor patient closely.

PATIENT TEACHING
- Instruct patient to take drug with 8 oz of water.
- If adverse GI reactions occur, patient may take drug with milk or meals.
- Teach patient signs and symptoms of GI bleeding, and tell him to notify doctor immediately if they occur.
- *Alert:* Use of aspirin, alcohol, or corticosteroids may increase risk of adverse GI reactions.
- Advise patient to use sunblock, wear protective clothing, and avoid prolonged exposure to sunlight because drug has been associated with photosensitivity reactions.
- Instruct patient to carefully read and follow package instructions and not to take drug for longer than 10 days for pain or 3 days for fever.

- Tell pregnant or breast-feeding patient to consult a doctor before taking ketoprofen.

magnesium salicylate tetrahydrate
Extra Strength Doan's

Pregnancy Risk Category C

HOW SUPPLIED
Caplets: 580 mg (equivalent to 467 mg magnesium salicylate anhydrous)

ACTION
Produces analgesia and anti-inflammatory effect by blocking prostaglandin synthesis (peripheral action). Salicylates may prevent the lowering of the pain threshold that occurs when prostaglandins sensitize pain receptors to stimulation; salicylates relieve fever by acting on the hypothalamic heat-regulating center to produce peripheral vasodilation.

Route	Onset	Peak	Duration
P.O.	Unknown	1.5-2 hr	Unknown

INDICATIONS & DOSAGES
Temporary relief from minor aches and pains associated

with backache and muscle aches—
Adults: 2 caplets q 6 hours while symptoms persist. Maximum 8 caplets in 24 hours.

ADVERSE REACTIONS
EENT: tinnitus, hearing loss.
GI: nausea, vomiting, *GI bleeding,* GI distress.
Hepatic: abnormal liver function tests, *hepatitis.*
Skin: rash, bruising.
Other: *hypersensitivity reactions (anaphylaxis,* asthma), *Reye's syndrome.*

INTERACTIONS
Drug-drug
ACE inhibitors, beta blockers, diuretics, uricosurics: may decrease effects of these drugs. Monitor patient closely.
Ammonium chloride, other urine acidifiers: increases blood levels of salicylates. Monitor patient for salicylate toxicity.
Antacids in high doses, other urine alkalinizers: decreases levels of salicylates. Monitor patient for decreased salicylate effect.
Anticoagulants: increases risk of bleeding. Advise patient to avoid using together.
Corticosteroids: enhances salicylate elimination. Monitor patient for decreased salicylate effect.

Methotrexate: increases risk of methotrexate toxicity. Advise patient to avoid using together.
Other NSAIDs, corticosteroids: increases risk of GI bleeding. Advise patient to avoid using together.

Drug-lifestyle
Alcohol use: increases risk of GI bleeding. Advise patient to avoid using together.

CONTRAINDICATIONS
Contraindicated in patients who are hypersensitive to drug or have aspirin-associated bleeding disorders or severe chronic renal insufficiency (risk of magnesium toxicity).

OVERDOSE & TREATMENT
Signs and symptoms of overdose include metabolic acidosis with respiratory alkalosis, hyperpnea, and tachypnea from increased carbon dioxide production and direct stimulation of the respiratory center.
  To treat overdose of magnesium salicylate, empty stomach immediately by inducing emesis with ipecac syrup if patient is conscious, or by gastric lavage. Administer activated charcoal via NG tube. Provide symptomatic and supportive measures, such as respiratory support and correction of fluid and electrolyte imbalances. Monitor labo-

ratory values and vital signs closely. Alkaline diuresis may enhance renal excretion.

NURSING CONSIDERATIONS
- Use cautiously in patient with hypoprothrombinemia and vitamin K deficiency.
- Therapeutic blood salicylate level in arthritis is 10 to 30 mg/100 ml. With long-term therapy, mild toxicity may occur at plasma levels of 20 mg/100 ml.
- Patient shouldn't use if taking a prescription drug for anticoagulation, diabetes, gout, or arthritis, unless directed by a doctor.
- Because of possible link to Reye's syndrome, the Centers for Disease Control and Prevention recommends not giving salicylates to children or teenagers with chickenpox or flu-like illness.

PATIENT TEACHING
- Advise patient that risk of GI irritation can be reduced by taking drug with food, milk, antacid, or a large glass of water.
- Instruct patient not to take the drug for longer than 10 days for pain, unless directed by a doctor.
- Tell patient who's allergic to salicylates or who has recurring problems such as heartburn, nausea, stomach pain, ulcers, or

bleeding problems to consult a doctor before using this drug.
- Tell patient to contact a doctor if pain persists or worsens or if new or unexpected symptoms occur.
- Tell pregnant or breast-feeding patient to consult a doctor before using this drug.

---

naproxen sodium
Aleve

Pregnancy Risk Category B

HOW SUPPLIED
Tablets, caplets, gelcaps:
220 mg (equivalent to 200 mg naproxen)

ACTION
Unknown. Produces anti-inflammatory, analgesic, and antipyretic effects, possibly by inhibiting prostaglandin synthesis.

Route	Onset	Peak	Duration
P.O.	1 hr	2-4 hr	7 hr

INDICATIONS & DOSAGES
Minor aches and pains caused by common cold, headache, toothache, muscle aches, backache, menstrual cramps, arthritis, fever—
Adults and children ages 12 years or older: 1 tablet (220 mg) P.O. q 8 to 12 hours, p.r.n. For the first dose, may take 2

tablets (440 mg) within the first
hour. Don't exceed 2 tablets
(440 mg) in any 8- to 12-hour
period or 3 tablets (660 mg) in
a 24-hour period.
**Elderly patients over age 65
years:** 1 tablet (220 mg) P.O., q
12 hours p.r.n. Don't exceed
220 mg in 12 hours.

ADVERSE REACTIONS
CNS: headache, drowsiness,
dizziness, vertigo.
CV: edema, palpitations.
EENT: visual disturbances, tinnitus, auditory disturbances.
GI: epigastric distress, occult
blood loss, nausea, peptic ulceration, constipation, dyspepsia,
heartburn, diarrhea, stomatitis,
thirst.
GU: elevated BUN and creatinine levels.
Hematologic: increases bleeding time.
Hepatic: elevated liver enzyme
levels.
Metabolic: hyperkalemia.
Respiratory: dyspnea.
Skin: pruritus, rash, urticaria,
ecchymosis, diaphoresis, purpura.

INTERACTIONS
Drug-drug
ACE inhibitors: may increase
risk of renal impairment. Advise patient to use together cautiously.

Antihypertensives, diuretics:
decreases effect of these drugs.
Monitor patient closely.
Aspirin, corticosteroids: increases risk of adverse GI reactions. Advise patient to avoid
using together.
Methotrexate: increases risk
of toxicity. Monitor patient
closely.
*Oral anticoagulants, other sul-
fonylureas, highly protein-
bound drugs:* increases risk
of toxicity. Monitor patient
closely.
Probenecid: decreases elimination of naproxen. Monitor patient for toxicity.

Drug-lifestyle
Alcohol use: increases risk of
adverse GI reactions. Advise
patient to avoid using together.

CONTRAINDICATIONS
Contraindicated in patients who
are hypersensitive to drug or
have syndrome of asthma,
rhinitis, and nasal polyps.

OVERDOSE & TREATMENT
Signs and symptoms of overdose include drowsiness, heartburn, indigestion, nausea, and
vomiting.
    To treat overdose of naprox-
en, empty patient's stomach immediately by inducing emesis
with ipecac syrup or by gastric
lavage. Administer activated

charcoal via NG tube. Provide symptomatic and supportive measures (respiratory support and correction of fluid and electrolyte imbalances). Monitor laboratory values and vital signs closely. Hemodialysis is ineffective in removing naproxen.

NURSING CONSIDERATIONS
• Use cautiously in elderly patient and in patient with renal disease, CV disease, GI disorders, hepatic disease, or a history of peptic ulcer disease.
• Pregnant patients should avoid use of drug during last trimester of pregnancy.
• Avoid use of NSAIDs in patient with preexisting renal failure, liver dysfunction, or heart failure; in elderly patient; and in patient taking diuretics. NSAIDs impair synthesis of renal prostaglandins and can decrease renal blood flow, causing reversible renal impairment.
• Watch carefully for signs and symptoms of infection; the antipyretic and anti-inflammatory actions can mask these signs and symptoms.
• Each tablet contains 20 mg of sodium.
• Because the drug appears in breast milk, breast-feeding patient should avoid its use.
• No age-related problems have been reported, but safety in children hasn't been established.

• The patient older than 60 is more sensitive to drug's adverse effects, especially GI toxicity.
• Drug's effect on renal prostaglandins may cause fluid retention and edema. Elderly patients with heart failure should avoid use.

PATIENT TEACHING
• Advise patient to take drug with food or milk to minimize GI upset. A full glass (8 oz) of water or other liquid should be taken with each dose.
• Serious GI toxicity, including peptic ulceration and bleeding, can occur in patient taking NSAIDs despite absence of GI symptoms. Teach patient signs and symptoms of GI bleeding and tell him to notify doctor immediately if they occur.
• Caution patient that use with aspirin, alcohol, or corticosteroids may increase risk of adverse GI reactions.
• Instruct patient to stop taking the medication and contact a doctor immediately if an allergic reaction occurs, if new or unexpected symptoms occur, if symptoms continue or worsen, or if patient has difficulty swallowing or develops heartburn.

nicotine polacrilex (nicotine-polacrilin resin complex)
Nicorette

Pregnancy Risk Category X

HOW SUPPLIED
Chewing gum: 2 mg/square, 4 mg/square

ACTION
Provides nicotine, which stimulates nicotinic acetylcholine receptors in the CNS, neuromuscle junction, autonomic ganglia, and adrenal medulla.

Route	Onset	Peak	Duration
Buccal	Unknown	15-30 min	Unknown

INDICATIONS & DOSAGES
Relief from nicotine withdrawal symptoms in patients undergoing smoking cessation—
Adults smoking fewer than 25 cigarettes per day: chew 2 mg (1 square) q 1 to 2 hours, weeks 1 to 6; chew 2 mg (1 square) q 2 hours, weeks 7 to 9; chew 2 mg (1 square) q 4 to 8 hours, weeks 10 to 12. Maximum 30 pieces per day.
Adults smoking more than 25 cigarettes per day: chew 4 mg (1 square) q 1 to 2 hours, weeks 1 to 6; chew 4 mg (1 square) q 2 hours, weeks 7 to 9; chew 4 mg (1 square) q 4 to 8 hours, weeks 10 to 12. Maximum 20 pieces per day.

ADVERSE REACTIONS
CNS: dizziness, irritability, insomnia, headache, lightheadedness.
CV: atrial fibrillation.
EENT: throat soreness, jaw muscle ache from chewing.
GI: nausea, vomiting, indigestion, eructation, anorexia, excessive salivation.
Respiratory: hiccups.

INTERACTIONS
Drug-drug
Beta blockers, methylxanthines, propoxyphene, propranolol: decreases metabolism of these drugs, increasing therapeutic effects. Dosage adjustments of these drugs may be needed.

Drug-food
Acidic beverages: interferes with buccal absorption before and during the chewing of nicotine gum. Advise patient to avoid eating and drinking 15 minutes before and while chewing gum.

Drug-lifestyle
Smoking: reduces effectiveness of drug. Advise patient not to smoke and use this drug.

CONTRAINDICATIONS

Contraindicated in patients with recent MI, life-threatening arrhythmias, severe or worsening angina pectoris, or active temporomandibular joint disorder. Also contraindicated in pregnant women and non-smokers.

OVERDOSE & TREATMENT

The risk of overdose is minimized by early nausea and vomiting that result from excessive nicotine intake. Poisoning causes nausea, vomiting, salivation, abdominal pain, diarrhea, cold sweats, headache, dizziness, disturbed hearing and vision, mental confusion, and weakness.

Treatment includes emesis; give ipecac syrup if vomiting hasn't occurred spontaneously. A saline cathartic will speed the gum's passage through the GI tract. Give gastric lavage followed by activated charcoal in unconscious patient. Provide supportive treatment of respiratory paralysis and CV collapse, as needed.

NURSING CONSIDERATIONS

• Use cautiously in patient with hyperthyroidism, pheochromocytoma, type 1 diabetes mellitus, peptic ulcer disease, history of esophagitis, oral or pharyngeal inflammation, or dental conditions that might be exacerbated by chewing gum.
• Smokers most likely to benefit from nicotine gum are those with high physical nicotine dependence—those who smoke more than 15 cigarettes daily, prefer brands of cigarettes with high nicotine levels, usually inhale the smoke, smoke the first cigarette within 30 minutes of rising, find the first morning cigarette the hardest to give up, smoke most frequently during the morning, find it difficult to refrain from smoking in places where it's forbidden, or smoke even when ill and confined to bed during the day.
• Nicotine replacement therapy works best when used together with a support program.
• Nicotine appears in breast milk and is readily absorbed by the infant after ingestion. Weigh infant's risk of exposure to nicotine from therapy against his risk of exposure from mother's continued smoking.

PATIENT TEACHING

• Make sure that patient reads and understands instructions included in the package.
• Instruct patient to chew gum slowly and intermittently until a "peppery" taste or tingling in the mouth occurs. Then "park"

the gum between cheek and gum (for approximately 1 minute) until this taste disappears. Repeat steps (chew and park) for about 30 minutes to promote slow and even buccal absorption of nicotine. Gum must be chewed to release nicotine. Swallowing gum is ineffective. Fast chewing tends to produce more adverse reactions.

- Tell patient to report to doctor any mouth, teeth, or jaw problems or an irregular heartbeat.
- Advise patient to gradually withdraw gum use after 3 months. Use of gum for longer than 6 months isn't recommended. Gradual withdrawal can be accomplished by shortening chewing time per piece while maintaining same frequency, or by reducing by 1 to 2 pieces per day while substituting missed dose with other sugarless gum.
- Instruct patient not to eat or drink anything 15 minutes before or while chewing gum.
- Advise patient to use at least 9 pieces a day to improve the chances of quitting smoking.
- Advise patient not to smoke or use other forms of nicotine while using nicotine replacement because of the increased risk for nicotine toxicity.

- Caution patient to stop using drug and notify doctor if nausea, vomiting, dizziness, weakness, or rapid heartbeat occurs. These may be symptoms of nicotine overdose.

nicotine transdermal system
Habitrol, NicoDerm CQ, Nicotrol, ProStep

Pregnancy Risk Category D

HOW SUPPLIED
Transdermal system: designed to release nicotine at a fixed rate.
Habitrol—21 mg/day, 14 mg/day, 7 mg/day
Nicoderm CQ—21 mg/day, 14 mg/day, 7 mg/day
Nicotrol—15 mg/16 hours
ProStep—22 mg/day, 11 mg/day

ACTION
Provides nicotine, which stimulates nicotinic acetylcholine receptors in the CNS, neuromuscle junction, autonomic ganglia, and adrenal medulla.

Route	Onset	Peak	Duration
Trans-dermal	Unknown	3-9 hr	Unknown

INDICATIONS & DOSAGES
Relief from nicotine withdrawal symptoms in patients undergoing smoking cessation—
Adults: initially, 1 transdermal system patch applied once daily to nonhairy part of body.
Habitrol, Nicoderm, and ProStep: patch replaced every 24 hours with new patch applied to a different skin site.
Nicotrol: patch applied upon awakening and removed h.s. After 4 to 12 weeks (depending on brand used), dose tapered to next lowest dose of nicotine in its dosage series, followed in 2 to 4 weeks by lowest nicotine dosage system in same series. Drug stopped after another 2 to 4 weeks.

ADVERSE REACTIONS
CNS: somnolence, dizziness, headache, insomnia, paresthesia, abnormal dreams, nervousness.
CV: hypertension.
EENT: pharyngitis, sinusitis.
GI: abdominal pain, constipation, dyspepsia, nausea, diarrhea, vomiting, dry mouth.
GU: dysmenorrhea.
Musculoskeletal: back pain, myalgia.
Respiratory: cough.
Skin: local or systemic erythema, pruritus, burning at application site, cutaneous hypersensitivity, rash, diaphoresis.

INTERACTIONS
Drug-drug
Acetaminophen, imipramine, oxazepam, pentazocine, propranolol, theophylline: may decrease induction of hepatic enzymes that help metabolize certain drugs. Lower doses may be needed.
Adrenergic agonists, such as isoproterenol and phenylephrine: may decrease circulating catecholamines. Higher doses may be needed.
Adrenergic antagonists such as labetalol and prazosin: may decrease circulating catecholamines. Lower doses may be needed.
Insulin: may increase amount of subcutaneous insulin absorbed. Lower dose of insulin may be needed.

Drug-herb
Blue cohosh: increases effects of nicotine. Advise patient to avoid using together.

Drug-food
Caffeine: may decrease induction of hepatic enzymes that help metabolize certain drugs. Lower doses of drug may be needed.

Drug-lifestyle
Smoking: increases risk of nicotine toxicity. Advise patient not to smoke and use drug.

Reactions may be *common*, uncommon, *life-threatening*, or COMMON AND LIFE-THREATENING.

CONTRAINDICATIONS

Contraindicated in patients who are hypersensitive to nicotine or any component of transdermal system; who have had a recent MI, life-threatening arrhythmias, or severe or worsening angina pectoris; and who are nonsmokers.

OVERDOSE & TREATMENT

Overdose may cause symptoms associated with acute nicotine poisoning, including nausea, vomiting, diarrhea, weakness, respiratory failure, hypotension, and seizures. Treat symptomatically.

NURSING CONSIDERATIONS

• Use cautiously in patient with hyperthyroidism, pheochromocytoma, hypertension, type 1 diabetes mellitus, or peptic ulcer disease.
• Avoid unnecessary contact with system, and wash hands with water alone because soap may enhance absorption, although health care workers' exposure to nicotine within transdermal systems is probably minimal.
• Nicotine replacement therapy works best when used together with a support program.
• Nicotine appears in breast milk and is readily absorbed by the infant after ingestion. Weigh infant's risk of exposure to nicotine from therapy against his risk of exposure from mother's continued smoking.
• The amount of nicotine in a patch could be fatal if ingested by a child. Even used patches contain a substantial amount of residual nicotine. Patients should make sure to keep used and unused transdermal patches away from children.

PATIENT TEACHING

• Advise patient to carefully read and follow package instructions.
• Inform patient that using transdermal system for longer than 3 months isn't recommended.
• Advise patient not to smoke or use other forms of nicotine while using nicotine replacement because of the increased risk for nicotine toxicity.
• Warn patient that continuation of smoking while using drug may cause serious adverse effects because peak serum nicotine levels will be substantially higher than those achieved by smoking alone.
• Teach patient to apply a new patch every day to a different area of the skin that is clean, dry, and hairless (usually the trunk or upper outer arm). Don't apply to skin that is burned, cut, or irritated.

• Instruct patient not to apply a new patch on a previously used area for at least 1 week.

• Instruct patient to wash hands with water after applying or removing a patch and not to touch eyes or mouth with hands before washing them.

• Suggest to patient wearing a 24-hour patch and having vivid dreams or disruptions of sleep that he try removing the patch at bedtime (after 16 hours) and applying a new one the next morning.

• Caution patient to dispose of patches properly to prevent accidental poisoning of children or pets caused by contact with patches (new or discarded).

• Tell patient who experiences persistent or severe local skin reactions or generalized rash to immediately discontinue use of patch and notify a doctor.

• Tell patient that swimming, bathing, or showering for short periods is allowed while using the patch.

Combination drugs

Brand name and active ingredients	Indications and dosages	Nursing considerations
Alka-Seltzer PM • aspirin 325 mg • diphenhydramine citrate 38 mg	*Temporary relief from occasional headaches and minor aches and pains with accompanying sleeplessness* **Adults:** 2 effervescent tablets, fully dissolved in 4 oz of water per tablet, P.O., h.s. if needed, or as directed by a doctor.	• Each tablet contains 503 mg of sodium and 4.04 mg of phenylalanine. • Because of possible link to Reye's syndrome, salicylates shouldn't be given to children or teenagers with chickenpox or flulike illness before a doctor is consulted. • Drug shouldn't be taken for longer than 10 days for pain or for longer than 3 days for fever, unless directed by a doctor. • Patient should consult a doctor if ringing in the ears or loss of hearing occurs. • Not for use in children younger than age 12. • Not for use by patient with breathing problems such as emphysema or chronic bronchitis, glaucoma, or difficult urination caused by enlargement of prostate gland, unless directed by a doctor. • Not for use by patient with ulcers or bleeding problems that persist or recur frequently. • Not for use by patient who is allergic to aspirin or has asthma, unless directed by a doctor. • Pregnant patient should avoid aspirin use, especially during third trimester of pregnancy, unless specifically directed by a doctor. • Breast-feeding patient should consult a doctor before taking this drug.

(continued)

Combination drugs *(continued)*

Brand name and active ingredients	Indications and dosages	Nursing considerations
Alka-Seltzer PM *(continued)*		• Patient should avoid alcoholic beverages while taking this drug. • Patient who takes sedatives or tranquilizers should consult a doctor before taking this drug. • Patient shouldn't take drug with a prescription drug for anticoagulation, diabetes, gout, or arthritis, unless directed by a doctor. • If sleeplessness persists for longer than 2 weeks, patient should consult a doctor.
Anacin • aspirin 400 mg • caffeine 32 mg	*Relief from minor aches and pains associated with headache, colds, muscle aches, backache, toothache, menstrual cramps, arthritis* **Adults and children ages 12 and older:** 2 tablets P.O. with a full glass (8 oz) of water q 6 hours while symptoms persist, or as directed by a doctor. Maximum 8 tablets in 24 hours.	• Patient who consumes 3 or more alcoholic drinks daily should consult a doctor about taking acetaminophen or other pain relievers. • Because of possible link to Reye's syndrome, salicylates shouldn't be given to children or teenagers with chickenpox or flulike illness. • Pregnant patient should avoid aspirin use, especially during third trimester of pregnancy, unless specifically directed by a doctor. • Patient shouldn't take drug for longer than 10 days for pain, unless directed by a doctor. • Pregnant or breast-feeding patient should seek advice from a doctor before taking this drug. • Patient shouldn't take drug with a prescription drug for anticoagulation, diabetes, gout, or arthritis, unless directed by a doctor.

Combination drugs *(continued)*

Brand name and active ingredients	Indications and dosages	Nursing considerations
Anacin *(continued)*		• Patient who is allergic to salicylates or has recurring stomach problems, such as heartburn, nausea, pain, ulcers, or bleeding, shouldn't use this drug before consulting a doctor. • If an allergic reaction occurs, patient should stop drug immediately and contact doctor.
Anacin Maximum Strength • aspirin 500 mg • caffeine 32 mg	*Relief from minor aches and pains associated with a cold, headache, muscle aches, backaches, toothache, menstrual cramps, arthritis* **Adults and children ages 12 and older:** 2 tablets q 6 hours while symptoms persist, or as directed by a doctor. Maximum 8 tablets in 24 hours.	• Patient who consumes 3 or more alcoholic drinks daily should consult a doctor about taking acetaminophen or other pain relievers. • Because of possible link to Reye's syndrome, salicylates shouldn't be given to children or teenagers with chickenpox or flulike illness. • Pregnant patient should avoid aspirin use, especially during third trimester of pregnancy, unless specifically directed by a doctor. • Patient shouldn't take for longer than 10 days for pain, unless directed by a doctor. • Pregnant or breast-feeding patient should seek advice from a doctor before taking this drug. • Patient shouldn't take this drug with a prescription drug for anticoagulation, diabetes, gout, or arthritis, unless directed by a doctor. • Patient who is allergic to salicylates or has recurring stomach problems, such as heartburn, nausea, pain, ulcers, or bleed-

(continued)

Combination drugs *(continued)*

Brand name and active ingredients	Indications and dosages	Nursing considerations
Anacin Maximum Strength *(continued)*		ing, shouldn't use this drug before consulting a doctor. • If an allergic reaction occurs, patient should stop drug immediately and contact doctor.
Aspirin Regimen Bayer Adult Low Strength with Calcium • aspirin 81 mg • buffered base of calcium carbonate 250 mg = 100 mg of elemental calcium	*Relief from minor aches and pain, or as recommended by a doctor* **Adults and children ages 12 and older:** 4 to 8 caplets P.O. with water q 4 hours, p.r.n., up to a maximum of 32 caplets in 24 hours.	• Patient who consumes 3 or more alcoholic drinks daily should consult a doctor about taking acetaminophen or other pain relievers. • Because of possible link to Reye's syndrome, salicylates shouldn't be given to children or teenagers with chickenpox or flulike illness. • Drug shouldn't be used for pain for longer than 10 days or for fever longer than 3 days, unless directed by a doctor. • Drug should be avoided by patient who is allergic to aspirin, who has asthma or persistent or recurring stomach problems, or who has gastric ulcers or bleeding problems, unless directed by a doctor. • Patient should consult a doctor if ringing in the ears or loss of hearing occurs. • Pregnant patient should avoid aspirin use, especially during last trimester of pregnancy, unless specifically directed by a doctor. • Not for use with a prescription drug for anticoagulation, diabetes, gout, or arthritis, unless directed by a doctor.

Combination drugs *(continued)*

Brand name and active ingredients	Indications and dosages	Nursing considerations
Aspirin-free Excedrin • acetaminophen 500 mg • caffeine 65 mg	*Relief from minor aches and pains associated with headache, sinusitis, cold, muscle aches, premenstrual and menstrual cramps, toothache, arthritis* **Adults and children older than age 12:** 2 geltabs or caplets P.O. q 6 hours while symptoms persist. Maximum 8 geltabs or caplets in 24 hours.	• Patient who consumes 3 or more alcoholic drinks daily should consult a doctor about taking acetaminophen or other pain relievers. • Pregnant or breast-feeding patient should consult a doctor before taking this drug. • Drug shouldn't be taken for longer than 10 days for pain or longer than 3 days for fever, unless directed by a doctor.
Aspirin-free Excedrin PM • acetaminophen 500 mg • diphenhydramine citrate 38 mg	*Relief from occasional headaches, minor aches and pains, with accompanying sleeplessness* **Adults and children ages 12 and older:** 2 tablets P.O. h.s. if needed, or as directed by a doctor.	• Pregnant or breast-feeding patient should consult a doctor before taking this drug. • Patient who consumes 3 or more alcoholic drinks daily should consult a doctor about taking acetaminophen or other pain relievers. • If symptoms persist or worsen, if new ones occur, or if sleeplessness persists continuously for longer than 2 weeks, patient should consult a doctor. • Drug shouldn't be used for longer than 10 days, unless directed by a doctor.

(continued)

Combination drugs *(continued)*

Brand name and active ingredients	Indications and dosages	Nursing considerations
Aspirin-free Excedrin PM *(continued)*		• Not for use by patient with breathing problems such as emphysema or chronic bronchitis, glaucoma, or difficult urination caused by enlargement of prostate gland, unless directed by a doctor.
Backaid Maximum Strength one dose (2 tablets) • acetaminophen 1 g • pamabrom 50 mg	*Relief from minor aches and pains associated with backaches, muscle aches, leg pain, joint aches, related discomfort* **Adults:** 2 tablets P.O. with a full glass (8 oz) of water. Repeat 2 tablets q 6 hours, p.r.n. Maximum 8 tablets in 24 hours.	• Advise patient not to exceed recommended dosage. • Drug shouldn't be used for longer than 10 days, unless directed by a doctor. • Patient who consumes 3 or more alcoholic drinks daily should ask a doctor about taking acetaminophen or other pain relievers. • Patient younger than age 18 should use only as directed by a doctor. • Pregnant or breast-feeding patient should seek advice from a doctor before taking this drug.
Extra Strength Bayer PM Caplets • aspirin 500 mg • diphenhydramine 25 mg	*Relief from occasional headaches and minor aches and pains with accompanying sleeplessness* **Adults and children ages 12 and older:** 2 caplets, with water, P.O. h.s. if needed, or as	• Patient should avoid alcoholic beverages while taking this drug. • Patient who consumes 3 or more alcoholic drinks daily should consult a doctor about taking aspirin or other pain relievers. • Because of possible link to Reye's syndrome, salicylates shouldn't be given to children or teenagers with chickenpox or flulike illness before a doctor is consulted.

Combination drugs *(continued)*

Brand name and active ingredients	Indications and dosages	Nursing considerations
Extra Strength Bayer PM Caplets *(continued)*	directed by a doctor.	• Pregnant patient should avoid aspirin use, especially during last trimester of pregnancy, unless specifically directed by a doctor. • Patient shouldn't take for longer than 10 days for pain, unless directed by a doctor. • Pregnant or breast-feeding patient should seek advice from a doctor before taking this drug. • Patient should consult a doctor if ringing in the ears or loss of hearing occurs. • Not for use in patient with breathing problems such as emphysema or chronic bronchitis, glaucoma, or difficult urination caused by enlargement of prostate gland, unless directed by a doctor. • Patient who takes sedatives or tranquilizers should consult a doctor before taking this drug. • Not for use by patient with stomach problems such as heartburn, nausea, pain, ulcers, or bleeding. • If sleeplessness persists continuously for longer than 2 weeks, patient should consult a doctor.
Excedrin Extra Strength • acetaminophen 250 mg • aspirin 250 mg • caffeine 65 mg	*Relief from minor aches and pains associated with headache, sinusitis, a cold, muscle aches, premenstrual and men-*	• Because of possible link to Reye's syndrome, salicylates shouldn't be given to children or teenagers with chickenpox or flulike illness. • Patient who consumes 3 or more alcoholic drinks daily *(continued)*

Combination drugs (continued)

Brand name and active ingredients	Indications and dosages	Nursing considerations
Excedrin Extra Strength *(continued)*	*strual cramps, toothache, arthritis* **Adults and children ages 12 and older:** 2 tablets P.O. with water q 6 hours while symptoms persist. Maximum 8 tablets in 24 hours, or as directed by a doctor.	should consult a doctor about taking acetaminophen or other pain relievers. • Pregnant patient should avoid aspirin, especially during third trimester of pregnancy, unless specifically directed by a doctor. • Breast-feeding patient should consult a doctor before taking this drug. • Drug shouldn't be used for longer than 10 days for pain or longer than 3 days for fever, unless directed by a doctor. • Patient should consult a doctor if ringing in the ears or loss of hearing occurs. • Not for use by patient who is allergic to aspirin, has asthma or persistent or recurring stomach problems, such as gastric ulcers or bleeding, unless directed by a doctor. • Not for use by patient taking a prescription drug for anticoagulation, diabetes, gout, or arthritis, unless directed by a doctor.
Excedrin Migraine • acetaminophen 250 mg • aspirin 250 mg • caffeine 65 mg	*Treatment of migraines* **Adults:** 2 tablets P.O. with a full glass (8 oz) of water. Maximum 2 tablets in 24 hours, unless directed by a doctor.	• Not for use by patient taking a prescription drug for anticoagulation, diabetes, gout, or arthritis, unless directed by a doctor. • Patient younger than age 18 should consult a doctor before use. • Patient should consult a doctor if ringing in the ears or loss of hearing occurs. • Pregnant patient should avoid aspirin use, especially during the third trimester of pregnancy,

Combination drugs *(continued)*

Brand name and active ingredients	Indications and dosages	Nursing considerations
Excedrin Migraine *(continued)*		unless specifically directed by a doctor. • Breast-feeding patient should consult a doctor before taking this drug. • Patient should stop taking the medicine and consult a doctor if migraine is not relieved or worsens after first dose or if new or unexpected symptoms occur. • Patient should consult doctor before using this drug if headache is different from the usual migraine, is "the worst headache ever," or is a migraine so severe it requires bed rest; if patient has never been diagnosed with migraines; or if patient has fever and stiff neck, daily headaches, bleeding, kidney disease, asthma, ulcers, or persistent or recurring liver or stomach problems. • Patient should limit the amount of drugs, foods, and beverages that contain caffeine while taking this drug.
Legatrin PM • acetaminophen 500 mg • diphenhydramine hydrochloride 50 mg	*Occasional relief from sleeplessness or minor aches and pains* **Adults and children ages 12 and older:** 1 caplet P.O. h.s. or as directed by a doctor.	• Patient shouldn't exceed recommended dosage. • Drug shouldn't be used for longer than 10 days, unless directed by a doctor. • Not for use by patient with asthma, glaucoma, emphysema, chronic pulmonary disease, shortness of breath, or difficult urination caused by enlargement of prostate gland, unless directed by a doctor.

(continued)

Combination drugs *(continued)*

Brand name and active ingredients	Indications and dosages	Nursing considerations
Legatrin PM *(continued)*		• Patient who takes sedatives or tranquilizers should consult a doctor before taking this drug. • Drug shouldn't be used with other drugs containing acetaminophen. • Patient should consult doctor if symptoms persist for longer than 3 days, or if sleeplessness persists for longer than 2 weeks.
Multi-Action Arthricare • capsicum oleo-resin 0.025% • menthol USP 1.25% • methyl nicotinate 0.25%	*Relief from minor aches and pains of muscles and joints caused by backache, arthritis, strains, or sprains* **Adults and children ages 2 and older:** apply to affected area t.i.d. to q.i.d.	• Drug shouldn't be used with a heating pad or immediately before or after showering or bathing. • Advise patient to avoid contact of drug with eyes. • Instruct patient not to bandage area tightly after applying drug. • Transient redness, burning, or stinging is usually evident at initial therapy but decreases with cautious use. This effect persists in patient who uses drug less often than t.i.d. If burning is severe, tell patient to stop using drug.
Percogesic • acetaminophen 325 mg • phenyltoloxamine citrate 30 mg	*Relief from minor aches and pains associated with headaches, muscle aches, backaches, premenstrual, menstrual discomfort, colds, flu, toothaches, arthritis; reduc-*	• Drug may cause drowsiness. Patient should use caution when driving a motor vehicle or operating machinery. • Alcoholic beverages, sedatives, and tranquilizers may increase the drowsiness effect. The drugs should be avoided while taking this drug. • May cause excitability, especially in children.

Combination drugs *(continued)*

Brand name and active ingredients	Indications and dosages	Nursing considerations
Percogesic *(continued)*	*tion of fever* **Adults and children ages 12 and older:** 1 or 2 tablets P.O. q 4 hours. Maximum 8 tablets daily. **Children ages 6 to 11 years:** 1 tablet q 4 hours. Maximum 4 tablets daily.	• Not for use by patient with breathing problems such as emphysema or chronic bronchitis, glaucoma, or difficult urination caused by enlargement of prostate gland, unless directed by a doctor. • If pain persists for longer than 5 days (children) or 10 days (adults), if fever persists longer than 3 days, or if condition worsens or new symptoms appear, patient should stop taking the drug and contact a doctor. • Pregnant or breast-feeding patient should seek advice from a doctor before taking this drug.
Tylenol PM • acetaminophen 500 mg • diphenhydramine hydrochloride 25 mg	*Relief from headaches and minor aches and pains with accompanying sleeplessness* **Adults and children ages 12 and older:** 2 caplets, geltabs, or gelcaps P.O., h.s., or as directed by a doctor.	• Patient should avoid alcoholic beverages while taking this drug. • Patient who takes sedatives or tranquilizers should consult a doctor before taking this drug. • Patient who consumes 3 or more alcoholic drinks daily should consult a doctor about taking acetaminophen or other pain relievers. • Drug shouldn't be used with other drugs containing acetaminophen. • Drug shouldn't be taken for longer than 10 days for pain or longer than 3 days for fever, unless directed by a doctor. • Not for use by patient with breathing problems such as emphysema or chronic bronchitis, glaucoma, or difficult urination caused by enlargement of pros-

(continued)

Combination drugs *(continued)*

Brand name and active ingredients	Indications and dosages	Nursing considerations
Tylenol PM *(continued)*		tate gland, unless directed by a doctor. • Pregnant or breast-feeding patient should consult a doctor before taking this drug. • Best results if taken at least 6 hours before patient needs to wake up.
Vanquish • aspirin 227 mg • acetaminophen 194 mg • caffeine 33 mg • buffered with aluminum hydroxide and magnesium hydroxide	*Relief from minor aches and pains associated with headaches, colds and flu, backaches, muscle aches, menstrual pain, arthritis* **Adults and children ages 12 and older:** 2 caplets P.O. with water q 4 hours, p.r.n. up to a maximum of 12 caplets in 24 hours, or as directed by a doctor.	• Because of possible link to Reye's syndrome, salicylates shouldn't be given to children or teenagers with chickenpox or flu-like illness. • Patient who consumes 3 or more alcoholic drinks daily should consult a doctor about taking acetaminophen or other pain relievers. • Pregnant patient should avoid aspirin use, especially during third trimester of pregnancy, unless specifically directed by a doctor. • Breast-feeding patient should seek advice from a doctor before taking this drug. • Not for use by patient who is allergic to aspirin, has asthma, or has persisting or recurring stomach problems, such as gastric ulcers, or bleeding, unless directed by a doctor. • Patient shouldn't take drug with a prescription drug for anticoagulation, diabetes, gout, or arthritis, unless directed by a doctor. • Drug shouldn't be used for longer than 10 days for pain or

Combination drugs *(continued)*

Brand name and active ingredients	Indications and dosages	Nursing considerations
Vanquish *(continued)*		longer than 3 days for fever, unless directed by a doctor. • If ringing in the ears or loss of hearing occurs, patient should consult a doctor.
Women's Tylenol • acetaminophen 500 mg • pamabrom 25 mg	*Relief from minor aches and pains caused by cramps, headache, backache; premenstrual or menstrual full feeling, waterweight gain, bloating, or swelling* **Adults and children ages 12 and older:** 2 caplets P.O. q 4 to 6 hours. Maximum 8 caplets in 24 hours, or as directed.	• Drug shouldn't be used with other drugs containing acetaminophen. • Pregnant or breast-feeding patient should seek advice from a doctor before taking this drug. • Patient who consumes 3 or more alcoholic drinks daily should consult a doctor about taking acetaminophen or other pain relievers.

4

Eyes, ears, nose, and throat

This chapter provides guidelines for recognizing and treating some of the eye, ear, nose, and throat (EENT) conditions that patients are likely to treat with OTC drugs. These conditions include allergic rhinitis, bad breath, canker sores, cerumen impaction, dry eyes, dry mouth, fever blisters, sinusitis, sore throat, and toothache. Although generally self-limiting, EENT conditions can become chronic, and they shouldn't be ignored. Furthermore, an apparently mild condition can be a symptom of a more severe underlying pathology; therefore, recommendations for follow-up care are also included.

Anatomy

Briefly review the anatomy of the eyes, ears, nose, and throat.

Eyes

The eye transmits visual images to the brain for interpretation. Every object reflects light. This reflected light, when intercepted by the eye, passes through numerous intraocular structures, ultimately creating an upside-down, reverse image on the retina. Specialized photoreceptor cells, known as cones and rods, send nerve impulses through the optic nerve to the visual cortex of the occipital lobe, which then interprets the image.

Normal anatomy of the eye includes intraocular and extraocular components. The intraocular structures include the sclera, cornea, anterior chamber, iris, pupil, aqueous humor, lens, ciliary body, vitreous humor, retina, and choroid. Extraocular structures include the lacrimal apparatus, the eyelids, and the conjunctivae, all serving to protect and lubricate the eye. The extraocular structures are most likely to be involved in acute, self-limiting problems. The lid margins contain hair follicles, which contain eyelashes and sebaceous glands.

Ears

The ear is divided into three parts: external, middle, and inner. The external ear gathers sound and directs it toward the middle ear. The tympanic membrane (eardrum) and three small bones (incus, malleus, and stapes) conduct sound vibrations from the external ear to the inner ear. The eustachian tube, which connects the middle ear and the nasopharynx cavity, allows air pressure in the middle ear to equilibrate with atmospheric pressure. The inner ear chamber (labyrinth) is encased in bone and filled with fluid. Movement of this fluid is interpreted by the brain as motion and thereby helps the body maintain balance. The cochlea, a snail-shaped bony organ, conducts signals to the acoustic nerve for interpretation by the brain.

Nose and throat
The nose is the site for the olfactory organ and serves as a conduit for breathing. The interior is lined with well-vascularized mucosa and a complex of folds and irregularities, which warm, filter, and humidify inspired air.

The sinuses are air-filled cavities within the facial bones; each is named for the bone that surrounds it—maxillary, frontal, ethmoid, and sphenoid. In addition to warming, filtering, and humidifying air, they contribute to voice resonance.

Tonsils and adenoids are made of lymph tissue and protect against infection. Tonsils and adenoids are most active during childhood; their role in adulthood isn't currently considered critical. Tonsils begin rather large and eventually shrink to almond size. Adenoids follow the same pattern, becoming almost nonexistent in adults.

Allergic rhinitis
Allergic rhinitis is an IgE-mediated reaction of the nasal mucous membranes to airborne allergens. Repeated exposure to an allergen triggers the release of histamine, which begins a cascade of immediate vasodilation of the mucous membranes, mucosal edema, and increased mucus production in an attempt to flush the allergen from the body.

Other forms of rhinitis are associated with exposure to odors, change of barometric pressure or air temperature, or animal dander; with aging or pregnancy, and with misuse of topical nasal decongestants.

Signs and symptoms
Sneezing, profuse clear watery rhinorrhea, nasal congestion, and itchy nose and eyes are usual characteristics. The patient may also have puffy red eyes, itchy or sore throat, headache, allergic shiners—the dark circles under the eyes

caused by venous congestion, postnasal drip, cough, malaise, fatigue, or fever. Perennial allergic rhinitis causes chronic nasal obstruction leading to eustachian tube obstruction.

Serious conditions

Allergic rhinitis can predispose the patient to chronic sinusitis, a high incidence of respiratory infections, or eustachian tube dysfunction. In young children, eustachian tube dysfunction can impair or delay speech development. Additional complications include otitis media, polyps, sleep apnea, diminished sense of smell, and asthma.

Complications

The use of antihistamines can cause drowsiness and, with overuse, dry eye or dry mouth syndrome. Decongestants can elevate blood pressure and can cause urinary retention in men with benign prostatic hypertrophy. Topical decongestants used for longer than 3 days can cause a rebound effect on the nasal mucosa.

Nursing considerations

• Evaluate relief from signs and symptoms.
• Monitor effectiveness of therapy.

• Assess the patient's nonpharmacologic methods to help control signs and symptoms.
• Make sure that any OTC drug use during pregnancy is approved by a doctor.
• Early control of signs and symptoms can prevent sinusitis or eustachian tube dysfunction.
• Monitor for adverse effects of OTC drugs.
• Refer the patient to specialist if signs and symptoms are severe.

Patient teaching

• Warn the patient not to use more than one antihistamine at a time.
• Warn the patient to use caution in driving or operating machinery if using antihistamines.
• Tell the patient not to use topical decongestants longer than 3 days.
• Tell the patient who has history of benign prostatic hypertrophy not to use antihistamines.
• Tell the patient with a history of hypertension or glaucoma not to use decongestants.
• Advise the patient that saline sprays will help counteract dryness of nasal passages or thick mucus.
• Advise the patient to wear a mask when doing yard work.
• Advise the patient to close windows and use air conditioning in the spring and summer.

• Instruct the patient on how to avoid the triggering allergen; for example, use polyester pillows, get rid of carpet, don't have plants or animals in bedroom, and vacuum and dust frequently.

Bad breath

Occasional bad breath (halitosis) is normal, especially first thing in the morning. There is cause for concern, however, if breath is offensive or chronically foul. Decaying food, plaque-covered teeth and tongue, cavities, dry mouth, and stomatitis can all contribute to offensive mouth odor. These are easily treated and should be attended to before they cause more serious problems.

Signs and symptoms

The usual characteristic is foul or offensive odor emanating from the oral cavity. Other signs and symptoms depend on the underlying cause.

Serious conditions

Bad breath itself doesn't have any serious consequences, except possibly on your social life. However, the underlying causes can lead to many potentially serious conditions if left untreated. Other problems that can cause bad breath include respiratory conditions such as chronic sinusitis, liver disease, lung disease, GI disorders, and kidney failure. Uncontrolled diabetes mellitus may cause a fruity-smelling breath.

Complications

No information available.

Nursing considerations

• Refer the patient for medical attention if his breath smells fishy, fruity, or like urine or feces.
• Patient should consult a doctor or dentist if the halitosis doesn't respond to home-care treatments.

Patient teaching

• Advise the patient that brushing teeth with a firm-bristle toothbrush may cause damage to teeth and gums.
• Encourage the patient to rinse with water or mouthwash, chew sugar-free gum or use floss after each meal, and always use a soft-bristle toothbrush.
• Advise the patient to have teeth professionally cleaned and examined, at least twice a year.
• Advise the patient to avoid eating pungent foods such as garlic, onion, hot peppers, or certain deli meats and cheeses.

• Suggest that the patient chew parsley, cloves, or fennel seeds after meals to freshen breath.

Canker sore

A canker sore (recurrent aphthous stomatitis) is an inflammation of the oral mucosa. Canker sores are slightly more common in women than in men, have familial tendencies, and occur most frequently during the winter and spring months. The cause is unknown.

Signs and symptoms

Canker sores usually cause superficial ulcerations on the mucous membranes of the lips, buccal surface, tongue, floor of the mouth, palate, and gums. Onset can start with localized burning sensation 1 to 48 hours before appearance of discrete painful vesicles, 2 to 5 mm in diameter. After 2 days, they rupture and form saucerlike ulcers with a red or grayish-red center and an elevated rimlike periphery. Ulcers may be single or multiple, and they usually heal spontaneously within 7 to 10 days.

Serious conditions

Canker sores are considered benign.

Complications

Canker sores can be confused with ulcers caused by other conditions, such as syphilis, herpes, vitamin or iron deficiencies, tobacco, carcinoma, leukemia, or food or drug allergies.

Nursing considerations

• Refer the patient to a dentist if lesion or ulceration persists longer than 2 weeks or if the patient's medical history suggests any other pathology.
• Canker sores may be difficult to treat in immunocompromised patients.

Patient teaching

• Explain to the patient that treatment will help to reduce the pain.
• Encourage the patient to consume sufficient amounts of nonirritating liquids or soft food to maintain hydration and nutrition.
• Suggest that the patient drink through a straw to avoid contact with the painful lesion.
• Encourage regular dental visits.
• Instruct the patient to call if ulcer hasn't resolved within 2 weeks.

Cerumen impaction

Cerumen impaction is obstruction of the external ear canal by cerumen, or ear wax. Cerumen is normally cleared but can become excessive and partially or totally occlude the canal.

Signs and symptoms

The patient with cerumen impaction usually has a feeling of fullness in the ear and impaired hearing. Hardened cerumen can also cause pain, itching, or vertigo.

Serious conditions

Conductive hearing loss can occur if the ear canal is totally occluded.

Complications

Improper attempts to remove the cerumen can damage the delicate structures of the ear or disrupt the integrity of the tympanic membrane allowing entry of water or pathogens.

Nursing considerations

- Rule out the presence of a foreign body.
- When irrigating the ear, stop immediately if the patient complains of pain or has bleeding.
- If the patient normally produces large amounts of wax, regularly scheduled ear irrigations may be warranted.

Patient teaching

- Remind the patient not to insert anything, including cotton-tipped swabs, into the ear canal.
- Advise the patient that ear wax should be removed only if it appears in the external auditory canal. He should do this using a damp washcloth wrapped around his finger.
- If the patient normally produces large amounts of cerumen, suggest that 1 or 2 drops of baby oil in each ear once or twice a week may help to soften the wax before removal is attempted.
- Tell the patient to administer a mixture of 3 drops of hydrogen peroxide and 3 drops of water in the external canal once or twice a week to decrease the likelihood of impaction.

Dry eye syndrome

Dry eye syndrome may result from any disease associated with deficiency of the tear film components, lid surface abnormalities, or epithelial abnormalities. The most likely causes are medications, such as antihistamines, beta blockers, or antimuscarinics. Other causes include eyelid abnormalities, such as ectropion or entropion, contact lens use, pterygium, hyperthyroidism, or decreased or absent blinking secondary to neurologic conditions. Dry eyes can also be a symptom of Sjögren's syndrome, Bell's palsy, or rheumatoid arthritis. Contributing environmental factors include dusty work conditions, smoke, and electric or forced-air heat.

Signs and symptoms
This syndrome is characterized by a scratchy or sandy (foreign body) sensation, itching, burning, photosensitivity, redness, pain, and difficulty moving the lids. Contrary to the name "dry eye," excessive tearing often occurs as well.

Serious conditions
If dry eye is left untreated, visual impairment, corneal ulceration, or corneal thinning with perforation can occur. Secondary bacterial infections also occasionally occur.

Complications
Most chemical preservatives in artificial tears produce a certain amount of toxicity to the tear film, corneal epithelium, or both. This may be a problem if the patient uses more than the recommended amount of the product.

Nursing considerations
• Assess environmental factors that may be contributing to the patient's condition.
• Discover which other non-pharmacologic treatment the patient uses to alleviate signs and symptoms.
• Note color and consistency of any discharge.
• Ask how long the patient has had this condition.
• Refer the patient to a doctor if condition looks like conjunctivitis.

Patient teaching
• Advise the patient that any abrasions, blunt trauma, and infections should be medically evaluated.
• Advise the patient that a humidifier may provide some relief from signs and symptoms.
• If the patient also uses a prescription eye medication, be sure he knows not to use the nonprescription medication immediately after instilling the prescription medication.

Dry mouth
Dry mouth, or xerostomia, is a partial or complete lack of saliva. Possible causes include head and neck radiation therapy, Sjögren's syndrome, chemotherapy, environmental conditions, stress, or drug therapy. The most likely candidates are

anticholinergics, antihistamines, decongestants, antipsychotics, and antihypertensive drugs.

Signs and symptoms

Cracking of the lips, difficulty swallowing, or changes in tongue texture may occur.

Serious conditions

Loss of the protective coating of the mucous membranes of the oral cavity can contribute to infections, severe dental caries, and denture problems.

Nursing considerations

• Make sure the patient is evaluated for use of medications or underlying medical conditions.
• Medications may need to be changed or adjusted to help alleviate the problem.

Patient teaching

• Explain that treatment is usually palliative.
• Explain that dental checks are imperative for anticaries control.
• Instruct the patient on irrigating the mouth regularly with OTC topical solutions.

Fever blisters

Herpes simplex type 1, more commonly called fever blisters or cold sores, is a recurrent viral infection, potentially transmissible to anyone who comes in direct contact with it. The vesicles are painful and occur in clusters around the oral mucous membrane. The virus travels to the dorsal root ganglia of the affected nerve and remains in a latent stage until reactivated by such conditions as fever, ultraviolet light, cold wind, systemic illness, menstruation, emotional stress, local trauma, or immunosuppression.

Signs and symptoms

Prodromal tingling can occur before the first vesicles appear. The lesions occur as grouped, uniform vesicles on an erythematous base. The pain is moderate to severe during the first 24 hours after the appearance of the first vesicle, and then rapidly diminishes. After 48 hours, the vesicles usually erode and are replaced by ulcer crusts. The lesions usually resolve within 7 to 10 days but can last as long as 2 weeks. Occasionally, fever or lymphadenopathy also occurs.

Serious conditions

Rarely, aseptic meningitis or herpes encephalitis, pneumonia, or septicemia can occur.

Complications

None reported.

Nursing considerations
- Assess whether the condition is recurrent and how long it has existed.
- Determine what factors generally precipitate an outbreak.
- Ask what method of treatment the patient uses.
- Transmission can occur through direct contact with active lesions or by contact with virus-containing saliva of a person with no evidence of active disease.
- Infected persons should avoid contact with immunocompromised patients during active outbreak.

Patient teaching
- Advise the patient that applying ice may help reduce swelling.
- Encourage use of sunscreen-containing lip protectants before sun exposure.
- Caution the patient to avoid direct physical contact while lesions are active.
- Instruct the patient to begin treatment at first sign of recurrence.

Sinusitis
Sinusitis is an inflammation or infection of the membrane lining the paranasal sinuses. It's usually bacterial but may be viral. Predisposing conditions include allergic rhinitis and sep-

tal deviation. Acute sinusitis is a short-term condition that responds well to antibiotics and decongestants. Chronic sinusitis is defined as at least four recurrences of acute sinusitis.

Signs and symptoms
Signs and symptoms of sinusitis are facial pain or pressure, nasal obstruction, thick green or yellow nasal discharge, diminished sense of smell, and cough. Other signs and symptoms include fever, bad breath, fatigue, dental pain, periorbital edema, and headache that becomes worse on bending forward.

Chronic sinusitis is usually characterized by nasal discharge and congestion lasting longer than 30 days, postnasal drip, dull ache or pressure across the face, headache, cough, fatigue, and bad breath. The patient may also have eye pain and "popping" of ears.

Serious conditions
Meningitis, orbital infection, and septic cavernous thrombosis may occur.

Complications
Complications can arise from the use of topical nasal decongestants for longer than 3 days. Systemic decongestants can

raise blood pressure and worsen glaucoma.

Nursing considerations
- Air travel can trigger acute sinusitis in a patient with an upper respiratory tract infection.
- Refer the patient with periorbital edema to the doctor immediately.
- Refer the patient to the doctor if his signs and symptoms haven't improved in 48 to 72 hours.

Patient teaching
- Advise the patient to seek medical evaluation if signs and symptoms haven't begun to resolve within 48 to 72 hours.
- Inform the patient that increased room humidity, steam inhalation, and warm compresses may help relieve signs and symptoms.
- Encourage increased fluid intake.
- Advise the patient to avoid airplane travel, swimming, and diving during the acute period.
- Advise the patient to avoid antihistamines, as they will thicken already thick secretions.
- Caution the patient that use of tobacco products can contribute to problem.

Sore throat
Sore throat, or pharyngitis, is an inflammation of the pharynx and surrounding lymph tissue (tonsils). The most common cause is viral, but can be bacterial. Sore throat may accompany mononucleosis, and sexually transmitted diseases, such as gonococcal or chlamydial infections, may manifest as pharyngitis. Noninfectious causes of pharyngitis include allergic rhinitis with postnasal drip, mouth breathing, and trauma, as from heat, alcohol, smoke, or sharp objects.

Signs and symptoms
The primary signs and symptoms of pharyngitis include redness, soreness, dryness, and scratchiness. Exudate or lesions may form on the tonsils. The patient often has fever, headache, and malaise, and may have tender, enlarged lymph nodes.

Serious conditions
Poststreptococcal glomerulonephritis can occur rarely. Rheumatic fever (less than 1% of group A streptococcal infections) can damage heart valves. Peritonsillar abscesses and suppurative adenitis can also occur.

Complications

Complications can arise from treatment choices. Long-term use of aspirin or ibuprofen can lead to GI upset or gastritis, and must be used cautiously by patients on anticoagulant therapy. Patients younger than age 18 shouldn't be given aspirin because of possible link to Reye's syndrome.

Nursing considerations

• Refer the patient to the doctor immediately if the pain is so severe the patient can't swallow; if the patient is drooling, can't open his mouth, or has difficulty breathing; or if the patient has stridor (especially in children). An accompanying red, slightly raised rash on the neck, arms, legs, or groin or red swollen tongue suggests scarlet fever.

Patient teaching

• Explain to patients or parents that an antibiotic is ineffective against viral sore throats, which are by far the most common.
• Advise the patient to notify the doctor if the sore throat persists longer than 3 to 5 days or if fever persists longer than 5 days. A temperature greater than 101° F (38.3° C) and enlarged tender lymph nodes with the sore throat strongly suggest that the pharyngitis is caused by *Streptococcus pyrogenes* (the cause of "strep throat").
• Advise the patient to read carefully and follow the directions on OTC drugs.

Toothache

A toothache (pulpitis) indicates that a portion of the pulp tissue is inflamed. Pulpitis may accompany dental lesion, loss of a dental filling, or trauma. The pain is usually severe and can occur in response to thermal stimuli, exposure to air, or exposure to foods, such as those containing sugar. The pain persists longer than 15 seconds after the stimulus is removed.

Signs and symptoms

Toothache is pain in a tooth that's exacerbated by stimuli. The pain may be accompanied by intraoral or extraoral swelling or fever. It may radiate to the suborbital area, side of the face, or the ear.

Serious conditions

Toothache can develop into meningitis with subsequent abscess or cellulitis formation.

Complications

If toothache is left untreated, localized abscess or cellulitis could develop.

Nursing considerations
• For afebrile patient with no evident swelling, give analgesics and refer the patient to a dentist within 24 hours.
• A patient with slight swelling or a low-grade fever probably needs antibiotic therapy; refer to dentist within 12 to 24 hours.
• Refer the patient for immediate medical attention if his temperature is greater than 101° F (38.3° C) or his face is asymmetrical because of swelling.

Patient teaching
• Advise the patient of the need for regular dental care as an adjunct to general health care.
• Advise the patient to read carefully and follow the directions on OTC drugs, including directive on when to contact a doctor.

benzocaine
carbamide peroxide
cromolyn sodium
epinephrine hydrochloride
hydrogen peroxide
isopropyl alcohol
levmetamfetamine
naphazoline
  hydrochloride
oxymetazoline
  hydrochloride
phenylephrine
  hydrochloride
propylhexedrine
pseudoephedrine
  hydrochloride
sodium chloride
sodium fluoride
tetrahydrozoline
  hydrochloride
xylometazoline
  hydrochloride

---

benzocaine
Baby Anbesol, Hurricaine,
Maximum Strength Anbesol,
Orabase B Gel, Orabase Gel,
Orajel Mouth-Aid,
SensoGARD, Tanac, Zilactin-
B, Zilactin Baby

Pregnancy Risk Category C

HOW SUPPLIED
Gel: 7.5%, 10%, 15%, 20%
Liquid: 6.3%, 9%, 20%
Paste: 10%
Spray: 20%

ACTION
Drug is an analgesic that acts at
sensory neurons to produce a
local anesthetic effect.

Route	Onset	Peak	Duration
Topical, buccal	Immediate	Unknown	20-30 min

INDICATIONS & DOSAGES
*Temporary relief from tooth-
ache pain—*
(Orajel)
Adults: apply a small amount
directly into the cavity and on
the gum surrounding the tooth.

*Temporary relief from pain of
canker sores, cold sores, fever
blisters, and minor irritations
of the mouth and gums—*
*(Orajel Mouth-Aid, Orabase B
Gel, SensoGARD, Tanac)*
**Adults and children ages 2
and older:** apply small amount
with fingertip or cotton swab
up to q.i.d.
(Zilactin-B)
**Adults and children ages 2
and older:** apply a thin coat
every 4 to 6 hours p.r.n. Allow
to dry for 30 to 60 seconds into
a protective film.

*Temporary relief from teething
pain—*
(Zilactin Baby)
**Infants and children ages 4
months and older:** apply small
amount with fingertip or cotton
swab up to q.i.d.

---

*Liquid contains alcohol.   **May contain tartrazine.   †Canada   ‡Australia   §U.K.

Temporary relief from canker sores, minor irritation or injury of mouth or gums, or mouth and gum irritation caused by dentures or orthodontics— (Anbesol, Orabase B paste)
Adults and children ages 2 and older: apply small amount gently at site of irritation up to q.i.d.

ADVERSE REACTIONS
Skin: urticaria, burning, stinging, tenderness, irritation, itching, erythema, rash.
Other: edema.

INTERACTIONS
Drug-drug
Antiarrhythmic drugs (Class I): Additive and synergistic, toxicity. Monitor patient closely.

CONTRAINDICATIONS
Contraindicated in patients who are hypersensitive to the drug or any of its components; also in patients with a history of allergy to local anesthetics such as procaine, butacaine, or benzocaine. This drug shouldn't be used in an ear with a perforated tympanic membrane or discharge, and it shouldn't be used in areas of infection. Benzocaine shouldn't be used in the eye; it's for external and mucous membrane use only.

OVERDOSE & TREATMENT
Maximum recommended dose is 5 g/day. Overdose is unlikely; however, methemoglobinemia has been reported after topical application for teething pain.

Treat symptomatically; if necessary, administer methylene blue 1% 0.1 ml/kg I.V. over at least 10 minutes.

NURSING CONSIDERATIONS
• Drug may mask more serious condition.
• Use cautiously in patients with severely traumatized mucosa or local sepsis.
• Avoid use in children younger than age 1.
• This drug isn't intended for prolonged use.
• Container must be kept tightly closed and away from moisture.

PATIENT TEACHING
• Advise patient to carefully read and follow instructions.
• Tell patient not to eat or chew gum until effect of local anesthetic has worn off, to avoid the risk of bite trauma.
• Advise patient to avoid smoking until the product is dry.
• Advise patient not to swallow the product.
• Tell patient that mild burning or stinging may occur. Applying ice may eliminate or decrease burning or stinging sensation.

Reactions may be *common*, uncommon, *life-threatening*, or COMMON AND LIFE-THREATENING.

• Tell patient using Orabase B Gel or Zilactin-B that a protective film will form 30 to 60 seconds after application. Tell patient not to peel off the film because this may irritate skin. To remove film, apply another coat of drug, then immediately wipe with moist gauze or tissue.

• Tell patient to contact doctor if pain lasts longer than 48 hours; if irritation, pain, or redness persists or worsens; or if swelling, rash, or fever develops.

• Tell patient not to use this product for longer than 1 week.

• Tell patient to avoid contact with eyes.

• Instruct patient to keep container tightly closed and away from moisture.

---

carbamide peroxide
Auro Eardrops, Bausch & Lomb Earwax Removal System, Debrox, Gly-Oxide Liquid, Murine Ear, Orajel Perioseptic Spot Treatment, Oral Cleanser Liquid, Proxigel

Pregnancy Risk Category NR

HOW SUPPLIED
Otic solution: 6.5% carbamide in glycerin or glycerin and propylene glycol
Oral solution: 10%

Oral liquid: 15%
Oral gel: 10%

ACTION
Otic: Emulsifies and disperses accumulated cerumen through effervescent activity.
Oral: Relieves pain and inflammation, cleanses and inhibits odor-forming bacteria through the release of oxygen on contact with mouth tissue.

Route	Onset	Peak	Duration
Otic	Immediate	Unknown	15-30 min
Oral	Immediate	Unknown	Unknown

INDICATIONS & DOSAGES
Impacted cerumen—
Adults and children ages 12 years and older: 5 to 10 drops into ear canal b.i.d. for up to 4 days. Allow solution to remain in ear canal for 15 minutes or longer; remove with warm water. Maximum use 4 days.

Temporary use to cleanse canker sores and minor wound or gum inflammation—
Adults and children ages 2 years and older: apply several undiluted drops of solution onto affected area and spit out after 2 to 3 minutes. Use up to 4 times daily after meals and at bedtime or as directed by dentist or doctor. Or, place 10 drops on tongue, mix with saliva, swish

for several minutes, and then spit out.

Gel: apply 4 times daily or as directed to affected area and massage in. Don't drink or rinse mouth for 5 minutes after use.

Everyday use to improve oral hygiene, as an adjunct to regular brushing or when regular brushing is inadequate or impossible—

Adults: apply solution to toothbrush, cover with toothpaste, brush normally, and spit out. Or, apply several undiluted drops of solution onto affected area and spit out after 2 to 3 minutes. Use up to q.i.d. after meals and h.s., or as directed by dentist or doctor. Or, place 10 drops on tongue, mix with saliva, swish for several minutes, and then spit out.

ADVERSE REACTIONS
None reported.

INTERACTIONS
None significant.

CONTRAINDICATIONS
Contraindicated in patients with perforated eardrum.

OVERDOSE & TREATMENT
Signs and symptoms of overdose include mild irritation to mucosal tissue or, if swallowed, irritation, inflammation, and burns in the mouth, throat, esophagus, or stomach. Gastric distention may result from liberation of oxygen. Accidental ocular exposure causes immediate pain and irritation, but severe injury is rare.

Irrigate eyes with large amounts of warm water for at least 15 minutes. Accidental dermal exposure bleaches the exposed area. Wash exposed skin twice with soap and water. Treat oral exposure by immediate dilution with water. Spontaneous vomiting may occur.

NURSING CONSIDERATIONS
• Use in children younger than age 12 only under direction of the doctor.
• Oral preparations shouldn't be self-administered by children younger than age 3; otic preparations shouldn't be self-administered by children younger than age 12.

PATIENT TEACHING
Otic administration
• Show patient or caregiver how to administer drug.
• Instruct patient to avoid inserting tip into the ear canal.
• Instruct patient to flush ear gently with warm water, using a rubber bulb syringe. Tell patient not to allow tip of ear syringe to obstruct the flow of water out of the ear.

Reactions may be *common,* uncommon, *life-threatening,* or COMMON AND LIFE-THREATENING.

• Advise patient to call doctor if self-treatment is unsuccessful after 4 days and at any time if redness, pain, or swelling occurs.

• Tell patient with ear discharge, ear pain, irritation or rash in ear, or dizziness to avoid use of drug.

• Tell patient to avoid use with perforated eardrum or after ear surgery.

Oral administration
• Instruct patient not to use products longer than 1 week unless otherwise directed.

• Tell patient not to swallow oral products.

• Tell patient to discontinue use and contact dentist or doctor if signs and symptoms last longer than 1 week; if irritation, pain, or redness persists or worsens; or if swelling, rash, or fever develops.

---

cromolyn sodium (sodium cromoglycate)
Nasalcrom, Nasalcrom Children's Allergy Prevention Nasal Spray

Pregnancy Risk Category B

HOW SUPPLIED
Nasal spray: 5.2 mg/metered spray (40 mg/ml)

ACTION
Inhibits the degranulation of sensitized mast cells that occurs after a patient's exposure to specific antigens. Also inhibits release of histamine and slow-reacting substance of anaphylaxis.

Route	Onset	Peak	Duration
Intranasal	Unknown	Unknown	Unknown

INDICATIONS & DOSAGES
Prevention and treatment of seasonal and perennial allergic rhinitis—
Adults and children ages 6 and older: 1 spray in each nostril t.i.d. or q.i.d. (q 4 to 6 hours). Maximum dosage is six times daily.

ADVERSE REACTIONS
CNS: dizziness, headache.
EENT: irritated throat and trachea, lacrimation, nasal congestion, pharyngeal irritation, sneezing, nasal burning and irritation, nosebleed.
GI: nausea, esophagitis, abdominal pain, bad taste in mouth.
GU: dysuria, urinary frequency.
Musculoskeletal: joint swelling and pain.
Respiratory: cough, wheezing, eosinophilic pneumonia.
Skin: rash, urticaria.
Other: swollen parotid gland, *angioedema.*

---

*Liquid contains alcohol.   **May contain tartrazine.   †Canada   ‡Australia   §U.K.

INTERACTIONS
None significant.

CONTRAINDICATIONS
Contraindicated in patients who are hypersensitive to the drug.

OVERDOSE & TREATMENT
No information available.

NURSING CONSIDERATIONS
• Drug should be used cautiously by patients with coronary artery disease or a history of arrhythmias. Note signs and symptoms, when they occur, and the pattern of drug use.
• Don't use to treat sinus infection, asthma, or cold signs and symptoms.
• Cromolyn use in children younger than age 5 is limited to the inhalation route of administration. Safety of nebulizer solution in children younger than age 2 and safety of nasal solution in children younger than age 6 haven't been established.

PATIENT TEACHING
• Tell patient with fever, discolored nasal discharge, sinus pain, or wheezing not to use drug.
• Advise patient to carefully read and follow product directions.
• Instruct patient that full effects of drug may not be noted for 1 to 2 weeks.

• To prevent allergic signs and symptoms, advise patient to use before contact with allergy triggers. Drug can be used up to 1 week before known contact.
• Advise patient to use every day while in contact with allergy triggers.
• Tell patient that esophagitis may be relieved by antacids or a glass of milk.
• Warn patient using nasal solution that stinging or sneezing may occur.
• Tell patient not to share drug with others, to prevent spread of infection.
• Tell patient to stop using drug if condition worsens, new signs and symptoms occur, or signs and symptoms don't improve within 2 weeks.

---

epinephrine hydrochloride
Adrenalin Chloride

Pregnancy Risk Category C

HOW SUPPLIED
Solution: 0.1%

ACTION
Causes local vasoconstriction of dilated arterioles, reducing blood flow and nasal congestion.

Route	Onset	Peak	Duration
Nasal	1-5 min	Unknown	1-3 hr

INDICATIONS & DOSAGES
Nasal congestion, local superficial bleeding—
Adults and children ages 6 years and older: Instill 1 or 2 drops with a sterile swab or gauze.

ADVERSE REACTIONS
CNS: nervousness, excitation.
CV: tachycardia.
EENT: rebound nasal congestion, stinging on application.
GU: increased BUN level.
Metabolic: hyperglycemia, lactic acidosis.

INTERACTIONS
None significant.

CONTRAINDICATIONS
Contraindicated in patients who are hypersensitive to the drug.

OVERDOSE & TREATMENT
Signs and symptoms of overdose include exaggeration of common adverse reactions, especially arrhythmias, extreme tremor or seizures, nausea and vomiting, fever, and CNS and respiratory depression.

Treatment requires supportive and symptomatic measures. Maintain airway and blood pressure. Don't administer vasopressors. Monitor vital signs closely. A beta blocker (such as propranolol) may be used to treat arrhythmias. A cardioselective beta blocker is recommended in asthmatic patients. Phentolamine may be used for hypertension, paraldehyde or diazepam for seizures, and dexamethasone for pyrexia.

NURSING CONSIDERATIONS
• Use with extreme caution in patients with long-standing bronchial asthma and emphysema who have developed degenerative heart disease.
• Use cautiously in elderly patients and in those with hyperthyroidism, CV disease, hypertension, psychoneurosis, and diabetes.
• Drug increases rigidity and tremor in patients with Parkinson's disease.

PATIENT TEACHING
• Advise patient to carefully read and follow product directions.
• Advise patient to clear nasal passages before administration.
• Teach patient how to instill nose drops. Tell patient to press finger against nasolacrimal duct gently for 1 to 2 minutes after instillation, to avoid excessive systemic absorption.
• Warn patient that slight stinging may occur.
• Advise patient to report bronchial irritation, nervousness, or

sleeplessness. Dosage may
need to be reduced.
• Tell patient that product should
only be used by one person to
prevent spread of infection.
• Tell patient not to exceed recommended dosage and to use
drug only when needed, for up
to 4 days.

---

hydrogen peroxide
Peroxyl Mouth Rinse, Peroxyl
Antiseptic Dental Rinse

Pregnancy Risk Category NR

HOW SUPPLIED
Concentrate: 30.5%
Gel: 1.5%
Solution: 1.5%, 3%

ACTION
A weak antibacterial agent and
a deodorant. Its pharmacologic
activity depends on the release
of nascent oxygen, causing a
powerful oxidizing effect that
destroys some microorganisms
and chemically alters many organic substances.

Route	Onset	Peak	Duration
Buccal, topical	Unknown	Unknown	Unknown

INDICATIONS & DOSAGES
*Pharyngitis, acute stomatitis,
gum irritation, gingivitis—*
Adults: dilute solution, rinse in
mouth, and spit out.

*Canker sores, minor wounds,
or gum inflammation from dental procedures, dentures, or orthodontic appliances; injury or
other irritations such as burns,
cheek bites, and toothbrush
abrasions—*
(Peroxyl Antiseptic Oral
Cleanser)
**Adults and children ages 2
and older:** rinse 2 tsp (½ cap-
ful) in mouth for 1 minute, and
spit out. Use up to q.i.d., after
meals, and h.s.

Breath freshener—
Adults: dilute solution, rinse in
mouth, and spit out.

Tooth whitener—
Adults: apply gel or solution
directly to teeth (dose and contact time vary according to
product).

ADVERSE REACTIONS
EENT: hairy tongue (hypertrophy of the papillae), irritation
of the buccal mucosa.

INTERACTIONS
None reported.

CONTRAINDICATIONS
None reported.

OVERDOSE & TREATMENT
In general, exposure to small
amounts of a dilute solution
won't result in serious compli-

Reactions may be *common,* uncommon, *life-threatening,* or COMMON AND LIFE-THREATENING.

cations and requires little treatment.

If the patient has ingested a 3% solution, force water ingestion to dilute; avoid emesis. Hospitalization may be required depending on volume ingested. If the patient has ingested a solution of more than 10% (concentrate), serious complications may result.

NURSING CONSIDERATIONS
• Solution must be diluted according to product directions; undiluted solution can be harsh to buccal tissue.

PATIENT TEACHING
• Advise patient not to swallow this medication, but instead to swish it around in the mouth and spit it out.
• Advise patient to carefully read and follow product instructions.
• Inform patient that overuse of product can be damaging.
• Advise patient to use for no longer than 1 week.
• Tell patient to call a doctor if no improvement occurs in 1 week; if irritation, pain, or redness persists or worsens; or if swelling, rash, or fever develops.

isopropyl alcohol
Auro-Dri, Dri/Ear, Ear-Dry, Swim Ear

Pregnancy Risk Category NR

HOW SUPPLIED
Liquid: 95% (in combination with other, inactive ingredients)

ACTION
Extracts moisture from ear canal by dehydration.

Route	Onset	Peak	Duration
Otic	Immediate	Unknown	Unknown

INDICATIONS & DOSAGES
Ear drying when water remains in ear after swimming, bathing, or showering—
Adults and children ages 2 years and older: 4 to 6 drops instilled in ear canal.

ADVERSE REACTIONS
EENT: local irritation, dryness.

INTERACTIONS
None reported.

CONTRAINDICATIONS
Contraindicated in patients with irritated ear canal, irritated or ruptured eardrum, or sensitivity to drug.

OVERDOSE & TREATMENT
None reported.

NURSING CONSIDERATIONS
• Long-term use of drug, as directed, doesn't cause harm.
• Product instructions aren't uniform and can't be used interchangeably.

PATIENT TEACHING
• Advise patient to carefully read and follow product instruction.
• Instruct patient to avoid use on mucous membranes or broken skin.
• Advise patient to avoid use with ear pain, ear discharge, irritation, perforated eardrum, or dizziness.
• Encourage patient to use earplugs to prevent entry of water while swimming.
• Instruct patient not to allow drug to come in contact with eyes.
• Advise patient that if signs and symptoms don't resolve within 4 days, he should discontinue use of product and contact doctor.

---

levmetamfetamine
Vicks Vapor Inhaler

Pregnancy Risk Category NR

HOW SUPPLIED
Nasal inhaler: 50 mg

ACTION
Decongestant that acts on the CNS, causing vasoconstriction and decongestion; consequent shrinkage of mucous membranes promotes drainage and improves ventilation.

Route	Onset	Peak	Duration
Nasal	Immediate	Unknown	Unknown

INDICATIONS & DOSAGES
Nasal congestion caused by the common cold, hay fever, upper respiratory tract allergies, or sinusitis—
Adults and children ages 12 and older: 2 inhalations per nostril, not more often than every 2 hours.
Children ages 6 to 11 years: 1 inhalation per nostril, not to exceed 1 dose every 2 hours.

ADVERSE REACTIONS
EENT: local burning, local stinging, sneezing, increased nasal discharge.

INTERACTIONS
None reported.

CONTRAINDICATIONS
Contraindicated in patients with heart disease, high blood pressure, thyroid disease, diabetes, or difficult urination caused by an enlarged prostate. Drug shouldn't be used by children

---

younger than age 6, unless directed by a doctor.

OVERDOSE & TREATMENT
No information available.

NURSING CONSIDERATIONS
• Patient shouldn't exceed 1 dose every 2 hours.
• Drug is effective for a minimum of 3 months after initial use.

PATIENT TEACHING
• Advise patient not to use this medication for longer than 3 days. If used for prolonged time, congestion may worsen.
• Instruct patient not to share inhalers because of the risk of spreading infection.
• Tell patient to keep the cap on when he's not using the medication.

---

naphazoline hydrochloride (optic)
AK-Con, Albalon Liquifilm, Allerest, Clear Eyes, Comfort Eyedrops, Degest 2, Nafazair, Naphcon, Naphcon Forte, VasoClear, Vasocon Regular

Pregnancy Risk Category C

HOW SUPPLIED
Ophthalmic solution: 0.012%, 0.02%, 0.03%, 0.1%

ACTION
Unknown. Thought to cause vasoconstriction by local adrenergic action on the blood vessels of the conjunctiva.

Route	Onset	Peak	Duration
Ophthalmic	10 min	Unknown	2-6 hr

INDICATIONS & DOSAGES
Ocular redness and irritation—
Adults: 1 to 3 drops of 0.1% solution per eye every 3 to 4 hours p.r.n. or 1 to 2 drops of 0.01% to 0.03% solution per eye up to q.i.d.

ADVERSE REACTIONS
CNS: headache, dizziness, nervousness, weakness.
EENT: transient eye stinging, pupillary dilation, eye irritation, photophobia, blurred vision, increased intraocular pressure, keratitis, lacrimation.
GI: nausea.
Skin: sweating.

INTERACTIONS
Drug-drug
MAO inhibitors, maprotiline, tricyclic antidepressants: hypertensive crisis if naphazoline is systemically absorbed. Advise patient to use together cautiously.

CONTRAINDICATIONS
Contraindicated in patients who are hypersensitive to the drug's

---

ingredients and in patients who have acute angle-closure glaucoma. Infants and small children shouldn't use the 0.1% (or higher) solution. Patients wearing soft contact lenses shouldn't use products containing benzalkonium chloride.

OVERDOSE & TREATMENT
Overdose may cause drowsiness, decreased body temperature, bradycardia, shocklike hypotension, and coma.

Treatment is symptomatic and supportive.

NURSING CONSIDERATIONS
• Use cautiously in patients with hyperthyroidism, cardiac disease, hypertension, or diabetes mellitus.
• Drug is the most widely used ocular decongestant.
• Soft contact lens use must be discontinued for the duration of treatment with drug.

PATIENT TEACHING
• Teach patient how to instill drug. Tell patient not to touch tip of dropper to eye or surrounding tissue.
• Warn patient not to exceed recommended dosages. Rebound congestion and conjunctivitis may occur with frequent or prolonged use.
• Tell patient to notify the doctor if photophobia, blurred vi-

sion, pain, or lid edema develops.
• Warn patient that headache, nausea, and decrease in body temperature may be signs of systemic absorption. Tell patient to notify the doctor if these signs and symptoms occur.
• Instruct patient to discontinue use of soft contact lenses during course of treatment and for a few hours after treatment has been discontinued.
• Instruct patient not to use if the solution is cloudy.

---

naphazoline hydrochloride (otic)
Privine

Pregnancy Risk Category NR

HOW SUPPLIED
Nose drops: 0.05% solution
Nasal spray: 0.05% solution

ACTION
Causes local vasoconstriction of dilated arterioles, reducing blood flow and nasal congestion.

Route	Onset	Peak	Duration
Nasal	10 min	Unknown	2-6 hr

INDICATIONS & DOSAGES
Nasal congestion—
Adults and children ages 12 and older: 1 or 2 drops or 1 to

2 sprays in each nostril no more than every 6 hours p.r.n.

ADVERSE REACTIONS
CNS: anxiety, restlessness.
EENT: rebound nasal congestion, sneezing, stinging, dryness of mucosa.
Other: systemic effects in children.

INTERACTIONS
Drug-drug
MAO inhibitors, maprotiline, tricyclic antidepressants: hypertensive crisis if naphazoline is systemically absorbed. Advise patient to use together cautiously.

CONTRAINDICATIONS
Contraindicated in patients who are hypersensitive to the drug.

OVERDOSE & TREATMENT
Signs and symptoms of overdose include CNS depression, sweating, decreased body temperature, bradycardia, shocklike hypotension, decreased respiration, CV collapse, and coma.

Activated charcoal or gastric lavage may be used initially to treat accidental ingestion (administer early before sedation occurs). Monitor vital signs and ECG, as ordered. Treat seizures with I.V. diazepam.

NURSING CONSIDERATIONS
• Use cautiously in patients with hyperthyroidism, heart disease, hypertension, or diabetes mellitus and in those who have difficulty urinating because of enlargement of prostate gland.
• Don't give to children younger than age 12 unless directed by a doctor.

PATIENT TEACHING
• Teach patient how to use drug. For nose drops, instruct patient to tilt head back as far as possible, instill drops, then lean head forward while inhaling; then repeat procedure for other nostril. Or, drops can be applied with patient's head down and turned to one side. Instruct patient to instill drops in lower nostril and remain in position for 5 minutes; then repeat with other nostril.
• For nasal spray, instruct patient to hold spray container and head upright. Tell him to blow his nose 3 to 5 minutes after spray is used.
• Tell patient that product should be used by only one person to prevent spread of infection.
• Warn patient not to exceed recommended dosage and not to use for longer than 3 to 5 days because of potential for rebound congestion.

• Instruct patient to call the doctor if nasal congestion persists after 3 days.

---

oxymetazoline hydrochloride (optic)
OcuClear, Visine L.R.

Pregnancy Risk Category C

HOW SUPPLIED
Ophthalmic solution: 0.025%

ACTION
A direct-acting sympathomimetic amine that acts on alpha-adrenergic receptors in the arterioles of the conjunctiva to produce vasoconstriction, resulting in decreased conjunctival congestion.

Route	Onset	Peak	Duration
Ophthalmic	5 min	Unknown	6 hr

INDICATIONS & DOSAGES
Relief from eye redness caused by minor eye irritations—
Adults and children ages 6 and older: 1 to 2 drops instilled into conjunctival sac b.i.d. to q.i.d. (at least 6 hours apart).

ADVERSE REACTIONS
CNS: anxiety, headáche, light-headedness, nervousness, restlessness, insomnia, trembling.
CV: palpitations, tachycardia, irregular pulse.

EENT: transient stinging on initial instillation; blurred vision, keratitis, lacrimation, increase in intraocular pressure; reactive hyperemia with excessive doses or prolonged use.

INTERACTIONS
Drug-drug
MAO inhibitors, maprotiline, tricyclic antidepressants: if significant systemic absorption of oxymetazoline occurs, concurrent use may potentiate pressor effect of oxymetazoline. Advise patient to avoid using together.

CONTRAINDICATIONS
Contraindicated in patients who are hypersensitive to the drug or its components and in patients with angle-closure glaucoma.

OVERDOSE & TREATMENT
Signs and symptoms of overdose include somnolence, sedation, sweating, CNS depression with hypertension, bradycardia, decreased cardiac output, rebound hypertension, CV collapse, depressed respirations, and coma.

If drug is ingested, onset of sedation is rapid, and emesis isn't recommended unless done immediately. Activated charcoal or gastric lavage may be used initially. Monitor vital

---

Reactions may be *common*, uncommon, *life-threatening*, or COMMON AND LIFE-THREATENING.

signs and ECG. Treat seizures with I.V. diazepam.

NURSING CONSIDERATIONS
• Use cautiously in patients with hyperthyroidism, cardiac disease, hypertension, eye disease, infection, or injury.
• Don't use if solution has become cloudy or has changed color.

PATIENT TEACHING
• Teach patient how to instill drops. Advise thorough hand washing before and after instillation, and tell patient not to touch tip of dropper to eye or surrounding tissue.
• Instruct patient to apply light finger pressure on lacrimal sac for 1 minute after drug instillation.
• Advise patient to stop drug and consult the doctor if eye pain occurs, if vision changes, or if redness or irritation continues, worsens, or lasts longer than 72 hours.
• Tell patient that overuse may cause increased eye redness.

---

oxymetazoline hydrochloride (otic)
Afrin, Afrin Children's Strength Nose Drops, Allerest 12 Hour Nasal Spray, Chlorphed-LA, Drixine Nasal‡, Duramist Plus, Duration, 4-Way 12-Hour Nasal Spray, Genasal Spray, Neo-Synephrine 12 Hour Nasal Spray, Nostrilla, NTZ Long Acting Decongestant Nasal Spray, Sinarest 12 Hour Nasal, Sinex 12-Hour Ultra Fine Nasal Mist, Twice-A-Day Nasal

Pregnancy Risk Category NR

HOW SUPPLIED
Nasal solution: 0.025%, 0.05%

ACTION
Unknown. Thought to cause local vasoconstriction of dilated arterioles, reducing blood flow and nasal congestion.

Route	Onset	Peak	Duration
Nasal	5-10 min	6 hr	< 12 hr

INDICATIONS & DOSAGES
Nasal congestion—
Adults and children ages 6 and older: 2 to 3 drops or sprays of 0.05% solution in each nostril b.i.d.
Children ages 2 to 5: 2 to 3 drops of 0.025% solution in each nostril b.i.d. Use no longer than 3 to 5 days.

ADVERSE REACTIONS
CNS: headache, drowsiness, dizziness, insomnia, sedation.
CV: palpitations, *CV collapse,* hypertension.

EENT: rebound nasal congestion or irritation, dryness of nose and throat, increased nasal discharge, stinging, sneezing. **Other:** systemic effects in children.

INTERACTIONS
None significant.

CONTRAINDICATIONS
Contraindicated in patients who are hypersensitive to the drug.

OVERDOSE & TREATMENT
Signs and symptoms of overdose include somnolence, sedation, sweating, CNS depression with hypertension, bradycardia, decreased cardiac output, rebound hypertension, CV collapse, depressed respirations, and coma.

If drug is ingested, emesis isn't recommended, unless used early, because of rapid onset of sedation. Activated charcoal or gastric lavage may be used initially. Monitor vital signs and ECG. Treat seizures with I.V. diazepam.

NURSING CONSIDERATIONS
• Use cautiously in patients with hyperthyroidism, cardiac disease, hypertension, diabetes mellitus, or difficult urination secondary to enlarged prostate.
• Use for longer than 2 to 3 days can lead to rebound congestion.

PATIENT TEACHING
• Teach patient how to apply drug. Tell him to hold head upright to minimize swallowing of drug and to sniff spray briskly.
• Advise patient that transient burning, stinging, sneezing, or increased nasal discharge may occur.
• Tell patient that drug should be used by only one person to prevent spread of infection.
• Tell patient not to exceed recommended dosage and to use only when needed for up to 3 days. Overuse may cause worsening congestion.
• Caution patient that excessive use may cause bradycardia, hypotension, dizziness, and weakness.

---

phenylephrine hydrochloride (optic)
AK-Nefrin, Isopto Frin, Ocu-Phrin, Prefrin Liquifilm, Relief

Pregnancy Risk Category NR

HOW SUPPLIED
Ophthalmic solution: 0.12%

ACTION
Causes local vasoconstriction of dilated arterioles, reducing blood flow and conjunctival congestion.

Route	Onset	Peak	Duration
Ophthalmic	Rapid	Unknown	0.5-1.5 hr

INDICATIONS & DOSAGES
Relief from ocular congestion, itching, and minor irritation caused by irritants; relief from redness—
Adults: 1 to 2 drops of 0.12% solution to affected eye every 3 to 4 hours p.r.n. Don't exceed four doses daily.

ADVERSE REACTIONS
EENT: transient stinging, blurred vision.

INTERACTIONS
None significant.

CONTRAINDICATIONS
Contraindicated in patients who are hypersensitive to the drug and in those with angle-closure glaucoma or aneurysm.

OVERDOSE & TREATMENT
Signs and symptoms of overdose include exaggeration of common adverse reactions, palpitations, paresthesia, vomiting, arrhythmias, and hypertension.

To treat an overdose, discontinue drug and provide symptomatic and supportive measures. Monitor vital signs closely. Use atropine sulfate to block reflex bradycardia; phentolamine to treat excessive hypertension; and propranolol to treat cardiac arrhythmias, or levodopa to reduce an excessive mydriatic effect of an ophthalmic preparation as necessary.

NURSING CONSIDERATIONS
• Don't use ophthalmic preparations in patients with glaucoma.
• Use cautiously in patients with hyperthyroidism, marked hypertension, type 1 diabetes mellitus, cardiac disease, or advanced arteriosclerotic changes and in patients who have trouble urinating because of an enlarged prostate.
• It's unknown whether drug appears in breast milk. Breast-feeding patients should use with caution.
• Infants and children may be more susceptible than adults to drug's effects. Because of the risk of causing severe hypertension, only ophthalmic solutions containing 0.5% or less should be used in infants younger than age 1. The 10% ophthalmic solution is contraindicated in infants.
• Effects may be exaggerated in elderly patients. In patients older than age 50, phenylephrine (ophthalmic solution) seems to change the response of the dilator muscle of the pupil, so that rebound miosis may occur the day after the drug is given.

PATIENT TEACHING
• Teach patient how to administer drug.
• Tell patient using eyedrops to apply pressure to the lacrimal sac for 1 to 2 minutes after instillation.
• Inform patient that drug should be used by only one person to prevent spread of infection.
• Tell patient not to touch tip of dropper to eye, to avoid contamination. Rinse with hot water after use.
• Tell patient not to exceed recommended dosage and to use only when needed. Frequent or prolonged use may worsen congestion.
• Advise patient not to use for longer than 2 to 3 days because of potential for rebound congestion.
• Tell patient to report ocular pain, vision changes, or continued redness or irritation; worsening condition; or signs and symptoms persisting longer than 3 days.
• Advise patient that overuse of eyedrops may cause increased redness.

phenylephrine hydrochloride (otic)
Alconefrin Nasal Drops 12, Alconefrin Nasal Drops 25, Alconefrin Nasal Drops 50, Doktors, Duration, Neo-Synephrine, Nostril, Rhinall, Rhinall-10 Children's Flavored Nose Drops, Sinex

Pregnancy Risk Category NR

HOW SUPPLIED
Nasal solution: 0.125%, 0.16%, 0.25%, 0.5%, 1%

ACTION
Causes local vasoconstriction of dilated arterioles, reducing blood flow and nasal congestion.

Route	Onset	Peak	Duration
Nasal	Rapid	Unknown	0.5-4 hr

INDICATIONS & DOSAGES
Nasal congestion—
Adults and children ages 12 and older: 2 to 3 drops or 2 to 3 sprays in each nostril q 4 hours, p.r.n.
Children ages 6 to 12: 2 to 3 drops or 1 to 2 sprays of 0.25% solution in each nostril q 3 to 4 hours, p.r.n.

ADVERSE REACTIONS
EENT: transient burning or stinging, sneezing, increased

nasal discharge, dryness of nasal mucosa; rebound nasal congestion.

INTERACTIONS
None significant.

CONTRAINDICATIONS
Contraindicated in patients who are hypersensitive to the drug.

OVERDOSE & TREATMENT
Signs and symptoms of overdose include exaggeration of common adverse reactions, palpitations, paresthesia, vomiting, arrhythmias, and hypertension.

To treat an overdose, discontinue drug and provide symptomatic and supportive measures. Monitor vital signs closely. Use atropine sulfate to block reflex bradycardia; phentolamine to treat excessive hypertension; and propranolol to treat cardiac arrhythmias, or levodopa to reduce an excessive mydriatic effect of an ophthalmic preparation as necessary.

NURSING CONSIDERATIONS
• Don't use nasal solution in patient with insomnia, tremors, asthenia, dizziness, or arrhythmias from previous dose.
• Use cautiously in elderly patient; patient with hyperthyroidism, marked hypertension, type 1 diabetes mellitus, cardiac disease, or advanced arteriosclerotic changes; and patient with difficulty urinating because of an enlarged prostate.
• It's unknown whether drug appears in breast milk. Breastfeeding patient should use with caution.
• Use cautiously in children of low body weight. Most manufacturers recommend that the 0.5% nasal solution not be used in children younger than age 12, except under medical supervision.
• Use cautiously in elderly patient.

PATIENT TEACHING
• Teach patient how to administer drug. For nose drops, instruct patient to tilt head back as far as possible, instill drops, then lean head forward while inhaling; then repeat procedure for other nostril. Or, drops can be applied with patient's head down and turned to one side. Instruct patient to instill drops in lower nostril and remain in position for 5 minutes; then repeat with other nostril.
• For nasal spray, instruct patient to hold spray container and head upright. Tell him to blow his nose 3 to 5 minutes after spray is used.
• Inform patient that nose drops or spray should be used by only one person, to avoid spreading infection.

• Tell patient not to touch tip of dropper to nose, to avoid contamination. Rinse dropper with hot water after use.
• Tell patient not to exceed recommended dosage and to use only when needed. Frequent or prolonged use may cause worsening congestion.
• Advise patient not to use for longer than 2 to 3 days because of potential for rebound congestion.
• Tell patient that transient burning, stinging, sneezing, or increased nasal discharge may occur with nose drops and sprays.
• Advise patient to contact doctor if nasal symptoms persist beyond 3 days.

propylhexedrine
Benzedrex

Pregnancy Risk Category NR

HOW SUPPLIED
Inhaler: 250 mg

ACTION
Believed to act as a sympathomimetic agent similar to amphetamine. Intranasal propylhexedrine is thought to stimulate alpha-adrenergic receptors, leading to constriction of dilated arterioles, reduction of nasal blood flow, reduced congestion, and increased lumen dimension of obstructed eustachian ostia. Through these processes, nasal ventilation and aeration are temporarily improved.

Route	Onset	Peak	Duration
Nasal	30 sec	5 min	30–120 min

INDICATIONS & DOSAGES
Nasal and sinus congestion—
Adults and children ages 6 to 12 years: 1 to 2 inhalations in each nostril, no more than every 2 hours. Maximum duration of therapy is 3 days.

ADVERSE REACTIONS
CNS: headache, nervousness.
CV: hypertension, increased ventricular rate.
EENT: transient burning, stinging, dryness of the mucosa, sneezing, rebound congestion.
Other: substance abuse.

INTERACTIONS
Drug-drug
Dihydroergotamines, furazolidone, methyldopa, reserpine: may cause extreme elevations in blood pressure. Advise patient to avoid using together; monitor blood pressure closely.
Guanethidine: may decrease the hypotensive effects of guanethidine and may potentiate decongestant effects of

propylhexedrine. Advise patient to avoid using together; monitor blood pressure closely.

MAO inhibitors: may result in severe headache, hypertension, and hyperpyrexia, possibly resulting in a hypertensive crisis. Advise patient to avoid using together; monitor blood pressure closely.

Phenothiazines: may antagonize or reverse the effects of the nasal decongestant. Monitor therapeutic response.

Theophylline: may increase risk or severity of side effects (nausea, nervousness, insomnia, and cardiotoxicity). Monitor patient closely.

Tricyclic antidepressants: may cause hypertension, dysrhythmias, or CNS stimulation, especially with overuse or prolonged use of the decongestant. Advise patient to avoid using together.

Urinary acidifiers: may reduce therapeutic effects of decongestant. Monitor therapeutic effects.

Urinary alkalinizers: may enhance therapeutic or toxic effects of decongestant. Advise patient to avoid using together.

Drug-herb
Ephedra, ginseng: may increase insomnia, headache, tremor. Advise patient to use together with caution.

Licorice: may cause severe headache, hypertension, hyperpyrexia, and hypertensive crisis. Advise patient to avoid using together.

Yohimbine: may increase insomnia, headache, tremor, hypertension. Advise patient to use together with caution.

Drug-food
Caffeine: enhances effect of drug. Advise patient to limit use together.

CONTRAINDICATIONS
Contraindicated in patients who are allergic to the drug, to lavender oil, or to menthol and in patients who participate in official athletic events. Use with extreme caution in patients with hyperthyroidism, heart disease, hypertension, diabetes mellitus, urinary incontinence, or glaucoma.

OVERDOSE & TREATMENT
Overuse of this product may lead to rebound congestion. The dose should be slowly tapered. Nasal saline or a nasal steroid can be used as treatment.

Abuse and toxicity of drug has been reported. The cotton pledgets are extracted from the inhaler, boiled, and prepared into a solution for I.V. injection or may be consumed orally by chewing. Pulmonary foreign body granulomas, pulmonary hypertension, cor pulmonale, pulmonary edema, diffuse fibrosis, cardiomegaly, psychosis, MI, ophthalmoplegia, hypertension, tachycardia, left ventricular hypertrophy, ischemic necrosis, brainstem dysfunction, thrombocytopenia, bleeding, and sudden death have been reported in persons taking the drug by the oral or I.V. route.

NURSING CONSIDERATIONS
• Propylhexedrine use shouldn't exceed 3 to 5 days.
• The inhaler is effective for a minimum of 3 months after first use.
• Use nasal saline as adjunctive therapy if patient experiences nasal dryness.
• Inhaler contains menthol and lavender oil.
• Information is insufficient to justify use by pregnant or breast-feeding women.

PATIENT TEACHING
• Advise patient who has trouble sleeping to limit use of propylhexedrine to daytime hours and to use an antihistamine alone before bedtime.
• Caution patient to carefully read and follow product instructions, including dose frequency and duration of treatment. Don't use for longer than 3 days. Frequent or prolonged use may cause worsening congestion.
• Advise patients with hyperthyroidism, heart disease, hypertension, diabetes mellitus, urinary incontinence, or glaucoma or those taking MAO inhibitors to consult a doctor before using this drug.
• Warn patients of the potential for abuse.
• Inform patient that inhaler should be used by only one person, to avoid spreading infection.

---

pseudoephedrine hydrochloride
Efidac/24, Pedia Care Infant's Decongestant, Sudafed, Sudafed 12 Hour

pseudoephedrine sulfate
Afrin, Drixoral Non-Drowsy Formula

Pregnancy Risk Category C

HOW SUPPLIED
pseudoephedrine hydrochloride
Tablets: 30 mg, 60 mg, 240 mg
Tablets (extended-release): 120 mg
Drops: 7.5 mg/0.8 ml
pseudoephedrine sulfate
Tablets (extended-release): 120 mg

Reactions may be *common*, uncommon, *life-threatening*, or COMMON AND LIFE-THREATENING.

ACTION
Stimulates alpha receptors in the respiratory tract, producing vasoconstriction, causing shrinkage of swollen nasal mucous membranes; reduction of tissue hyperemia, edema, and nasal congestion; and an increase in airway patency.

Route	Onset	Peak	Duration
P.O.	0.5 hr	0.5-1 hr	4-12 hr

INDICATIONS & DOSAGES
Nasal and eustachian tube decongestion—
Adults and children older than age 12: 60 mg P.O. q 4 to 6 hours; or 120 mg extended-release tablet P.O. q 12 hours; or 240 mg (Efidac/24) once daily. Maximum dose is 240 mg daily.
Children ages 6 to 12: 30 mg P.O. regular-release form q 4 to 6 hours. Maximum dose is 120 mg daily.
Children ages 2 to 5: 15 mg P.O. regular-release form q 4 to 6 hours. Maximum dose is 60 mg daily.
Children ages 2 to 3 (24 to 35 lb): 2 droppers (1.6 ml) q 4 to 6 hours up to q.i.d.
Children ages 12 to 23 months (18 to 23 lb): 1½ droppers (1.2 ml) q 4 to 6 hours up to q.i.d.
Children ages 4 to 11 months (12 to 17 lb): 1 dropper (0.8 ml) q 4 to 6 hours up to q.i.d.

Children ages 0 to 3 months (6 to 11 lb): ½ dropper (0.4 ml) q 4 to 6 hours up to q.i.d.

ADVERSE REACTIONS
CNS: anxiety, transient stimulation, tremor, dizziness, headache, insomnia, nervousness.
CV: arrhythmias, palpitations, tachycardia, *CV collapse.*
GI: anorexia, nausea, vomiting, dry mouth.
GU: dysuria.
Respiratory: respiratory difficulties.
Skin: pallor.

INTERACTIONS
Drug-drug
Antihypertensives: may attenuate hypotensive effect. Monitor blood pressure closely.
MAO inhibitors: may cause severe hypertension (hypertensive crisis). Advise patient to avoid using together.
Methyldopa: may result in increased pressor response. Monitor patient closely.

Drug-food
Caffeine: has an additive effect. Advise patient to avoid using together.

CONTRAINDICATIONS
Contraindicated in breast-feeding patients, patients with severe hypertension or severe coronary artery disease, and pa-

tients who use MAO inhibitors; extended-release preparations are contraindicated in children younger than age 12.

OVERDOSE & TREATMENT
Signs and symptoms of overdose include exaggeration of common adverse reactions, particularly seizures, arrhythmias, and nausea and vomiting.

Treatment may include an emetic and gastric lavage within 4 hours of ingestion. Charcoal is effective only if administered within 1 hour, unless extended-release form was used. If renal function is adequate, forced diuresis may be used in severe overdose. Monitor vital signs, cardiac state, and electrolyte levels. I.V. propranolol may control cardiac toxicity; I.V. diazepam may be helpful to manage delirium or seizures; dilute I.V. potassium chloride solutions may be given for hypokalemia.

NURSING CONSIDERATIONS
• Drug should be used cautiously by patients with hypertension, cardiac disease, diabetes, glaucoma, hyperthyroidism, or prostatic hyperplasia.
• Drug appears in breast milk. Breast-feeding patients should avoid use; infant may be susceptible to drug effects.

• Children younger than age 12 shouldn't use the extended-release form.
• Because the elderly patient is more sensitive to drug's effects, he shouldn't use extended-release tablets unless safety with short-acting preparations has been established.

PATIENT TEACHING
• Tell patient not to crush or break extended-release forms.
• Advise patient to carefully read and follow product instructions.
• Instruct patient not to take drug within 2 hours before bedtime because it can cause insomnia.
• Warn patient to stop drug if he becomes unusually restless, and to notify doctor promptly.

---

sodium chloride, hypertonic
Adsorbonac, Ak-NaCl, Muro-128, Muroptic-5

Pregnancy Risk Category NR

HOW SUPPLIED
Ophthalmic ointment: 5%
Ophthalmic solution: 2%, 5%

ACTION
Removes excess fluid from cornea by osmosis.

Route	Onset	Peak	Duration
Ophthalmic	Unknown	Unknown	Unknown

INDICATIONS & DOSAGES
Temporary relief from corneal edema—
Adults and children: 1 to 2 drops in affected eye q 3 to 4 hours or as directed, or ¼ inch (6 mm) of ointment applied q 3 to 4 hours or as directed.

ADVERSE REACTIONS
EENT: slight eye stinging.
Other: hypersensitivity reactions.

INTERACTIONS
None significant.

CONTRAINDICATIONS
Contraindicated in patients who are hypersensitive to the drug or its components.

OVERDOSE & TREATMENT
No information available.

NURSING CONSIDERATIONS
• Ophthalmic solution isn't interchangeable with other saline solutions.
• Check expiration date before use.

PATIENT TEACHING
• Teach patient how to instill drug. Advise him to wash hands before and after instillation and to apply light finger pressure on lacrimal sac for 1 minute after drops are instilled.
• Warn patient not to touch dropper to eye or surrounding tissue.
• Tell patient to prevent caking on dropper bottle tip by putting a few drops of sterile irrigation solution inside bottle cap.
• Warn patient that ointment may cause blurred vision.
• Instruct patient to discontinue drug and notify doctor if he experiences severe headache, pain, rapid change in vision, acute redness of eyes, sudden appearance of floating spots, pain on exposure to light, or double vision.
• Advise patient to store drug in tightly closed container.
• Advise patient not to use solution if it changes color or becomes cloudy.

sodium chloride, nasal
Afrin Moisturizing Saline Mist, Afrin Saline Mist with Eucalyptol & Menthol, Ary Saline Nasal Mist, Ayr Baby Saline Spray/Drops, Breathe Free, Dristan Saline Spray, HuMist Nasal Mist, Mycinaire Saline Nasal Mist, NaSal Moist, Natru-Vent Nasal Spray, Ocean, Pretz, Saline, SeaMist, 4-Way Saline Nasal Spray

Pregnancy Risk Category NR

HOW SUPPLIED
Solution: 0.6 %, 0.64%, 0.65%
Mist: 0.4%, 0.69%
Drops: 0.4%, 0.65%

ACTION
By creating an osmotic gradient, nasal saline may relieve nasal edema and dryness and, by removing dried, encrusted, thick mucus, may allow for enhanced nasal drainage.

Route	Onset	Peak	Duration
Nasal	Immediate	Immediate	30 min-1 hr

INDICATIONS & DOSAGES
Relief from dry, irritated nasal passages—
Adults and children: 1 to 6 sprays or drops in each nostril p.r.n.

ADVERSE REACTIONS
EENT: burning, stinging, sneezing, increased nasal discharge.

INTERACTIONS
None reported.

CONTRAINDICATIONS
None reported.

OVERDOSE & TREATMENT
No information available.

NURSING CONSIDERATIONS
• Bottle of nasal saline should be discarded once symptoms are relieved.
• Can be used in combination with cold, allergy, and sinus products.
• Product isn't habit-forming.

PATIENT TEACHING
• Advise patient to blow nose or wipe infant's or child's nose before using product.
• Tell patient to keep head upright and inhale while dispensing sprays.
• Advise parent to place infant in supine position and instill drops in each nostril. Keep child supine for 1 to 2 minutes after instilling drops. Can be used with bulb syringe.
• Tell patient to avoid touching tip of container to nose, nasal mucosa, or nasal discharge and

---

Reactions may be *common*, uncommon, *life-threatening*, or COMMON AND LIFE-THREATENING.

to rinse container with warm water after use.
• Advise patient to always check the expiration date before using drug.
• Instruct patient to discard the product if it's discolored or if he suspects deterioration.
• Caution patient not to share the same container with another person.
• Instruct patient to discard product once symptoms are relieved.

---

sodium fluoride, topical
ACT, Fluorigard, Gel-Tin, Minute-Gel, Mouth Kote F/R, Stop Gel

Pregnancy Risk Category NR

HOW SUPPLIED
Gel: 0.1%
Rinse: 0.02%, 0.04%

ACTION
Stabilizes the apatite crystal of bone and teeth. Increases tooth resistance to acid breakdown.

Route	Onset	Peak	Duration
Topical	Unknown	30-60 min	Unknown

INDICATIONS & DOSAGES
Prevention of dental caries—
Adults and children ages 6 and older: 5 to 10 ml of rinse or thin ribbon of gel applied to teeth with toothbrush or mouth trays for at least 1 minute h.s.

ADVERSE REACTIONS
None reported.

INTERACTIONS
Drug-drug
Aluminum hydroxide, calcium, iron, magnesium: may decrease absorption. Tell patient to separate administration times.

Drug-food
Dairy products: decreases absorption. Advise patient to avoid using together.

CONTRAINDICATIONS
Contraindicated in patients who are hypersensitive to the fluoride.

OVERDOSE & TREATMENT
In children, acute ingestion of 10 to 20 mg of sodium fluoride may cause excessive salivation and GI disturbances; 500 mg may be fatal. GI disturbances include salivation, nausea, abdominal pain, vomiting, and diarrhea. CNS disturbances include CNS irritability, paresthesias, tetany, hyperactive reflexes, seizures, and respiratory or cardiac failure (from the calcium-binding effect of fluoride). Hypoglycemia and hypocalcemia are frequent laboratory findings.

Gastric lavage with 1% to 5% calcium chloride solution may precipitate the fluoride. Administer glucose I.V. in saline solution; parenteral calcium administration may be indicated for tetany. Adequate urine output should be maintained.

NURSING CONSIDERATIONS
● Use of OTC product shouldn't replace regular dental checkups.
● Levels of sodium fluoride in breast milk increase only when daily intake exceeds 1.5 mg of sodium fluoride. Breast-feeding patient should consult her doctor before taking sodium fluoride.
● Young children usually can't perform the rinse process necessary with oral solutions.
● Because prolonged ingestion or improper techniques may result in dental fluorosis and osseous changes, the dosages must be carefully adjusted according to the amount of fluoride ion in drinking water.

PATIENT TEACHING
● Advise patient that product shouldn't be used if water supply is fluorinated.
● Advise patient that topical rinses and gels shouldn't be swallowed.
● Drug is most effective when used right after brushing teeth or flossing. Tell patient to rinse around and between teeth for 1 minute; then spit out.
● Tell patient not to eat, drink, or rinse mouth for 30 minutes after application.
● Tell patient to dilute drops or rinses in plastic, not glass, containers.
● Advise patient to notify dentist if tooth mottling occurs.
● Instruct patient not to exceed recommended dosage.
● Advise parent to supervise child to prevent excessive swallowing.

tetrahydrozoline hydrochloride
Collyrium Fresh, Eyesine, Murine Plus, Optigene 3, Tetrasine, Visine, Visine Moisturizing

Pregnancy Risk Category C

HOW SUPPLIED
Ophthalmic solution: 0.05%

ACTION
Unknown. Thought to cause vasoconstriction by local adrenergic action on the blood vessels of the conjunctiva.

Route	Onset	Peak	Duration
Ophthalmic	Few min	Unknown	1-4 hr

INDICATIONS & DOSAGES
Temporary relief from redness and pain caused by minor eye irritation—
Adults: 1 to 2 drops of 0.05% solution instilled up to q.i.d. or as directed by doctor.

ADVERSE REACTIONS
CNS: headache, drowsiness, insomnia, dizziness, tremor.
CV: *arrhythmias.*
EENT: transient eye stinging, pupillary dilation, increased intraocular pressure, keratitis, lacrimation, eye irritation.

INTERACTIONS
Drug-drug
Guanethidine, MAO inhibitors, tricyclic antidepressants: hypertensive crisis if tetrahydrozoline is systemically absorbed. Advise patient to avoid using together.

CONTRAINDICATIONS
Contraindicated in patients who are hypersensitive to the drug or its components and in those with angle-closure glaucoma or other serious eye diseases.

OVERDOSE & TREATMENT
Signs and symptoms of overdose include bradycardia, decreased body temperature, shocklike hypotension, apnea, drowsiness, CNS depression and coma.

Because of rapid onset of sedation, emesis isn't recommended unless induced early. Activated charcoal or gastric lavage may be used initially. Monitor vital signs and ECG. Treat seizures with I.V. diazepam.

NURSING CONSIDERATIONS
• Use cautiously in patients with hyperthyroidism, heart disease, hypertension, or diabetes mellitus.
• Rebound congestion may occur with frequent or prolonged use.
• Don't use in elderly patient to treat redness and inflammation, which may represent a more serious eye condition in this population.
• Elderly patients are more likely than younger patients to react adversely to sympathomimetics.

PATIENT TEACHING
• Teach patient how to instill drug, and advise washing hands before and after instillation.
• Instruct patient to apply light finger pressure on lacrimal sac for 1 minute after drops are instilled and not to touch tip of dropper to eye or surrounding tissue.
• Warn patient not to exceed recommended dosage.

• Tell patient to stop drug and notify a doctor if redness or irritation continues or if no relief occurs within 2 days.

• Warn patient not to share ophthalmic drugs.

---

xylometazoline hydrochloride
Otrivin Nasal Spray, Otrivin Pediatric Nasal Drops

Pregnancy Risk Category NR

HOW SUPPLIED
Nasal solution: 0.05%, 0.1%

ACTION
Unknown. Thought to cause local vasoconstriction of dilated arterioles, reducing blood flow and nasal congestion.

Route	Onset	Peak	Duration
Nasal	5-10 min	Unknown	5-6 hr

INDICATIONS & DOSAGES
Nasal congestion—
Adults and children ages 12 and older: 2 to 3 drops or sprays of 0.1% solution in each nostril q 8 to 10 hours, not to exceed three times in 24 hours. Tell patient to use for no longer than 3 consecutive days.
Children ages 2 to 12 years: 2 to 3 drops of 0.05% solution in each nostril q 8 to 10 hours, not to exceed three times in 24 hours. Tell patient to use for no longer than 3 consecutive days.

ADVERSE REACTIONS
EENT: transient burning, stinging; dryness or ulceration of nasal mucosa; sneezing; rebound nasal congestion, or irritation.

INTERACTIONS
None significant.

CONTRAINDICATIONS
Contraindicated in patients who are hypersensitive to the drug and in patients with angle-closure glaucoma.

OVERDOSE & TREATMENT
Signs and symptoms of overdose include somnolence, sedation, sweating, CNS depression with hypertension, bradycardia, decreased cardiac output, rebound hypotension, CV collapse, depressed respirations, and coma.

Because of rapid onset of sedation, emesis isn't recommended unless induced early. Activated charcoal or gastric lavage may be used initially. Monitor vital signs and ECG. Treat seizures with I.V. diazepam.

NURSING CONSIDERATIONS
• Use cautiously in patients with hyperthyroidism, cardiac dis-

ease, hypertension, diabetes mellitus, difficulty urinating because of enlarged prostate, or advanced arteriosclerosis.
• It's unknown whether drug appears in breast milk, so breast-feeding patients should consult doctor before using.
• Children may be prone to greater system absorption, with resultant increase in adverse effects. Use cautiously in children.
• Use with caution in elderly patients who have CV disease, diabetes mellitus, or poorly controlled hypertension.

PATIENT TEACHING
• Teach patient how to apply drug. Have patient hold head upright to minimize swallowing of drug, then sniff spray briskly.
• Tell patient that drug may cause burning, stinging, sneezing, or increased nasal discharge.
• Tell patient that drug should be used by only one person to prevent spread of infection.
• Advise patient not to exceed recommended dosage and to use only as needed for 3 days. Frequent or prolonged use may increase congestion.
• Tell parent not to give 0.1% solution to children younger than age 12 unless directed by a doctor.

Combination products

Brand name and active ingredients	Indications and dosages	Nursing considerations
Actifed Cold & Sinus • pseudoephedrine hydrochloride 30 mg • acetaminophen 500 mg • triprolidine 1.25 mg	*Nasal congestion from common cold or sinusitis; aches, pains, headache, and fever with a cold; rhinorrhea, sneezing, itchy nose and throat, and itchy, watery eyes from allergies* **Adults and children ages 12 and older:** 2 caplets P.O. q 6 hr.	• Tell patient not to exceed recommended dosage. • Warn patient to discontinue use and notify the doctor if he becomes nervous, dizzy, or sleepless. • Avoid use in patient with heart disease, hypertension, thyroid disease, diabetes, or difficulty urinating because of enlarged prostate, unless directed by the doctor. • Drug shouldn't be taken for longer than 10 days. • Patient should notify the doctor if condition doesn't improve, or if sore throat is severe, lasts longer than 2 days, or is accompanied by fever lasting longer than 3 days, headache, rash, nausea, or vomiting. • Patient who consumes more than 3 alcoholic drinks per day should consult the doctor before taking this product. • Drug shouldn't be taken within 2 weeks of an MAO inhibitor.
Advil Cold & Sinus, Advil Flu, & Body Ache • pseudoephedrine hydrochloride 30 mg • ibuprofen 200 mg	*Nasal congestion, fever, headache, body aches, and pain from common colds, sinusitis, or flu* **Adults and children ages 12 and older:** 1 tablet P.O. q 4 to 6 hr. Can increase to 2 tablets if	• Drug shouldn't be taken by patient who's allergic to aspirin. • Patient who consumes more than 3 alcoholic drinks per day should contact the doctor before taking this product. • Drug shouldn't be taken for longer than 10 days for pain or longer than 3 days for fever. • Instruct patient to notify the doctor if pain or fever persists or worsens, if new symptoms

Combination products *(continued)*

Brand name and active ingredients	Indications and dosages	Nursing considerations
Advil Cold & Sinus, Advil Flu, & Body Ache *(continued)*	needed. Maximum dose is 6 tablets in 24 hr.	occur, or if painful area becomes red or swollen. • Warn patient not to take with products containing aspirin or acetaminophen. • Patient who is under care for a serious medical condition should contact the doctor before taking this product. • Drug shouldn't be used during the third trimester of pregnancy, unless directed.
Aleve Cold & Sinus • naproxen sodium 220 mg • pseudoephedrine 120 mg	*Sinus pressure, minor aches and pains, headache, congestion, fever* **Adults and children ages 12 and older:** 1 caplet P.O. q 12 hr. Maximum 2 doses in 24 hr.	• Instruct patient to swallow caplet whole; don't crush or chew. • Advise patient that naproxen may cause severe allergic reaction, including hives, facial swelling, asthma, and shock. • Advise patient who is allergic to other pain relievers or fever reducers to avoid this drug. • Warn patient to discontinue use and notify the doctor if he becomes nervous, dizzy, or sleepless. • Instruct patient to notify the doctor if congestion lasts longer than 1 week, if symptoms worsen, if he has difficulty swallowing, or if new or unexplained symptoms or stomach pain occurs. • Patient who is taking other pain relievers, is receiving care for a serious medical condition, or is taking other medications should avoid this drug, unless directed by the doctor.

(continued)

Combination products (continued)

Brand name and active ingredients	Indications and dosages	Nursing considerations
Aleve Cold & Sinus (continued)		• Instruct patient in the third trimester of pregnancy to avoid taking this drug. • Patient who consumes more than 3 alcoholic drinks per day should consult the doctor before taking this product. • Drug shouldn't be taken within 2 weeks of an MAO inhibitor.
Anbesol Cold Sore Therapy • allantoin 1% • benzocaine 20% • white petrolatum 64.9%	*Relief from pain associated with cold sores and fever blisters* **Adults and children ages 2 and older:** apply to affected area t.i.d. to q.i.d.	• Warn patient that product must not be swallowed. • Mild burning or stinging may occur. Applying ice may eliminate or decrease burning or stinging sensation. • Instruct patient to contact doctor if pain lasts longer than 48 hours; if irritation, pain, or redness persists or worsens; or if swelling, rash, or fever occurs. • Drug shouldn't be used longer than 1 week. • Tell patient not to let product get in his eyes.
Clear Eyes ACR • naphazoline hydrochloride 0.012% • zinc sulfate 0.25%	*Relief from redness from minor irritation; protection against further irritation* **Adults:** 1 to 2 drops in affected eye, up to q.i.d.	• Overuse may cause increased redness. • Instruct patient to discard solution if discolored or cloudy • Instruct patient to report eye pain, vision changes, or continued redness or irritation to the doctor. • Advise patient with glaucoma not to use this drug. • Instruct patient to avoid contamination. Tell him not to touch tip of dropper to eye or surrounding tissue.

Combination products *(continued)*

Brand name and active ingredients	Indications and dosages	Nursing considerations
Dristan Sinus • pseudoephedrine hydrochloride 30 mg • ibuprofen 200 mg	*Nasal congestion, fever, headache, body aches and pains from common colds, sinusitis, or flu* **Adults and children ages 12 and older:** 1 tablet P.O. q 4 to 6 hr. Can increase to 2 tablets if needed. Maximum dose is 6 tablets in 24 hr.	• Tell patient not to exceed recommended dosage. • Warn patient to discontinue use and notify the doctor if he becomes nervous, dizzy, or sleepless. • If heartburn, upset stomach, or stomach pain occur, patient should take drug with food or milk. • Drug shouldn't be taken by patient who's allergic to aspirin. • Drug shouldn't be taken for cold symptoms lasting longer than 1 week or fever lasting longer than 3 days. • Instruct patient to notify the doctor if symptoms are persistent or worsening, or if new symptoms appear. • Patient who is taking prescription drugs or is under care for a serious medical condition should consult the doctor before taking drug. • Drug shouldn't be taken by patient who has heart disease, hypertension, thyroid disease, diabetes, or difficulty urinating because of enlarged prostate, unless directed by the doctor. • Drug shouldn't be taken with other OTC pain relievers. • Drug shouldn't be used during the third trimester of pregnancy. • Drug shouldn't be taken within 2 weeks of an MAO inhibitor.

(continued)

Combination products *(continued)*

Brand name and active ingredients	Indications and dosages	Nursing considerations
Drixoral Allergy-Sinus • dexbromphen-iramine maleate 3 mg • pseudoephedrine sulfate 60 mg	*Rhinorrhea, sneezing, itchy nose and throat, itchy watery eyes from allergies; headache, aches, pains, and nasal congestion from sinusitis, colds, and allergies* **Adults and children ages 12 and older:** 2 tablets P.O. q 12 hr. Maximum 4 tablets in 24 hr.	• Tell patient not to exceed recommended dosage. • Warn patient to discontinue use and notify the doctor if he becomes nervous, dizzy, or sleepless. • Instruct patient to notify the doctor if symptoms are accompanied by a fever or not improved in 1 week, symptoms worsen, new symptoms occur, or painful area becomes red or swollen. • Drug shouldn't be taken by patient with heart disease, hypertension, thyroid disease, diabetes, or difficulty urinating because of enlarged prostate, unless directed by the doctor. • Warn parents that drug may make children excitable. • Tell patient that drug may cause drowsiness. • Instruct patient to avoid use with alcohol, sedatives, and tranquilizers, because they may increase drowsiness. • Instruct patient to use caution when driving or operating heavy machinery. • Patient who consumes more than 3 alcoholic drinks per day should consult the doctor before taking this product. • Drug shouldn't be taken within 2 weeks of an MAO inhibitor.

Combination products *(continued)*

Brand name and active ingredients	Indications and dosages	Nursing considerations
Motrin Cold & Flu **Motrin Sinus Headache** • ibuprofen 200 mg • pseudoephedrine hydrochloride 30 mg	*Congestion, headache, body aches and pains, fever from sinusitis, colds, and flu* **Adults and children ages 12 and older:** 1 caplet P.O. q 4 to 6 hr. May take 2 caplets if needed. Maximum 6 caplets in 24 hr.	• Tell patient not to exceed recommended dosage. • Warn patient to discontinue use and notify the doctor if he becomes nervous, dizzy, or sleepless. • Drug shouldn't be taken by patient with heart disease, hypertension, thyroid disease, diabetes, or difficulty urinating because of enlarged prostate, unless directed by the doctor. • If heartburn, upset stomach, or stomach pain occurs, patient should take drug with food or milk and notify the doctor if symptoms worsen or persist. • Instruct patient to notify the doctor if condition doesn't improve, if symptoms are accompanied by fever lasting longer than 3 days, or if new symptoms occur. • Patient should consult the doctor before taking this drug if under care for a serious medical condition or if taking prescription drugs. • Patient who consumes more than 3 alcoholic drinks per day should consult the doctor before taking this product. • Warn patient not to take this drug with other products containing ibuprofen. • Drug shouldn't be used by patient in third trimester of pregnancy. • Drug shouldn't be taken within 2 weeks of an MAO inhibitor.

(continued)

Combination products *(continued)*

Brand name and active ingredients	Indications and dosages	Nursing considerations
Naphcon-A • naphazoline hydrochloride 0.025% • pheniramine maleate 0.3%	*Relief from redness and itching from ragweed, pollen, grass, animal hair, and dander* **Adults:** 1 to 2 drops in affected eye, up to q.i.d.	• Overuse may cause increased redness. • Instruct patient to report eye pain, vision changes, or continued redness or irritation to the doctor. • Drug shouldn't be used by patient with heart disease, hypertension, or glaucoma. • Instruct patient to remove contact lenses before using product. • Instruct patient to discard solution if cloudy or discolored. • Instruct patient to avoid contamination of product. Tell him not to touch tip of dropper to eye or surrounding tissue.
Opcon-A • naphazoline hydrochloride 0.027% • pheniramine maleate 0.315%	*Relief from redness and itching from pollen, ragweed, grass, animal hair, and dander* **Adults:** 1 to 2 drops in affected eye up to q.i.d.	• Overuse may cause increased redness. • Instruct patient to report eye pain, vision changes, or continued redness or irritation to the doctor. • Drug shouldn't be used by patient with heart disease, hypertension, or glaucoma. • Instruct patient to discard solution if cloudy or discolored. • Instruct patient to avoid contamination of product. Tell him not to touch tip of dropper to eye or surrounding tissue.
Sine-Aid • acetaminophen 500 mg • pseudoephedrine 30 mg	*Sinus headache, congestion* **Adults and children ages 12 and older:**	• Tell patient not to exceed recommended dosage. • Warn patient to discontinue use and notify the doctor if he becomes nervous, dizzy, or sleepless.

Combination products (continued)

Brand name and active ingredients	Indications and dosages	Nursing considerations
Sine-Aid *(continued)*	2 caplets P.O. q 4 to 6 hr. Maximum 8 caplets in 24 hr.	• Patient with heart disease, diabetes, or difficulty urinating because of enlarged prostate shouldn't take this drug unless directed by the doctor. • Tell patient not to take this drug for pain lasting longer than 1 week or fever lasting longer than 3 days, unless directed by the doctor. • Instruct patient to notify the doctor if pain or fever persists or worsens, if new symptoms occur, or if painful area becomes red and swollen. • Patient who consumes more than 3 alcoholic drinks per day should consult the doctor before taking this product. • Drug shouldn't be taken within 2 weeks of an MAO inhibitor.
Sinutab Sinus Non-Drowsy, Sudafed Sinus Relief • acetaminophen 500 mg • pseudoephedrine 30 mg	*Minor aches and pains, headache, and congestion from sinusitis* **Adults and children ages 12 and older:** 2 caplets q 6 hr. Maximum 8 caplets in 24 hr.	• Tell patient not to exceed recommended dosage. • Warn patient to discontinue use and notify the doctor if he becomes nervous, dizzy, or sleepless. • Drug shouldn't be taken by patient with heart disease, hypertension, thyroid disease, diabetes, or difficulty urinating because of enlarged prostate, unless directed by the doctor. • Tell patient not to take drug for longer than 10 days. • Advise patient to notify the doctor if symptoms are unimproved or accompanied by a

(continued)

Combination products *(continued)*

Brand name and active ingredients	Indications and dosages	Nursing considerations
Sinutab Sinus Non-Drowsy, Sudafed Sinus Relief *(continued)*		fever lasting longer than 3 days, or if new symptoms occur. • Patient who consumes more than 3 alcoholic drinks per day should consult the doctor before taking this product. • Drug shouldn't be used within 2 weeks of an MAO inhibitor.
Sudafed Cold & Sinus • acetaminophen 325 mg • pseudoephedrine 30 mg	*Congestion, aches, pains, headache, muscle aches, sore throat, and fever from common cold; congestion from sinusitis* **Adults and children ages 12 and older:** 2 liquicaps q 4 to 6 hr. Maximum 8 caplets in 24 hr.	• Tell patient not to exceed recommended dosage. • Warn patient to discontinue use and notify the doctor if he becomes nervous, dizzy, or sleepless. • Drug shouldn't be taken by patient with heart disease, hypertension, thyroid disease, diabetes, or difficulty urinating because of enlarged prostate, unless directed by the doctor. • Drug shouldn't be taken longer than 10 days. • Instruct patient to notify the doctor if condition doesn't improve, if symptoms are accompanied by a fever lasting longer than 3 days, if new symptoms occur, or if sore throat is severe, lasts longer than 2 days, or is accompanied by fever, headache, rash, nausea, and vomiting. • Patient who consumes more than 3 alcoholic drinks per day should consult the doctor before taking this product. • Drug shouldn't be used within 2 weeks of an MAO inhibitor.

Combination products *(continued)*

Brand name and active ingredients	Indications and dosages	Nursing considerations
Sudafed Non-Drowsy Non-Drying Sinus Liquid • guaifenesin 200 mg • pseudoephedrine 30 mg	*Congestion from sinusitis; loosening of phlegm and thinning of bronchial secretions* **Adults and children ages 12 and older:** 2 liquicaplets P.O. q 4 hr. Maximum 8 caplets in 24 hr.	• Tell patient not to exceed recommended dosage. • Warn patient to discontinue use and notify the doctor if he becomes nervous, dizzy, or sleepless. • Tell patient to notify the doctor if symptoms are accompanied by a fever or aren't improved in 1 week. • Patient with heart disease, hypertension, thyroid disease, diabetes, or difficulty urinating because of enlarged prostate shouldn't take this drug, unless directed by the doctor. • Instruct patient to notify the doctor if cough lasts longer than 1 week or is accompanied by fever, rash, or persistent headache. • Drug shouldn't be taken for persistent or chronic cough associated with smoking, asthma, chronic bronchitis, or emphysema, or for cough accompanied by excessive mucus. • Drug shouldn't be taken within 2 weeks of an MAO inhibitor.
Vasocon-A • naphazoline hydrochloride 0.05% • antazoline phosphate 0.5%	*Relief from redness and itching from pollen and animal hair* **Adults:** 1 to 2 drops in affected eye up to q.i.d.	• Overuse may cause increased redness. • Transient burning and stinging may occur. • Instruct patient to remove contact lenses before using product. • Instruct patient to report eye pain, vision changes, or continued redness or irritation to the doctor. • Drug shouldn't be used by patient with heart disease, hypertension, or glaucoma.

(continued)

Combination products (continued)

Brand name and active ingredients	Indications and dosages	Nursing considerations
Vasocon-A *(continued)*		• Instruct patient to discard solution if cloudy or discolored. • Instruct patient to avoid contamination of product. Tell him not to touch tip of dropper to eye or surrounding tissue.
Visine A. C. • tetrahydrozoline 0.05% • zinc sulfate 0.25% **Visine Advanced Relief** • dextran 70 0.1% • polyethylene glycol 400 1% • povidone 1% • tetrahydrozoline hydrochloride 0.05%	*Relief from redness and pain from minor eye irritation* **Adults and children ages 6 and older:** 1 to 2 drops in affected eye up to q.i.d.	• Warn patient to discontinue use and notify the doctor if eye pain, vision change, or continued redness, irritation, or worsening symptoms occurs, or if condition doesn't improve in 3 days. • Instruct patient to remove contact lenses before use. • Overuse may cause increased redness. • Patient with glaucoma shouldn't use this drug, unless directed by the doctor. • Instruct patient to discard a cloudy or discolored solution. • Visine A. C. may cause a brief, tingling sensation when instilled. • Instruct patient to avoid contamination of product. Tell him not to touch tip of dropper to eye or surrounding tissue.
Visine-A • naphazoline hydrochloride 0.025% • pheniramine maleate 0.3%	*Relief from redness and itching of eyes* **Adults:** 1 to 2 drops in affected eye up to q.i.d.	• Instruct patient to report eye pain, vision changes, or continued redness or irritation to the doctor. • Transient tingling may occur. • Instruct patient to discard solution if cloudy or discolored. • Instruct patient to avoid contamination of product. Tell him not to touch tip of dropper to eye or surrounding tissue.

5

Gastrointestinal system

The main function of the gastrointestinal (GI), or digestive, system, is to convert ingested nutrients and fluids into forms the body can use. This conversion is accomplished by ingestion, digestion, absorption, and elimination. The GI system consists of the GI tract, which includes the mouth, esophagus, stomach, and small and large intestines, ending with the anus. The associated structures are the teeth, tongue, salivary glands, liver, pancreas, and gallbladder.

After food is ingested, it comes in contact with several secretions, which help break down the food. The ingested materials are propelled through the digestive tract by involuntary muscle contractions known as peristalsis.

The central nervous system (CNS) or the cardiac system may affect GI function. The parasympathetic and sympathetic branches of the CNS innervate the GI system. The GI tract receives 20% to 30% of the total cardiac output, and this increases significantly after a meal. Therefore, if the CNS or cardiac system is altered in any way, the digestive system can be affected in turn.

Regular GI function is needed to maintain a healthy body. A patient can experience changes in digestion at any age and from various causes. These changes may result from illness, diagnostic testing, or surgical intervention. Many GI problems begin with diarrhea, constipation, or heartburn. Often, rather than seeking medical attention for such conditions, a patient treats himself using alternative methods, such as OTC drugs. You should be prepared to answer questions appropriately and offer education as necessary regarding OTC treatment of these GI problems.

Diarrhea

Diarrhea, the frequent passage of loose, unformed stools, usually with an increase in volume, is not a disease but rather a symptom of an underlying disorder. Digestion, absorption, and secretion of the GI tract are all affected by diarrhea. Causes of diarrhea may include increased osmotic pressure in the intestines, which draws water into the stool; excessive secretion of water and electrolytes into the bowel; or increased motility of the bowel, which leads to rapid emptying without water absorption.

Diarrhea stools contain increased water and increased mucus, which contributes to the usual increase in volume of stools.

Acute diarrhea, which is self-limited, is most often caused by an infection of the intestine. Symptoms remain until the toxin is excreted. Chronic diarrhea lasts for at least 2 weeks and can be life threatening.

Signs and symptoms

The signs and symptoms of diarrhea vary depending on the cause, severity, and general overall health of the patient. Abdominal cramping, nausea (with or without vomiting), anal soreness, generalized weakness, intestinal rumbling (borborygmus), and anorexia commonly accompany diarrhea. You may also assess hyperactive bowel sounds, abdominal distention, anal excoriation, and fluid deficit signs (poor skin turgor, dry mouth, muscle weakness, altered electrolytes). Often a patient with diarrhea will be homebound because of the uncertainty of this condition and the need to stay close to a bathroom.

Serious conditions

A patient with diarrhea loses body fluid, causing a loss of essential electrolytes. If left untreated, this loss can lead to altered fluid and electrolyte balance. This balance is necessary for the human body to maintain homeostasis.

Fluid volume deficit can occur rapidly without the patient realizing its severity. A severe loss of fluids can lead to vascular collapse and hypovolemic shock. Often a patient will treat his diarrhea by drinking water to replace the fluids lost in the stool, but this doesn't replace the lost essential nutrients, which provide the necessary electrolytes. The most serious electrolytes lost with diarrhea are sodium and potassium. Both are critical for nerve transmission, and potassium also functions to maintain cardiac rhythm.

Complications

If a patient tries to treat himself at home with minimal fluid intake, malabsorption and malnutrition (with weight loss) may occur. The patient may also be taking an OTC antidiarrheal. These drugs may slow down or even stop the diarrhea temporarily, but they don't treat the underlying cause or prevent fluid and electrolyte imbalances. The guidelines for some of these drugs recommend not using them for longer than 2 days. If these drugs haven't resolved the problem in 2 days, the patient should consult his doctor to rule out a more serious condition.

Nursing considerations
• Explore the patient's history by asking specific questions about the change in bowel functioning.
• Monitor all output and its characteristics.
• Accurately assess the abdomen.
• Watch for signs and symptoms of fluid and electrolyte deficits.
• Monitor the use of OTC drugs.
• Help the patient to gradually replenish fluids and introduce soft foods.
• Monitor the patient for any weight loss.

Patient teaching
• Teach the patient the necessary information for all antidiarrheals.
• Educate the patient regarding the serious complications that

can occur if diarrhea isn't treated properly and quickly.
• Review with the patient dietary considerations to prevent fluid and electrolyte deficits.
• Teach the patient the importance of good handwashing after each bowel movement.
• Review with the patient steps to prevent or manage diarrhea in the future: drink 8 glasses of water a day, limit fatty foods, increase intake of fiber, avoid alcohol, limit caffeine.
• Encourage the patient to identify any causative agents that may be contributing to episodes of diarrhea. Sometimes it's helpful to keep a daily diet diary to discover any unidentified irritants.
• Instruct the patient to follow all manufacturer and doctor guidelines for taking OTC drugs.

Constipation
Constipation is defined as difficulty in defecation or the infrequent or incomplete passage of firm stools. Because bowel patterns vary from person to person, individual normal bowel habits must be explored so that a bowel elimination problem is not misinterpreted. Usually, a diagnosis of constipation is considered when a patient has fewer than three bowel movements per week, but any varia-

tion from usual bowel habits may be viewed as a problem. Constipation isn't a disease itself but rather a symptom of an underlying disorder.

If feces aren't expelled soon after the patient feels the urge to defecate, then water is further absorbed into the large intestine, thus creating dry, hard stools. Either slow transit through the GI tract or difficulty with expulsion could lead to firm stools. Organic reasons for constipation occur with diseases of the GI tract or the nervous system, whereas functional constipation occurs with failure to respond to the urge to defecate or personal habits. Constipation can also result from weakened abdominal muscles or drug side effects.

Signs and symptoms
The signs and symptoms of constipation are dry, hard stools that are infrequent or difficult to pass, accompanied by fullness in the rectum, abdominal distention, back pain, headache, anorexia, malaise, and sensation of incomplete rectal emptying. The severity of these will depend on the length of time between bowel movements.

Serious conditions
Constipation is often accompanied by straining (Valsalva maneuver), which can lead to vagal stimulation. This stimulation may result in reflex changes in blood pressure and heart rate. This could be detrimental to individuals with cardiac disorders. Intestinal perforation rarely occurs from an obstruction originating from constipation.

Complications
Prolonged retention of stool can result in fecal impaction, thereby making independent passage of stool nearly impossible. Impaction may also result from dependence on laxatives, which patients frequently use to treat constipation. Over time, an impaction may cause ulcerations in the colon from the pressure of the stool mass on the mucosa. Hemorrhoids can occur from perianal vascular congestion that accompanies straining. Passage of hard stool can cause anal fissures or tears.

If left untreated, constipation can cause any or all of these complications. The length of time for these to occur varies with each person. Patients who treat themselves with OTC drugs may become dependent on laxatives; or, the OTC laxative they're using may become ineffective.

Nursing considerations

• Ask the patient when the constipation started and how long it has lasted.
• Explore the patient's lifestyle, and note any changes.
• Monitor the use of any drugs or self-treatments for relief of constipation.
• Explore food and fluid intake.
• Monitor all stool output.
• Ask about the patient's medication history.

Patient teaching

• Educate the patient on the side effects and potential long-term effects of laxatives and enemas.
• Teach the patient how to establish a bowel routine by having a regular time for defecation.
• Provide and review with the patient dietary information helpful for the prevention and treatment of constipation (high-fiber, bran, increased fluids).
• Teach the patient the importance of daily exercise to stimulate bowel movement.
• Emphasize the importance to act in a timely manner at the urge to defecate.

Heartburn

Heartburn is a burning sensation in the lower esophagus over the sternum or the mid-epigastric area. It's also called gastroesophageal reflux, dyspepsia, or pyrosis. Heartburn is a symptom of a disease and one of the most frequent complaints of patients, especially the elderly. Abnormal functioning or incompetency of the lower esophageal sphincter (LES) leads to heartburn. Often the patient has transient episodes of ineffective relaxation of the LES, leading to reduced LES pressure. This weakened relaxation can occur spontaneously or be induced by smoking, alcohol, overeating, pregnancy, chocolate, peppermint, or certain drugs. The incompetent sphincter allows gastric contents to ascend into the esophagus, which causes the burning sensation.

Local esophageal or gastric irritants can also cause heartburn. The causative irritant can lead to an inflammatory process on the surface mucosa, depending on the nature of the causative agent and the amount and duration of exposure to it. This burning sensation can also be from a hyperacidic condition in the stomach.

Heartburn, the primary symptom of gastroesophageal

reflux disease (GERD) and hiatal hernia, often accompanies peptic ulcer disease (PUD). Self-treatment is common with heartburn because of the vast number of OTC drugs available for this purpose.

Signs and symptoms

The burning sensation or irritation of heartburn can occur in the esophagus and upper epigastric regions and can radiate between the two areas. Heartburn can be accompanied by reflux of gastric secretions (backward flow) into the esophagus. Along with reflux, the patient may complain of bad breath (halitosis) and belching.

Serious conditions

If heartburn is accompanied by reflux, esophageal tissue damage may occur, which could impair swallowing and lead to aspiration. Further tissue damage can lead to Barrett's metaplasia (Barrett's esophagus). In this disease, chronic tissue injury induces transformation of the cells, which is considered a premalignant condition.

Recurring heartburn can be a symptom of PUD. Once the tissue erosion has started, continual exposure to gastric acids will cause further ulceration

and can even lead to perforation or hemorrhage.

Complications

Heartburn is easily treated with OTC drugs, specifically antacids, H_2 blockers, and low-dose antiulcer drugs. But if the heartburn persists and the patient continues to treat it with OTC drugs, complications may result from the treatment. Many antacid preparations interfere with drug absorption and can cause a change in bowel habits. Thus, a patient may experience malabsorption, dehydration, or fecal impaction from the use of OTC drugs to treat his heartburn. Because many antacid products contain electrolytes, they can lead to fluid and electrolyte imbalances, especially in elderly patients. Most importantly, many people mistake the pain of angina for heartburn; continued self-treatment for the incorrect problem could, in this case, be life threatening.

Nursing considerations

• Investigate the frequency and timing of heartburn episodes.
• Explore the treatment the patient uses to relieve heartburn, and its effectiveness.
• Watch for symptoms of fluid and electrolyte imbalance.

- Accurately assess the patient's abdomen.
- Monitor the patient's use of OTC drugs.
- Monitor the patient for any weight changes.
- Explore the patient's lifestyle, including any current stressors.

Patient teaching
- Teach the patient why heartburn may occur.
- Teach the patient the proper timing and dosing for the administration of antacids.
- Inform the patient of the serious complications that may occur without treatment.
- Teach the patient dietary changes that may reduce the occurrence of heartburn.
- Review with the patient any lifestyle changes that may help reduce the occurrence of heartburn.
- Advise the patient to seek medical evaluation if the problem is ongoing.

The GI system plays a vital role in the nutritional status of patients. Diarrhea, constipation, and heartburn can indicate serious GI disorders. Often a patient attempts to self-treat because of OTC treatment availability, busy lifestyles, financial concerns of medical treatment, and fear of the unknown. It's imperative for health care professionals to be knowledgeable about these issues, as well as the wide range of treatment options available today.

activated charcoal
alpha-D-galactosidase
  enzyme
aluminum carbonate
aluminum hydroxide
attapulgite
benzocaine
bisacodyl
bismuth subsalicylate
calcium carbonate
calcium polycarbophil
cascara sagrada
castor oil
cimetidine
cyclizine hydrochloride
dimenhydrinate
docusate calcium
docusate sodium
famotidine
glycerin
ipecac syrup
kaolin and pectin
lactase enzyme
loperamide
magaldrate
magnesium citrate
magnesium hydroxide
magnesium oxide
magnesium sulfate
malt soup extract
meclizine hydrochloride
methylcellulose
mineral oil
nizatidine
pancreatin
phosphorated
  carbohydrate solution
psyllium
pyrantel pamoate
ranitidine hydrochloride

senna
simethicone
sodium citrate
sodium phosphates
witch hazel

---

activated charcoal
Actidose, Actidose-Aqua,
Charcoaid, Charcoaid 2000,
Charcoal Plus DS,
CharcoCaps, Insta-Char
Adult, Insta-Char Pediatric,
Liqui-Char

Pregnancy Risk Category C

HOW SUPPLIED
Tablets: 250 mg/L
Tablets (delayed-release):
200 mg
Capsules: 260 mg
Powder: 15 g, 30 g, 40 g, 50 g,
120 g, 240 g
Oral suspension: 15 g, 25 g,
30 g, 50 g

ACTION
An adsorbent that adheres to
many drugs and chemicals, inhibiting their absorption from
the GI tract. Antiflatulent effects occur through absorptive
properties, reducing intestinal
volume.

Route	Onset	Peak	Duration
P.O.	Immediate	Unknown	Unknown

INDICATIONS & DOSAGES

Flatulence, dyspepsia—
Adults: 0.6 g to 5 g P.O. as single dose or 0.975 g to 3.9 g P.O. t.i.d. after meals.

Poisoning—
Adults and children: initially, 1 to 2 g/kg (30 to 100 g) P.O. or 10 times the amount of poison ingested as a suspension in 120 to 240 ml (4 to 8 oz) of water.

ADVERSE REACTIONS

GI: black stools, nausea, constipation, intestinal obstruction.

INTERACTIONS

Drug-drug
Acetylcysteine, ipecac: inactivates drugs. Charcoal should be given after vomiting has been induced by ipecac; remove charcoal by nasogastric (NG) tube before giving acetylcysteine.
Acetaminophen, barbiturates, carbamazepine, digitoxin, digoxin, furosemide, glutethimide, hydantoins, methotrexate, nizatidine, phenothiazines, phenylbutazone, propoxyphene, salicylates, sulfonamides, sulfonylureas, tetracyclines, theophyllines, tricyclic antidepressants, valproic acid: may reduce absorption of these drugs. Charcoal should be given at least 2 hours before or 1 hour after other drugs.

Drug-food
Milk products: decreases effectiveness of activated charcoal. Advise patient to avoid using together.

CONTRAINDICATIONS

None known.

OVERDOSE & TREATMENT

No information available.

NURSING CONSIDERATIONS

• Drug is commonly used for treating poisoning or overdose with acetaminophen, aspirin, atropine, barbiturates, dextropropoxyphene, digoxin, poisonous mushrooms, oxalic acid, phenol, phenytoin, propantheline, propoxyphene, strychnine, or tricyclic antidepressants.
• *Alert:* Drug is ineffective for poisoning or overdose of cyanide, mineral acids, caustic alkalis, and organic solvents; not very effective with ethanol, lithium, methanol, and iron salts.
• Check with poison control center for use in other types of poisonings or overdoses.
• Give after emesis is complete because activated charcoal absorbs and inactivates ipecac syrup.
• Mix powder (most effective form) with tap water to consistency of thick syrup. Adding a small amount of fruit juice or

---

flavoring will make mix more palatable. Don't mix with ice cream, milk, or sherbet because these will decrease absorptive capacity of activated charcoal.

• Give by large-bore NG tube after lavage, if needed.

• If patient vomits shortly after administration, be prepared to repeat dose.

• Space doses at least 1 hour apart from other drugs if treatment is for indications other than poisoning.

• Follow treatment with stool softener or laxative, as ordered, to prevent constipation unless sorbitol is part of product ingredients.

• Preparations made with sorbitol have a laxative effect that lessens risk of severe constipation or fecal impaction.

• Don't use charcoal with sorbitol in fructose-intolerant patients or children younger than age 1.

PATIENT TEACHING

• Tell patient to call poison control center or emergency department before taking activated charcoal as an antidote.

• Explain use and administration of drug to patient (if awake) and family.

• Warn patient that stools will be black.

• Advise patient not to mix drug with milk products.

alpha-D-galactosidase enzyme
Beano

Pregnancy Risk Category NR

HOW SUPPLIED
Beano: *Liquid:* 150 galactosidase U/5 drops
Tablets: 150 galactosidase U/tablet

ACTION
Alpha-D-galactosidase is derived from *Aspergillus niger* mold and is classified as a food. This enzyme hydrolyzes raffinose, verbascose, and stachyose into the sugars sucrose, fructose, glucose, and galactose, which may be metabolized by colonic bacteria. Alpha-D-galactosidase has no effect on fiber.

Route	Onset	Peak	Duration
P.O.	Immediate	Minutes	Duration of meal

INDICATIONS & DOSAGES
Treatment of flatulence or bloating as a result of eating a variety of grains, cereals, nuts, seeds, or vegetables containing sugars, raffinose, stachyose, or verbascose—
Adults: 3 tablets swallowed, chewed, or crumbled onto food for a normal meal that consists

of three servings of problem foods; or 5 drops added to the first portion of food consumed. This dose should be sufficient for all subsequent portions of the meal. Numbers of tablets or drops may be adjusted up or down, depending on the quantity of food eaten, levels of alpha-linked sugars, gas-producing propensity, and individual tolerance.

ADVERSE REACTIONS
GI: intestinal perforation, cramping, diarrhea.
Skin: rash, pruritus.
Other: *hypersensitivity reactions.*

INTERACTIONS
None reported.

CONTRAINDICATIONS
Because this product produces galactose, patients with galactosemia should avoid it.

OVERDOSE & TREATMENT
No information available.

NURSING CONSIDERATIONS
• Give cautiously to diabetic patient because the enzyme may produce 2 to 6 g of carbohydrates per 100 g of food.
• Advise caution in patient who may be allergic to molds because Beano is derived from molds.

• The safety of alpha-D-galactosidase hasn't been determined.
• This enzyme has been used in food processing for years and is regarded as safe by the FDA; however, the amount contained in Beano is probably much greater than what may be found in processed foods.
• Mix in offending foods only after foods have cooled to less than 130° F (54° C).

PATIENT TEACHING
• Instruct patient who is diabetic or has been told that he has a problem with glucose breakdown to check with his doctor before using Beano.
• Inform patient that Beano should be taken with foods to prevent intestinal gas from forming.
• Instruct patient not to cook with this product.
• Instruct patient who is using Beano drops to add drug only after the food has cooled.
• Instruct patient taking tablet form to either swallow, chew, or crumble tablets onto food.
• Advise patient that he may adjust the number of drops or tablets based on quantity of food eaten or signs and symptoms of gas or bloating.
• Advise patient to have regular checkups with his doctor.

*Liquid contains alcohol.   **May contain tartrazine.   †Canada   ‡Australia   §U.K.

• Instruct patient to report new or worsened signs and symptoms promptly to his doctor.
• Tell patient who is pregnant or planning to become pregnant not to use this drug and to contact her doctor if she becomes pregnant or suspects pregnancy while using this product.

aluminum carbonate
Basaljel

Pregnancy Risk Category NR

HOW SUPPLIED
Tablets or capsules: equivalent to aluminum hydroxide 500 mg
Oral suspension: equivalent to aluminum hydroxide 400 mg/ 5 ml

ACTION
Antacid that reduces total acid load in the GI tract, elevates gastric pH to reduce pepsin activity, strengthens the gastric mucosal barrier, and increases esophageal sphincter tone.

Route	Onset	Peak	Duration
P.O.	20 min	Unknown	20-180 min

INDICATIONS & DOSAGES
Antacid—
Adults: 5 to 10 ml of suspension P.O. q 2 hours, p.r.n.; or 1 to 2 tablets or capsules P.O. q 2 hours, p.r.n. Maximum dose is 24 capsules, tablets, or teaspoonfuls per 24 hours.

Management of hyperphosphatemia (in conjunction with low-phosphate diet)—
Adults: 30 to 40 ml P.O. t.i.d. to q.i.d.; or 2 to 6 tablets or capsules 1 hour after meals and h.s.

ADVERSE REACTIONS
CNS: encephalopathy.
GI: constipation, intestinal obstruction.
Metabolic: hypophosphatemia, increased serum gastrin levels.
Musculoskeletal: osteomalacia.

INTERACTIONS
Drug-drug
Allopurinol, antibiotics (including quinolones, tetracyclines), corticosteroids, diflunisal, digoxin, ethambutol, H_2 antagonists, iron salts, isoniazid, penicillamine, phenothiazines, thyroid hormones, ticlopidine: decreases pharmacologic effect because of possible impaired absorption. Advise patient to separate administration times by 1 to 2 hours.
Enteric-coated drugs: may be released prematurely in stomach. Advise patient to separate doses by at least 1 hour.

CONTRAINDICATIONS
None known.

OVERDOSE & TREATMENT
No information available.

NURSING CONSIDERATIONS
• Use cautiously in patients with chronic renal disease.
• Use cautiously in children younger than age 6.
• When administering through NG tube, make sure tube is placed correctly and is patent; after instilling, flush tube with water to ensure passage to stomach and to clear tube.
• *Alert:* Monitor long-term, high-dose use in patients on restricted sodium intake. Each tablet, capsule, or 5 ml of suspension contains about 3 mg of sodium.
• Record stool amount and consistency. Manage constipation with laxatives or stool softeners, as ordered. Alternate with magnesium-containing antacids (unless patient has renal disease).
• Monitor serum calcium and phosphate levels.
• Watch for signs and symptoms of hypophosphatemia (anorexia, mal-aise, muscle weakness) with prolonged use; can also lead to resorption of calcium and bone demineralization.
• Because drug contains aluminum, it's used in patients with renal failure to help control hyperphosphatemia by binding with phosphate in the GI tract.
• Patients with impaired renal function are at a higher risk of aluminum toxicity to brain, bone, and parathyroid glands.
• Basaljel liquid contains no sugar.
• Aluminum carbonate may interfere with imaging techniques using sodium pertechnetate Tc99m and thus impair evaluation of Meckel's diverticulum.
• The drug may interfere with reticuloendothelial imaging of liver, spleen, or bone marrow using technetium Tc99m sulfur colloid.
• The drug may antagonize pentagastrin's effect during gastric acid secretion tests.

PATIENT TEACHING
• Warn patient not to take aluminum carbonate indiscriminately or to switch antacids without medical advice.
• Tell patient to shake suspension well and to take with small amount of water or fruit juice to facilitate passage.
• Instruct patient to report signs and signs and symptoms of bleeding, tarry stools, or coffee-ground vomitus.
• Instruct pregnant patient to seek medical advice before taking drug.

• Warn elderly patient with decreased GI motility that drug may cause constipation.

---

aluminum hydroxide
AlternaGEL, Alu-Cap§, Aluminum Hydroxide Gel, Aluminum Hydroxide Gel Concentrated, Alu-Tab, Amphojel, Dialume, Nephrox Suspension

Pregnancy Risk Category NR

HOW SUPPLIED
Tablets: 300 mg, 500 mg, 600 mg
Capsules: 400 mg, 500 mg
Oral suspension: 320 mg/5 ml, 450 mg/5 ml, 600 mg/5 ml, 675 mg/5 ml

ACTION
Antacid that reduces total acid load in the GI tract, elevates gastric pH to reduce pepsin activity, strengthens the gastric mucosal barrier, and increases esophageal sphincter tone.

Route	Onset	Peak	Duration
P.O.	Variable	Unknown	20-180 min

INDICATIONS & DOSAGES
Antacid—
Adults: 500 to 1,500 mg P.O. (5 to 30 ml of most suspension products) 1 hour after meals and h.s.; or, 300- or 600-mg tablet (chewed before swallowing) taken with milk or water five to six times daily after meals and h.s.

ADVERSE REACTIONS
CNS: encephalopathy.
GI: constipation, intestinal obstruction.
Metabolic: hypophosphatemia, increased serum gastrin levels.
Musculoskeletal: osteomalacia.

INTERACTIONS
Drug-drug
Allopurinol, antibiotics (including quinolones, tetracyclines), corticosteroids, diflunisal, digoxin, ethambutol, H_2 antagonists, iron salts, isoniazid, penicillamine, phenothiazines, thyroid hormones, ticlopidine: decreases pharmacologic effect because of possible impaired absorption. Advise patient to separate administration times by 1 to 2 hours.
Enteric-coated drugs: may release prematurely in stomach. Advise patient to separate doses by at least 1 hour.

Reactions may be *common*, uncommon, *life-threatening*, or COMMON AND LIFE-THREATENING.

CONTRAINDICATIONS
None known.

OVERDOSE & TREATMENT
No information available.

NURSING CONSIDERATIONS
• Use cautiously in patients with chronic renal disease.
• When administering through NG tube, make sure tube is placed correctly and is patent; after instilling, flush tube with water to ensure passage to stomach and to clear tube.
• *Alert:* Monitor long-term, high-dose use in patient on restricted sodium intake. Each tablet, capsule, or 5 ml of suspension contains 2 to 3 mg of sodium.
• Record amount and consistency of stools. Manage constipation with laxatives or stool softeners, as ordered; alternate with magnesium-containing antacids (if patient doesn't have renal disease).
• Monitor serum phosphate levels.
• Watch for signs and symptoms of hypophosphatemia (anorexia, malaise, and muscle weakness) with prolonged use; can also lead to resorption of calcium and bone demineralization.
• Because drug contains aluminum, it's used in patients with renal failure to help control hyperphosphatemia by binding with phosphate in the GI tract.
• Patient with impaired renal function is at higher risk for aluminum toxicity to brain, bone, and parathyroid glands.
• Aluminum hydroxide therapy may interfere with imaging techniques using sodium pertechnetate Tc99m and thus impair evaluation of Meckel's diverticulum.
• The drug may interfere with reticuloendothelial imaging of liver, spleen, or bone marrow using technetium Tc99m sulfur colloid.
• The drug may antagonize pentagastrin's effect during gastric acid secretion tests.

PATIENT TEACHING
• Instruct patient to shake suspension well and to follow with small amount of milk or water to facilitate passage.
• Advise patient not to take aluminum hydroxide indiscriminately or to switch antacids without medical advice.
• Instruct patient to notify doctor if signs and symptoms of bleeding, tarry stools, or coffeeground vomitus occur.
• Instruct pregnant patient to consult a doctor before taking drug.
• Warn elderly patient with decreased GI motility that this drug may cause constipation.

*Liquid contains alcohol.   **May contain tartrazine.   †Canada   ‡Australia   §U.K.

• This drug should be used with caution in children younger than age 6.

---

attapulgite
Diasorb, Donnagel, Fowler's†, Kaopectate Advanced Formula, Kaopectate Maximum Strength, K-Pek, Parepectolin, Rheaban Maximum Strength

Pregnancy Risk Category NR

HOW SUPPLIED
Tablets: 300 mg, 600 mg, 630 mg , 750 mg
Oral suspension: 600 mg/15 ml, 750 mg/5 ml, 750 mg/15 ml, 900 mg/15 ml
Caplets: 750 mg

ACTION
Hydrated magnesium aluminum silicate that's thought to adsorb large numbers of bacteria and toxins and reduce water loss.

Route	Onset	Peak	Duration
P.O.	Unknown	Unknown	Unknown

INDICATIONS & DOSAGES
Acute, nonspecific diarrhea—
Adults and children older than age 12: 1.2 to 1.5 g (up to 3 g if using Diasorb) P.O. after each loose bowel movement, not to exceed 9 g in 24 hours.
Children ages 6 to 12: 600 mg (suspension) or 750 mg (tablet) P.O. after each loose bowel movement, not to exceed 4.2 g (suspension) or 4.5 g (tablet) in 24 hours.
Children ages 3 to 6: 300 mg P.O. after each loose bowel movement, not to exceed 2.1 g in 24 hours.

ADVERSE REACTIONS
GI: constipation.

INTERACTIONS
Drug-drug
Oral drugs: potential for impaired absorption of oral drugs. Advise patient to take attapulgite not less than 2 hours before or 3 hours after other oral drugs, and monitor for decreased effectiveness.

CONTRAINDICATIONS
Contraindicated in patients with dysentery or suspected bowel obstruction.

OVERDOSE & TREATMENT
Because attapulgite isn't absorbed, an overdose is unlikely to pose a significant health problem.

NURSING CONSIDERATIONS
• Use cautiously in patients with dehydration. Promote adequate

---

fluid intake to compensate for fluid loss from diarrhea.

• Drug shouldn't be used if diarrhea is accompanied by fever or blood or mucus in the stool. If these signs and symptoms occur during treatment, withhold drug and notify doctor.

• This drug should be used in elderly patient only with extreme caution and while under medical supervision.

• For children younger than age 3, this drug should be administered only under medical supervision.

PATIENT TEACHING
• Tell patient to take drug after each loose bowel movement until diarrhea is controlled.

• Instruct patient to consult a doctor if diarrhea isn't controlled within 48 hours, if fever develops, or if blood or mucus are in stool.

• Advise patient also taking prescription drugs to notify doctor before taking this drug.

• Tell patient not to crush or chew tablets, but to swallow them whole.

---

benzocaine
Americaine, Lanacane, Medicone

Pregnancy Risk Category C

HOW SUPPLIED
Cream: 6%, 20%
Ointment: 20%

ACTION
Benzocaine temporarily relieves itching, burning, and pain by reversibly blocking the transmission of nerve impulses.

Route	Onset	Peak	Duration
Topical	Unknown	Unknown	Unknown

INDICATIONS & DOSAGES
Temporary relief from pain and itching associated with episiotomy, pruritus vulvae, hemorrhoids—
Adults and children ages 2 and older: apply 5% to 20% strength to affected areas t.i.d. to q.i.d.

ADVERSE REACTIONS
Skin: rash, irritation.

INTERACTIONS
None reported.

CONTRAINDICATIONS
Avoid drug in patients with known allergy to ester- or PABA-derivative local anesthetics (tetracaine, procaine, or butamben). Don't use benzocaine in patients with congenital or idiopathic methemoglobinemia or in children younger than age 12 who are receiving methemoglobin-inducing drugs.

---

*Liquid contains alcohol.   **May contain tartrazine.   †Canada   ‡Australia   §U.K.

Because of insufficient data, benzocaine should be avoided in pregnant and breast-feeding women.

OVERDOSE & TREATMENT
Systemic absorption of benzocaine may result in CV depression (increased sweating, low blood pressure, pale skin, slow or irregular heartbeat); cardiac arrest; CNS toxicity (blurred or double vision, confusion, convulsions, dizziness, lightheadedness, drowsiness, feeling hot or cold or numb, ringing or buzzing in the ears, unusual anxiety, excitement, nervousness, restlessness); methemoglobinemia (difficulty in breathing on exertion, dizziness, headache, tiredness, weakness).

Treat patient symptomatically. Securing and maintaining a patent airway, administering 100% oxygen, and instituting assisted or controlled respiration may be needed. For circulatory collapse, an I.V. vasopressor or fluid bolus may be administered and a benzodiazepine may be given for convulsions. For methemoglobinemia, methylene blue or ascorbic acid may also be administered.

NURSING CONSIDERATIONS
• *Alert:* Because of insufficient data, the use of benzocaine in breast-feeding women should be avoided. Caution is warranted in pediatric, elderly, or debilitated patients, as well as patients with local infection or traumatized mucosa at area of treatment or bleeding hemorrhoids.
• Avoid drug in patients with known allergy to ester- or PABA-derivative local anesthetics (tetracaine, procaine, or butamben).
• Benzocaine topical creams and ointments should be stored in tight containers and protected from light; prolonged exposure to temperatures higher than 86° F (30° C) should be avoided.

PATIENT TEACHING
• Advise patient that if condition doesn't improve or if redness, irritation, swelling, pain, or other signs and symptoms develop or increase, he should discontinue the product and consult a doctor.
• Instruct patient to notify doctor immediately if bleeding occurs.
• Inform patient that if he has had an allergic reaction to local anesthetic in the past (especially tetracaine or butamben), he should avoid these products.
• Instruct patient to contact doctor if signs and symptoms of hemorrhoids worsen or don't

improve after 7 days of treatment.

• Instruct patient to apply sparingly and only to the external perianal area.

• Instruct patient not to apply benzocaine to children or infants.

• Instruct pregnant or breastfeeding patient not to use benzocaine unless specifically instructed to by doctor.

• Teach patient how to properly administer the rectal ointment or cream:

– Cleanse the area with mild soap and water or use a cleansing wipe.

– Rinse the perianal area thoroughly.

– Dry area gently.

– Apply only a thin film of ointment or cream to the external perianal area.

bisacodyl
Alophen, Bisac-Evac, Bisacodyl Uniserts, Bisacolax†, Bisalax‡, Bisco-Lax**, Carter's Little Pills, Correctol, Dulcagen, Dulcolax, Durolax‡, Feen-A-Mint, Fleet Bisacodyl, Fleet Bisacodyl Prep, Fleet Laxative, Laxit†, Modane

Pregnancy Risk Category NR

HOW SUPPLIED
Tablets (enteric-coated): 5 mg
Enema: 0.33 mg/ml, 10 mg/5 ml (microenema)‡
Powder for rectal solution (bisacodyl tannex): 1.5 mg bisacodyl and 2.5 g tannic acid
Suppositories: 5 mg, 10 mg

ACTION
Unknown. Stimulant laxative that increases peristalsis, probably by direct effect on smooth muscle of the intestine. It's thought to either irritate the musculature or stimulate the colonic intramural plexus. Drug also promotes fluid accumulation in colon and small intestine.

Route	Onset	Peak	Duration
P.O.	6-12 hr	Variable	Variable
P.R.	15-60 min	Variable	Variable

INDICATIONS & DOSAGES
Preparation for delivery, surgery, or rectal or bowel examination—
Adults and children ages 12 and older: up to 30 mg P.O. p.r.n. and as ordered; or 10 mg P.R. for evacuation before examination or surgery; or 1 packet of bisacodyl tannex dissolved in 1 L of lukewarm water P.R. as enema on day of procedure.

Chronic constipation—
Adults and children ages 12 and older: 5 to 15 mg P.O. daily in the evening; or 10 mg P.R. daily as a single dose.
Children younger than age 2: 5 mg P.R. daily as a single dose.
Children ages 2 to 11: 5 to 10 mg P.R. daily as a single dose.
Children older than age 3: 5 to 10 mg P.O. daily as a single dose.

ADVERSE REACTIONS
CNS: muscle weakness with excessive use, dizziness, faintness.
CV: palpitations.
GI: nausea, vomiting, abdominal cramps, diarrhea with high doses, burning sensation in rectum (with suppositories), laxative dependence with long-term or excessive use, excessive bowel activity.
Metabolic: alkalosis, hypokalemia, fluid and electrolyte imbalance, protein-losing enteropathy in excessive use.
Other: tetany.

INTERACTIONS
Drug-drug
Antacids: gastric irritation or dyspepsia from premature dissolution of enteric coating. Advise patient to avoid using together.

Drug-food
Milk: gastric irritation or dyspepsia from premature dissolution of enteric coating. Advise patient to avoid using together.

CONTRAINDICATIONS
Contraindicated in patients who are hypersensitive to drug or its components and in those with rectal bleeding, gastroenteritis, intestinal obstruction, abdominal pain, nausea, vomiting, or other signs and symptoms of appendicitis or acute surgical abdomen. Bisacodyl tannex is contraindicated in children younger than age 10.

OVERDOSE & TREATMENT
Long-term use or overdose may cause hypokalemia, hypocalcemia, metabolic acidosis or alkalosis, abdominal pain, diarrhea, malabsorption, weight loss, and protein-losing enteropathy. Electrolyte disturbances may cause vomiting, muscle weakness, osteomalacia, secondary aldosteronism, and tetany. Pathologic changes of the colon may occur.

Treatment is symptomatic and supportive.

NURSING CONSIDERATIONS
• Use bisacodyl tannex cautiously in patients receiving multiple enemas and in those

---

Reactions may be *common*, uncommon, *life-threatening*, or COMMON AND LIFE-THREATENING.

with extensive ulceration of the colon.

• Time administration of drug so as not to interfere with scheduled activities or sleep. Soft, formed stools are usually produced 15 to 60 minutes after rectal administration.

• Before giving for constipation, determine if patient has adequate fluid intake, exercise, and diet.

• Tablets and suppositories are used together to clean the colon before and after surgery and before barium enema.

• Insert suppository as high as possible into the rectum, and try to position suppository against the rectal wall. Avoid embedding within fecal material because this may delay onset of action.

• *Alert:* Drug may be habit forming. Long-term use may result in laxative dependence.

PATIENT TEACHING

• Advise patient to swallow enteric-coated tablet whole to avoid GI irritation. Advise patient to avoid using within 1 hour of milk or antacid intake.

• Tell patient that drug is for short-term (1 week) treatment only (stimulant laxatives are frequently abused). Discourage excessive use.

• Advise patient not to start using this drug if he is experiencing abdominal pain, nausea, or vomiting.

• Advise patient to report adverse effects, sudden changes in bowel patterns lasting longer than 2 weeks, or no effect with laxative use after 1 week.

• Teach patient about dietary sources of bulk, including bran and other cereals, fresh fruit, and vegetables.

• Tell patient to take drug with a full glass (8 oz) of water or juice.

• Drug shouldn't be administered to children younger than age 6 unless ordered by health care provider.

• Tell pregnant and breast-feeding patient to use this drug only if advised to by doctor.

---

bismuth subsalicylate
Bismatrol, Bismatrol Extra Strength, Pepto-Bismol, Pepto-Bismol Maximum Strength, Pink Bismuth

Pregnancy Risk Category NR

HOW SUPPLIED
Tablets (chewable): 262 mg
Oral suspension: 262 mg/ 15 ml, 524 mg/15 ml

ACTION
Unknown. Has a mild water-binding capacity; may adsorb

---

toxins and provide protective coating for mucosa.

Route	Onset	Peak	Duration
P.O.	1 hr	Unknown	Unknown

INDICATIONS & DOSAGES
Mild, nonspecific diarrhea—
Adults: 30 ml or 2 tablets P.O. q 30 minutes to 1 hour, up to maximum of eight doses and for no longer than 2 days.
Children ages 9 to 12: 15 ml or 1 tablet P.O.
Children ages 6 to 9: 10 ml or ⅔ tablet P.O.
Children ages 3 to 6: 5 ml or ⅓ tablet P.O.

ADVERSE REACTIONS
GI: temporary darkening of tongue and stools.
Other: salicylism with high doses.

INTERACTIONS
Drug-drug
Aspirin, other salicylates: risk of salicylate toxicity. Monitor closely; if ringing in the ears occurs, discontinue drug and notify doctor immediately.
Corticosteroids: may decrease salicylate levels, decreasing effectiveness of bismuth. Avoid using together.
Oral anticoagulants, oral antidiabetics: theoretical risk of increased effects of these drugs after high doses of bismuth

subsalicylate. Monitor patient closely.
Tetracycline: decreases tetracycline absorption. Advise patient to separate administration times by at least 2 hours.

CONTRAINDICATIONS
Contraindicated in patients who are hypersensitive to salicylates.

OVERDOSE & TREATMENT
Overdose hasn't been reported. Probable signs and symptoms of overdose include CNS effects, such as tinnitus, and fever.
   Treatment of overdose is supportive.

NURSING CONSIDERATIONS
●Use cautiously in patient taking aspirin. Discontinue if tinnitus occurs.
●Salicylate absorption may occur from bismuth subsalicylate. Use cautiously in patient with bleeding disorders or salicylate sensitivity and in children.
●Monitor patient for signs and symptoms of bleeding.
●Avoid use before GI radiologic procedures because bismuth is radiopaque and may interfere with X-ray examination of GI tract.
●If drug is being administered by tube, flush tube via NG tube to clear it and ensure passage of drug to stomach.

Reactions may be *common*, uncommon, *life-threatening*, or COMMON AND LIFE-THREATENING.

• Bismuth subsalicylate has used experimentally to treat peptic ulcer disease.

• Drug is useful for indigestion without causing constipation, for nausea, and for relief of flatulence and abdominal cramps.

• Small amounts of drug are excreted in breast milk. Patient should consult her doctor before using this drug.

PATIENT TEACHING

• Advise patient that bismuth subsalicylate contains salicylate (each tablet has 102 mg salicylate; the regular-strength liquid has 130 mg/15 ml, and the extra-strength liquid has 230 mg/15 ml).

• Instruct patient to chew tablets well before swallowing or to shake liquid before measuring dose.

• Tell patient to call doctor if diarrhea persists for longer than 2 days or is accompanied by high fever.

• Tell patient to consult with doctor before giving bismuth subsalicylate to children or teenagers during or after recovery from the flu or chickenpox.

• Inform patient that all forms of Pepto-Bismol are effective against traveler's diarrhea. Tablets and caplets may be more convenient to carry.

• Tell patient that small amounts of drug are excreted in breast milk. Patient should seek approval from her doctor before using this drug.

• Warn patient that bismuth may temporarily darken stools and tongue.

---

calcium carbonate
Alka-Mints, Amitone, Cal-Sup‡, Children's Mylanta, Chooz, Dicarbosil, Maalox Antacid Caplets, Rolaids Calcium Rich, Titralac Extra Strength, Titralac Instant Relief, Tums, Tums E-X, Tums Ultra

Pregnancy Risk Category NR

HOW SUPPLIED
Calcium carbonate contains 40% calcium; 20 mEq calcium/g
Tablets (chewable): 350 mg, 420 mg, 500 mg, 750 mg, 850 mg, 1,000 mg, 1,250 mg‡
Tablets: 500 mg, 600 mg, 650 mg, 1,000 mg, 1,250 mg
Chewing gum: 500 mg/piece
Oral suspension: 1,250 mg/ 5 ml
Lozenges: 600 mg

ACTION
Antacid that reduces total acid load in the GI tract, elevates gastric pH to reduce pepsin activity, strengthens the gastric

---

mucosal barrier, and increases esophageal sphincter tone.

Route	Onset	Peak	Duration
P.O.	20 min	Unknown	20-180 min

INDICATIONS & DOSAGES
Antacid, calcium supplement—
Adults: 350 mg to 2 g P.O. or 2 pieces of chewing gum 1 hour after meals and h.s., p.r.n.
Children ages 6 to 11 years or 22 to 43 kg (48 to 95 lb): 2 tablets or 2 tsp Children's Mylanta P.O. up to t.i.d. Maximum 6 tablets or 6 tsp in 24 hours.
Children ages 2 to 5 years or 11 to 21 kg (24 to 47 lb): 1 tablet or 1 tsp Children's Mylanta P.O. up to t.i.d. Maximum 3 tablets or 3 tsp in 24 hours.

ADVERSE REACTIONS
CNS: headache, irritability, weakness.
CV: *arrhythmias, cardiac arrest.*
GI: rebound hyperacidity, hemorrhage, nausea, vomiting, thirst, abdominal pain, constipation.
GU: polyuria, renal calculi.
Metabolic: altered serum phosphate levels, hypercalcemia.

INTERACTIONS
Drug-drug
Antibiotics (including quinolones, tetracyclines), hydantoins, iron salts, isoniazid, salicylates: decreases pharmacologic effect because of possible impaired absorption. Advise patient to separate administration times.
Enteric-coated drugs: may be released prematurely in stomach. Advise patient to separate doses by at least 1 hour.

Drug-food
Milk, other foods high in vitamin D: possible milk-alkali syndrome (headache, confusion, distaste for food, nausea, vomiting, hypercalcemia, hypercalciuria). Advise patient to avoid using together.

CONTRAINDICATIONS
Contraindicated in patients with ventricular fibrillation or hypercalcemia.

OVERDOSE & TREATMENT
Acute hypercalcemia syndrome is characterized by a markedly elevated plasma calcium level, lethargy, weakness, nausea and vomiting, and coma, and may lead to sudden death.

In case of overdose, calcium should be discontinued immediately. After oral ingestion of calcium overdose, treatment includes removal by emesis or gastric lavage, followed by supportive therapy, as needed.

Reactions may be *common,* uncommon, *life-threatening,* or COMMON AND LIFE-THREATENING.

NURSING CONSIDERATIONS

• Use cautiously, if at all, in patients with sarcoidosis or renal or cardiac disease, and in patients receiving cardiac glycosides.

• Record amount and consistency of stools. Manage constipation with laxatives or stool softeners, as ordered.

• Monitor serum calcium levels, especially in patients with mild renal impairment.

• Watch for signs and symptoms of hypercalcemia (nausea, vomiting, headache, confusion, and anorexia).

• If GI upset occurs, administer drug 2 to 3 hours after meals.

• Maalox products may contain phenylalanine.

PATIENT TEACHING

• Advise patient not to take calcium carbonate indiscriminately or to switch antacids without medical advice.

• Tell patient taking chewable tablets to chew thoroughly before swallowing and follow with an 8-oz glass of water.

• Tell patient using suspension form to shake well and take with a small amount of water to facilitate passage.

• Tell patient not to use maximum dose for longer than 2 weeks.

• Instruct patient to report signs and symptoms of bleeding, tarry stools, or coffee-ground vomitus.

• Warn patient not to use bone meal or dolomite as a source of calcium, as they may contain lead.

• Inform elderly patient that calcium absorption may be decreased.

• Advise patient taking prescription drugs to consult a doctor before taking calcium carbonate.

• Inform the pregnant patient to consult doctor before taking antacids.

• Instruct patient to keep all medication out of reach of children and pets.

---

calcium polycarbophil
Equalactin, Fiberall, FiberCon, Fiber-Lax, Konsyl, Mitrolan

Pregnancy Risk Category NR

HOW SUPPLIED
Tablets: 500 mg, 625 mg
Tablets (chewable): 500 mg, 1,250 mg

ACTION
Bulk-forming laxative that absorbs water and expands to increase bulk and moisture content of stools. The increased bulk encourages peristalsis and bowel movement. As an an-

---

tidiarrheal, drug absorbs free fecal water, thereby producing formed stools.

Route	Onset	Peak	Duration
P.O.	12-24 hr	3 days	Variable

INDICATIONS & DOSAGES
Constipation and diarrhea associated with conditions such as irritable bowel syndrome and diverticulosis; acute nonspecific diarrhea—
Children younger than age 6: use must be directed by doctor.
Children ages 6 to younger than 12: 500 mg P.O. less than or equal to q.i.d., p.r.n. Maximum dose is 2 g in 24-hour period.
Adults and children ages 12 and older: 1 g P.O. once daily to q.i.d., p.r.n. Maximum dose is 4 g in 24-hour period.

ADVERSE REACTIONS
GI: abdominal fullness and increased flatus, intestinal obstruction.
Other: laxative dependence with long-term or excessive use.

INTERACTIONS
Drug-drug
Tetracyclines: impairs absorption of tetracyclines. Advise patient to avoid using together.

CONTRAINDICATIONS
Contraindicated in patients with signs and symptoms of appendicitis, which include dysphagia, abdominal pain, nausea, and vomiting.

OVERDOSE & TREATMENT
Long-term use or overdose may cause persistent diarrhea, hypokalemia, loss of essential nutritional factors, and dehydration. Treatment is symptomatic and supportive.

NURSING CONSIDERATIONS
• Before giving for constipation, determine if patient has adequate fluid intake, exercise, and diet.
• *Alert:* Rectal bleeding or failure to respond to therapy may indicate need for surgery.
• Monitor patient for adverse effects, such as fever, nausea, vomiting, or abdominal pain.
• Instruct patient regarding dosing guidelines.

PATIENT TEACHING
• Advise patient to chew Equalactin or Mitrolan tablets thoroughly before swallowing and to drink a full glass of water with each dose. When drug is used as an antidiarrheal, tell patient not to drink a glass of water.

- Tell patient to take with an 8-oz glass of water to prevent choking.
- Teach patient about dietary sources of bulk, including bran and other cereals, fresh fruit, and vegetables.
- For severe diarrhea, advise patient to repeat dose every 30 minutes, but not to exceed maximum daily dose.
- Tell patient not to use for longer than 2 days for diarrhea or if diarrhea is accompanied by fever.
- Instruct patient to contact doctor if he experiences chest pain, regurgitation, vomiting, or difficulty swallowing or breathing; if signs and symptoms are not relieved in 7 days; if sudden changes in bowel patterns last for longer than 2 weeks; or if rectal bleeding occurs.
- Advise patient to avoid use if vomiting, nausea, or abdominal pain occurs.

---

cascara sagrada

cascara sagrada aromatic fluidextract*

cascara sagrada fluidextract*
Pregnancy Risk Category C

HOW SUPPLIED
Tablets: 325 mg
Aromatic fluidextract: 1 g/ml
Fluidextract: 1 g/ml

ACTION
Unknown. Stimulant laxative that increases peristalsis, probably by direct effect on smooth muscle of the intestine. It's thought to either irritate the musculature or stimulate the colonic intramural plexus. Drug also promotes fluid accumulation in colon and small intestine.

Route	Onset	Peak	Duration
P.O.	6-10 hr	Variable	Variable

INDICATIONS & DOSAGES
Acute constipation, preparation for bowel or rectal examination—
Adults and children ages 12 and older: one 325-mg tablet of cascara sagrada P.O. once daily h.s.; 0.5 to 1.5 ml of cascara sagrada fluidextract P.O. once daily, or 2 to 6 ml of aromatic cascara fluidextract P.O. once daily.
Children ages 2 to 12: ½ adult dosage.
Children younger than age 2: ¼ adult dosage.

ADVERSE REACTIONS
GI: nausea; vomiting; diarrhea; loss of normal bowel function with excessive use; abdominal cramps, especially in severe constipation; malabsorption of

---

nutrients; cathartic colon (syndrome resembling ulcerative colitis radiologically and pathologically) with long-term misuse; discoloration of rectal mucosa after long-term use; protein enteropathy; laxative dependence with long-term or excessive use.

Metabolic: hypokalemia, electrolyte imbalance with excessive use.

INTERACTIONS
None reported.

CONTRAINDICATIONS
Contraindicated in patients with abdominal pain, nausea, vomiting, or other symptoms of appendicitis or acute surgical abdomen; acute surgical delirium; fecal impaction; or intestinal obstruction or perforation.

OVERDOSE & TREATMENT
Long-term use or overdose may cause hypokalemia, hypocalcemia, metabolic acidosis or alkalosis, abdominal pain, diarrhea, malabsorption, weight loss, and protein-losing enteropathy. Electrolyte disturbances may cause vomiting, muscle weakness, osteomalacia, secondary aldosteronism and tetany. Pathologic changes of the colon may occur. Treatment is symptomatic and supportive.

NURSING CONSIDERATIONS
• *Alert:* Use cautiously when patient has rectal bleeding.
• Before giving for constipation, determine if patient has adequate fluid intake, exercise, and diet.
• Monitor serum electrolyte levels during prolonged use.
• Cascara sagrada aromatic fluidextract is less active and less bitter than the nonaromatic fluidextract.
• Liquid preparations are more reliable than solid dosage forms.
• Cascara may be excreted in breast milk, which may result in increased incidence of diarrhea in infant.
• Depending on urine pH, drug may color urine reddish pink (alkaline) or yellowish brown (acidic).
• Drug turns alkaline urine pink to red, red to violet, or red to brown in the phenolsulfonphthalein excretion test.

PATIENT TEACHING
• Warn patient that drug may turn alkaline urine red-pink and acidic urine yellow-brown.
• Tell patient to report sudden changes in bowel patterns that last longer than 2 weeks, or lack of effect of laxative after 1 week.
• Teach patient about dietary sources of bulk, including bran

and other cereals, fresh fruit, and vegetables.
- Tell patient to take drug with an 8-oz glass of water.
- Inform pregnant patient that bulk-forming or surfactant laxatives are preferred during pregnancy. Patient should consult doctor.
- Tell patient that cascara may be excreted in breast milk, which may result in increased incidence of diarrhea in infant.

---

castor oil
Emulsoil, Fleet Flavored Castor Oil, Purge

Pregnancy Risk Category X

HOW SUPPLIED
Capsules: 0.62 ml
Oral liquid: 67% (Fleet), 95% (Emulsoil, Purge)

ACTION
Unknown. Stimulant laxative that increases peristalsis, probably by direct effect on smooth muscle of the intestine. It's thought to either irritate the musculature or stimulate the colonic intramural plexus. Drug also promotes fluid accumulation in colon and small intestine.

Route	Onset	Peak	Duration
P.O.	2-6 hr	Variable	Variable

INDICATIONS & DOSAGES
Preparation for rectal or bowel examination or for surgery—
Adults and children ages 12 and older: 15 to 60 ml P.O.
Children ages 2 to 12: 5 to 15 ml P.O.
Children younger than age 2: 1 to 5 ml P.O. Increased dosage produces no greater effect.
   For all patients, administer as a single dose about 16 hours before surgery or procedure.

ADVERSE REACTIONS
GI: nausea; vomiting; diarrhea; loss of normal bowel function with excessive use; abdominal cramps, especially in severe constipation; malabsorption of nutrients; cathartic colon (syndrome resembling ulcerative colitis radiologically and pathologically) with long-term misuse; protein-losing enteropathy; laxative dependence with long-term or excessive use; constipation after catharsis.
Metabolic: hypokalemia, other electrolyte imbalances with excessive use.

INTERACTIONS
Drug-drug
Intestinally absorbed drugs: may decrease the absorption of these drugs. Avoid using together.

---

*Liquid contains alcohol.   **May contain tartrazine.   †Canada   ‡Australia   §U.K.

Drug-herb
Male fern: may increase absorption and increase risk of toxicity. Advise patient to avoid using together.

CONTRAINDICATIONS
Contraindicated in patients with ulcerative bowel lesions; abdominal pain, nausea, vomiting, or other symptoms of appendicitis or acute surgical abdomen; anal or rectal fissures, fecal impaction, or intestinal obstruction or perforation; also contraindicated during menstruation or pregnancy.

OVERDOSE & TREATMENT
Long-term use or overdosage may cause hypokalemia, hypocalcemia, metabolic acidosis or alkalosis, abdominal pain, diarrhea, malabsorption, weight loss, and protein-losing enteropathy. Electrolyte disturbances may cause vomiting, muscle weakness, osteomalacia, secondary aldosteronism and tetany. Pathologic changes of the colon may occur.
   Treatment is symptomatic and supportive.

NURSING CONSIDERATIONS
• *Alert:* Use cautiously in patient with rectal bleeding.
• To prepare for surgery or procedures, patient should receive a residue-free diet the day before surgery or procedure and a cleansing enema the day of the procedure.
• Give castor oil with juice or carbonated beverage to mask oily taste. Have patient stir mixture and drink it promptly. Ice held in the mouth before taking drug will help prevent tasting it.
• Shake emulsion well before measuring dose. Emulsion is better tolerated but is more expensive. Store below 40° F (4.4° C). Don't freeze.
• Give on empty stomach for best results.
• Time drug administration so that it doesn't interfere with scheduled activities or sleep.
• Increased intestinal motility lessens absorption of oral drugs administered at the same time. Advise patient to separate administration times.
• *Alert:* Failure of patient to respond to drug may indicate acute condition requiring surgery.
• Observe patient for signs and symptoms of dehydration.

PATIENT TEACHING
• Tell patient not to expect another bowel movement for 1 to 2 days after castor oil has emptied bowel.
• Warn patient about potential adverse reactions.
• Tell patient to report sudden changes in bowel patterns that

---

Reactions may be *common*, uncommon, *life-threatening*, or COMMON AND LIFE-THREATENING.

last longer than 2 weeks or if no effect with laxative use after 1 week.
• Instruct patient not to take drug at bedtime.
• Instruct patient to shake emulsion well.
• Warn elderly patient that, with long-term use, he may experience electrolyte depletion resulting in weakness, incoordination, and orthostatic hypotension.
• Instruct breast-feeding patient to consult doctor before taking this drug.

---

cimetidine
Tagamet HB

Pregnancy Risk Category B

HOW SUPPLIED
Tablets: 200 mg

ACTION
Competitively inhibits action of H_2 at receptor sites of the parietal cells, decreasing gastric acid secretion.

Route	Onset	Peak	Duration
P.O.	Unknown	45-90 min	4-5 hr

INDICATIONS & DOSAGES
Heartburn—
Adults and children ages 12 and older: 200 mg P.O. with water as symptoms occur, or as directed, up to b.i.d. Maximum daily dose is 400 mg. Drug shouldn't be taken daily for longer than 2 weeks.

ADVERSE REACTIONS
CNS: confusion, dizziness, headache, peripheral neuropathy, somnolence, hallucinations.
GI: mild and transient diarrhea.
GU: transient elevations in serum creatinine levels, impotence, mild gynecomastia if used longer than 1 month.
Hepatic: increased serum alkaline phosphatase levels.
Musculoskeletal: muscle pain, arthralgia.
Other: *hypersensitivity reactions.*

INTERACTIONS
Drug-drug
Antacids: interference with cimetidine absorption. Advise patient to separate administration by at least 1 hour, if possible.
Lidocaine, phenytoin, propranolol, some benzodiazepines, theophylline, warfarin: inhibits hepatic microsomal enzyme metabolism of these drugs. Monitor serum levels.

Drug-herb
Guarana: may increase caffeine serum levels or prolong serum caffeine half-life. Discourage using together.

Pennyroyal: may change rate of formation of toxic metabolites of pennyroyal. Discourage using together.

Yerba maté: may decrease clearance of yerba maté methylxanthines and cause toxicity. Discourage using together.

Drug-lifestyle
Smoking: may increase gastric acid secretion and worsen disease. Discourage patient from smoking.

CONTRAINDICATIONS
Contraindicated in patients who are hypersensitive to drug.

OVERDOSE & TREATMENT
Clinical effects of overdose include respiratory failure and tachycardia. Overdose is rare; intake of up to 10 g has caused no untoward effects.

Support respiration and maintain a patent airway. Induce emesis or use gastric lavage; follow with activated charcoal to prevent further absorption. Treat tachycardia with propranolol, if necessary.

NURSING CONSIDERATIONS
• Use cautiously in elderly or debilitated patients because they may be more susceptible to cimetidine-induced confusion.

• Assess for abdominal pain. Note blood in emesis, stool, or gastric aspirate.

• Schedule cimetidine dose at end of hemodialysis treatment because hemodialysis reduces blood levels of cimetidine. Adjust dosage, as ordered, for patients with renal failure.

• Drug may antagonize pentagastrin's effect during gastric acid secretion tests.

• Drug may cause false-negative results in skin tests that use allergen extracts.

• FD and C blue dye #2 used in Tagamet tablets may impair interpretation of Hemoccult and Gastroccult tests on gastric content aspirate. Wait at least 15 minutes after tablet administration before drawing sample and follow test manufacturer's instructions closely.

• *Alert:* Don't confuse cimetidine with simethicone.

PATIENT TEACHING
• Instruct patient not to exceed recommended dosage and not to take daily for longer than 14 days.

• Instruct patient to notify doctor if signs and symptoms worsen or persist for 14 or more days.

• Urge patient to avoid cigarette smoking because it may increase gastric acid secretion and worsen disease.

- Advise patient to report abdominal pain, blood in stools, emesis, or difficulty swallowing.
- Inform patient that drug is excreted in breast milk and shouldn't be taken while breast-feeding.
- Warn elderly patient or caregiver of potential CNS effects.
- Tell patient that drug can help to prevent heartburn if taken up to 30 minutes before eating food or drinking beverages that cause heartburn.
- Tell patient with kidney disease to consult a doctor before taking drug.

cyclizine hydrochloride
Marezine

Pregnancy Risk Category B

HOW SUPPLIED
Tablets: 50 mg

ACTION
Cyclizine probably inhibits nausea and vomiting by centrally depressing sensitivity of the labyrinth apparatus that relays stimuli to the chemoreceptor trigger zone and thus stimulates the vomiting center in the brain. Drug depresses conduction in vestibular-cerebellar pathways and reduces labyrinth excitability.

Route	Onset	Peak	Duration
P.O.	30-60 min	Unknown	4-6 hr

INDICATIONS & DOSAGES
Motion sickness (prophylaxis and treatment)—
Adults and children older than age 12: 50 mg P.O. 30 minutes before travel, then q 4 to 6 hours, p.r.n., to maximum of 200 mg daily.
Children ages 6 to 12: 25 mg P.O. every 6 to 8 hours to maximum of 1½ tablets in 24 hours. For prevention, take the first dose 30 minutes before departure.

ADVERSE REACTIONS
CNS: drowsiness, auditory and visual hallucinations, restlessness, excitation, nervousness.
CV: hypotension, palpitations, tachycardia.
EENT: blurred vision, diplopia, tinnitus, dry nose and throat.
GI: constipation, dry mouth, anorexia, nausea, vomiting, diarrhea, cholestatic jaundice.
GU: urine retention, urinary frequency.
Skin: urticaria, rash.

INTERACTIONS
Drug-drug
Other CNS depressants, such as anxiolytics, barbiturates, sleeping agents, or tranquilizers: additive sedative and CNS depressant effects may occur when

---

used together. Monitor patient closely.

Ototoxic drugs, such as amino-glycosides, cisplatin, loop diuretics, salicylates, and vancomycin: may mask signs and symptoms of ototoxicity. Advise patient to avoid using together.

Drug-lifestyle
Alcohol use: additive sedative and CNS depressant effects may occur when cyclizine is used with alcohol. Advise patient to avoid using together.

CONTRAINDICATIONS
Contraindicated in patients hypersensitive to drug.

OVERDOSE & TREATMENT
Signs and symptoms of overdose may include either CNS depression (sedation, reduced mental alertness, apnea, and CV collapse) or CNS stimulation (insomnia, hallucinations, tremors, or seizures). Anticholinergic signs and symptoms, such as dry mouth, flushed skin, fixed and dilated pupils, and GI symptoms, are common, especially in children.

Treat overdose with gastric lavage to empty stomach contents; inducing emesis with ipecac syrup may be ineffective. Treat hypotension with vasopressors and control seizures with diazepam or phenytoin. Don't give stimulants.

NURSING CONSIDERATIONS
● Use cautiously in patients with heart failure or who have recently had surgery, benign prostatic hypertrophy, asthma, glaucoma, emphysema, chronic pulmonary disease, shortness of breath, or difficulty breathing.
● Be aware of potential additive CNS effects when coadministered with other CNS depressants.
● Monitor patient for adverse CNS effects.
● Monitor patient and vital signs closely.
● Encourage patient to discuss signs and symptoms with doctor.
● Obtain allergy history before giving patient this or any other drug.
● Breast-feeding patient should avoid the use of antihistamines such as cyclizine. Most antihistamines are excreted in breast milk, exposing the infant to risks of unusual excitability; premature infants are at particular risk for seizures.
● Cyclizine may inhibit lactation.
● Drug may prevent, reduce, or mask response to diagnostic skin tests. Patient should discontinue drug 4 days before tests.

- Elderly patient may be more sensitive to adverse effects of antihistamines; he's more likely to experience a greater degree of dizziness, sedation, hyperexcitability, dry mouth, and urine retention than a younger patient.

PATIENT TEACHING
- Instruct patient to position himself in places of minimal motion (such as in the middle, not front or back, of ship), to avoid excessive intake of food or drink, and not to read while in motion.
- Tell patient to avoid hazardous activities that required mental alertness until CNS reaction is determined.
- Advise elderly patient that he may be more sensitive to adverse effects of antihistamines and is more likely to experience a greater degree of dizziness, sedation, hyperexcitability, dry mouth, and urine retention than a younger patient.
- Inform parent or caregiver that this drug isn't indicated for use in children younger than age 6; they may experience paradoxical hyperexcitability.
- Inform breast-feeding patient that antihistamines such as cyclizine shouldn't be used during breast-feeding. Most antihistamines are excreted in breast milk, exposing the infant to risks of unusual excitability;

premature infants are at particular risk for seizures.
- Tell breast-feeding patient that cyclizine may inhibit lactation.

dimenhydrinate
Andrumin‡, Apo-Dimenhydrinate†, Calm-X, Children's Dramamine, Dimetabs, Dinate, Dramamine*, Dramamine Chewable**, Dramamine Liquid*, Dramanate, Dymenate, Gravol†, Gravol L/A†, Hydrate, PMS-Dimenhydrinate†, Triptone Caplets

Pregnancy Risk Category B

HOW SUPPLIED
Tablets: 50 mg
Tablets (chewable): 50 mg
Syrup: 12.5 mg/4 ml

ACTION
Unknown. Antihistamine that may affect neural pathways originating in the labyrinth to inhibit nausea and vomiting.

Route	Onset	Peak	Duration
P.O.	15-30 min	Unknown	3-6 hr

INDICATIONS & DOSAGES
Prevention and treatment of motion sickness—
Adults and children ages 12 and older: 50 to 100 mg P.O. q

4 to 6 hours. Maximum dose is 400 mg daily. For prevention, take 30 minutes before motion exposure.
Children ages 6 to 12: 25 to 50 mg P.O. q 6 to 8 hours, not to exceed 150 mg in 24 hours.
Children ages 2 to 6: 12.5 to 25 mg P.O. q 6 to 8 hours, not to exceed 75 mg in 24 hours.

ADVERSE REACTIONS
CNS: drowsiness; headache; dizziness; confusion; nervousness; vertigo; tingling and weakness of hands; lassitude; excitation; insomnia, especially in children.
CV: palpitations, hypotension, tachycardia.
EENT: blurred vision, dry respiratory passages, diplopia, nasal congestion.
GI: dry mouth, nausea, vomiting, diarrhea, epigastric distress, constipation, anorexia.
Respiratory: wheezing, thickened bronchial secretions, tightness of chest.
Skin: photosensitivity, urticaria, rash.
Other: *anaphylaxis.*

INTERACTIONS
Drug-drug
CNS depressants: additive CNS depression. Avoid using together.

Drug-lifestyle
Alcohol use: additive CNS depression. Avoid using together.

CONTRAINDICATIONS
Contraindicated in patients who are hypersensitive to drug or its components.

OVERDOSE & TREATMENT
Signs and symptoms of overdose may include either CNS depression (sedation, reduced mental alertness, apnea, and CV collapse) or CNS stimulation (insomnia, hallucinations, tremors, or seizures). Anticholinergic signs and symptoms, such as dry mouth, flushed skin, fixed and dilated pupils, and GI symptoms are likely to occur, especially in children.
  Use gastric lavage to empty stomach contents; emesis may be ineffective. Diazepam or phenytoin may be used to control seizures. Provide supportive treatment.

NURSING CONSIDERATIONS
• Use cautiously in patients with seizures, acute angle-closure glaucoma, or enlarged prostate gland, and in patients receiving ototoxic drugs.
• Elderly patients may be more susceptible to CNS adverse effects.

Reactions may be *common*, uncommon, *life-threatening*, or COMMON AND LIFE-THREATENING.

• Drug may prevent, reduce, or mask response to diagnostic skin tests. Patient should discontinue drug 4 days before tests.

• Drug may alter test results for xanthines (caffeine, aminophylline) because of its 8-chlorotheophylline content.

• *Alert:* Drug may mask signs and symptoms of ototoxicity, brain tumor, or intestinal obstruction.

• *Alert:* Don't confuse dimenhydrinate with diphenhydramine.

• To prevent motion sickness, patient should take drug 30 minutes before traveling and again before meals and at bedtime.

PATIENT TEACHING
• Advise patient to avoid activities that require alertness until CNS effects of drug are known.

• Instruct patient to report adverse reactions promptly.

• Tell patient to take drug 30 minutes before exposure.

• Inform elderly patient that he may be more sensitive to adverse effects of histamines than younger patients. He is especially likely to experience a greater degree of dizziness, sedation, hyperexcitability, dry mouth, and urine retention.

• Advise parent or caregiver not to administer this drug to children without approval of doctor.

• Inform breast-feeding patient that many antihistamines are excreted in breast milk. Instruct her to consult doctor before taking this or any drug.

---

docusate calcium (dioctyl calcium sulfosuccinate)
DC Softgels, Pro-Cal-Sof, Sulfalax Calcium, Surfak

docusate sodium (dioctyl sodium sulfosuccinate)
Colace, Coloxyl‡, Coloxyl Enema Concentrate 1 in 24‡, Diocto, Dioctyl§, Dioeze, Diosuccin, Disonate, Di-Sosul, DOS, D-S-S, Duosol, Fletchers' Enemette§, Modane Soft, Regulax SS, Regulex, Therevac-SB

Pregnancy Risk Category C

HOW SUPPLIED
docusate calcium
Capsules: 50 mg, 240 mg

docusate sodium
Tablets: 100 mg, 50 mg
Capsules: 50 mg, 100 mg, 240 mg, 250 mg
Oral liquid: 150 mg/15 ml
Oral solution: 50 mg/ml, 10 mg/ml
Syrup: 20 mg/5 ml, 50 mg/15 ml, 60 mg/15 ml
Enema concentrate: 18 g/100 ml (must be diluted)‡

ACTION
Stool softener that reduces surface tension of interfacing liquid contents of the bowel. This detergent activity promotes incorporation of additional liquid into stools, thus forming a softer mass.

Route	Onset	Peak	Duration
P.O., P.R.	24-72 hr	24-72 hr	24-72 hr

INDICATIONS & DOSAGES
Stool softener—
Adults and children older than age 12: 50 to 500 mg P.O. daily until bowel movements are normal. Or, give enema (where available). Dilute 1:24 with sterile water before administration, and give 100 to 150 ml (retention enema), 300 to 500 ml (evacuation enema), or 0.5 to 1.5 L (flushing enema) P.R.
Children ages 6 to 12: 40 to 120 mg docusate sodium P.O. daily.
Children ages 3 to 6: 20 to 60 mg docusate sodium P.O. daily.
Children younger than age 3: 10 to 40 mg docusate sodium P.O. daily.
  Higher dosage may be used for initial therapy. Dosage is adjusted to individual response.

ADVERSE REACTIONS
GI: bitter taste, mild abdominal cramping, diarrhea, laxative dependence with long-term or excessive use.

INTERACTIONS
Drug-drug
Mineral oil: may increase mineral oil absorption and cause toxicity and lipoid pneumonia. Advise patient to separate administration times.

CONTRAINDICATIONS
Contraindicated in patients who are hypersensitive to drug and in those with intestinal obstruction, undiagnosed abdominal pain, vomiting, or other signs and symptoms of appendicitis, fecal impaction, or acute surgical abdomen.

OVERDOSE & TREATMENT
No information available.

NURSING CONSIDERATIONS
• *Alert:* Don't use laxatives in patient experiencing abdominal pain.
• Avoid using docusate sodium in sodium-restricted patients.
• Give liquid in milk, fruit juice, or infant formula to mask bitter taste.
• Before giving for constipation, determine if patient has adequate fluid intake, exercise, and diet.
• Drug isn't for use in treating existing constipation but pre-

vents constipation from developing.

• Drug is laxative of choice for patients who shouldn't strain during defecation, including patients recovering from MI or rectal surgery, those with rectal or anal disease that makes passage of firm stools difficult, and those with postpartum constipation.

• Drug should be stored at 59° to 86° F (15° to 30° C), and the liquid protected from light.

PATIENT TEACHING
• Teach patient about dietary sources of bulk, including bran and other cereals, fresh fruit, and vegetables.

• Advise patient to increase fluid intake as tolerated and allowed.

• Instruct patient to use drug only occasionally and not for longer than 1 week without medical advice.

• Tell patient to discontinue drug if severe cramping occurs and to notify doctor.

• Notify patient that it may take from 1 to 3 days to soften stools.

• Advise breast-feeding patient to consult doctor before taking drug; however, it's thought that docusate salts are minimally absorbed.

• Inform elderly patient that docusate salts are usually a good choice, because they cause fewer side effects and rarely cause laxative dependency.

---

famotidine
Pepcid AC, Pepcid AC Gelcaps

Pregnancy Risk Category B

HOW SUPPLIED
Tablets: 10 mg
Gelcaps: 10 mg
Chewable tablets: 10 mg

ACTION
Competitively inhibits action of H_2 at receptor sites of the parietal cells, decreasing gastric acid secretion.

Route	Onset	Peak	Duration
P.O.	1 hr	1-3 hr	12 hr

INDICATIONS & DOSAGES
Prevention or treatment of heartburn—
Adults: 10 mg P.O. 1 hour before meals (prevention), or 10 mg P.O. with water when signs and symptoms occur. Maximum daily dose is 20 mg.

ADVERSE REACTIONS
CNS: headache, dizziness, vertigo, malaise, paresthesia.
CV: palpitations, flushing.
EENT: tinnitus, orbital edema.

GI: diarrhea, constipation, anorexia, taste perversion, dry mouth.
GU: increased BUN and creatinine levels.
Hepatic: elevated hepatic enzyme levels.
Musculoskeletal: bone and muscle pain.
Skin: acne, dry skin.
Other: fever.

INTERACTIONS
Drug-drug
Enteric-coated drugs: may cause enteric coating to dissolve too rapidly because of increased gastric pH. Advise patient to avoid using together.
Ketoconazole: decreases absorption of ketoconazole when administered together. Monitor patient closely; may require increased dose of ketoconazole.

Drug-lifestyle
Smoking: may increase gastric acid secretion and worsen disease. Advise patient to avoid smoking.

CONTRAINDICATIONS
Contraindicated in patients who are hypersensitive to drug.

OVERDOSE & TREATMENT
Overdose hasn't been reported.
If overdose does occur, treatment should include gastric lavage or induced emesis, followed by activated charcoal to prevent further absorption, and supportive and symptomatic therapy. Hemodialysis doesn't remove famotidine.

NURSING CONSIDERATIONS
• Assess for abdominal pain. Note blood in emesis, stool, or gastric aspirate.
• Discuss lifestyle changes that may help patient lessen signs and symptoms.
• Patient may be receiving antacids at the same time.
• Drug may antagonize pentagastrin during gastric acid secretion tests.
• In skin tests using allergen extracts, drug may cause false-negative results.

PATIENT TEACHING
• Instruct patient on proper use of product.
• Advise patient to limit use of drug to no longer than 2 weeks, and to consult a doctor if signs and symptoms persist.
• With medical advice, patient may take antacids at the same time, especially at beginning of therapy when pain is severe.
• Urge patient to avoid cigarette smoking because it may increase gastric acid secretion and worsen disease.
• Advise patient to report abdominal pain, emesis, or blood in stools.

- Advise elderly patient or caregiver that drug may cause adverse effects, especially CNS effects.
- Advise breast-feeding patient that drug may be excreted in breast milk and to consult doctor before taking this drug.

---

glycerin
Fleet Babylax, Fleet Glycerin Suppositories, Sani-Supp

Pregnancy Risk Category NR

HOW SUPPLIED
Enema (pediatric): 4 ml/applicator
Suppositories: adult, children, and infant size

ACTION
Hyperosmolar laxative that draws water from the tissues into the feces, thus stimulating evacuation.

Route	Onset	Peak	Duration
P.R.	15-60 min	15-60 min	15-60 min

INDICATIONS & DOSAGES
Constipation—
Adults and children ages 6 and older: 2 to 3 g as rectal suppository; or 5 to 15 ml as enema.
Children younger than age 6: 1 to 1.7 g as rectal suppository; or 2 to 5 ml as enema.

ADVERSE REACTIONS
GI: cramping pain, rectal discomfort, hyperemia of rectal mucosa.

INTERACTIONS
Drug-drug
Diuretics: use together may result in additive effects. Monitor patient closely.

CONTRAINDICATIONS
Contraindicated in patients who are hypersensitive to drug and in those with intestinal obstruction, undiagnosed abdominal pain, vomiting, or other signs and symptoms of appendicitis, fecal impaction, or acute surgical abdomen.

OVERDOSE & TREATMENT
No information available.

NURSING CONSIDERATIONS
- Drug is used mainly to reestablish proper toilet habits in laxative-dependent patients.
- Discuss dietary habits and ways to improve, if necessary, so that patient doesn't resume laxative consumption.
- Monitor for localized adverse effects, if necessary.

PATIENT TEACHING
- Advise patient to avoid forcing product into the rectum because injury may occur.

• Tell patient that drug must be retained for at least 15 minutes and that it usually acts within 1 hour. Entire suppository need not melt to be effective.

• Warn patient about adverse GI reactions.

• Instruct patient to contact doctor if adverse effects occur.

• Tell patient that rectal discomfort or burning may occur.

• Advise patient to avoid use if nausea, vomiting, or abdominal pain is present, unless directed by doctor.

• Tell patient to discontinue use and notify doctor if rectal bleeding occurs or if no bowel movement occurs after use.

• Tell patient not to use for longer than 1 week unless directed by doctor.

• Advise elderly patient who is dehydrated that he may be more prone to adverse CNS effects.

• Advise breast-feeding patient to consult doctor before using this drug, as safety in breast-feeding infants hasn't been established.

---

ipecac syrup

Pregnancy Risk Category C

HOW SUPPLIED
Syrup*: 70 mg powdered ipecac/ml (contains glycerin 10% and alcohol 1% to 2.5%)

ACTION
Induces vomiting by acting locally on the gastric mucosa and centrally on the chemoreceptor trigger zone.

Route	Onset	Peak	Duration
P.O.	20-30 min	Unknown	20-25 min

INDICATIONS & DOSAGES
To induce vomiting in poisoning—
Adults and children older than age 12: 30 ml P.O.; then 240 to 480 ml (8 to 16 oz) of water.
Children ages 1 to younger than 12: 15 ml P.O.; then 240 to 480 ml (8 to 16 oz) of water. Dose may be repeated in patients older than age 1 if vomiting doesn't occur within 20 to 30 minutes. If no vomiting occurs within 30 to 45 minutes after second dose, gastric lavage should be performed.
Infants and children ages 6 months to younger than 1 year: 5 ml P.O.; then 120 to 240 ml (4 to 8 oz) of water.

ADVERSE REACTIONS
CNS: depression, drowsiness.
CV: *arrhythmias, bradycardia,* hypotension; atrial fibrillation, *fatal myocarditis* (with excessive doses).
GI: diarrhea.

Reactions may be *common*, uncommon, *life-threatening*, or COMMON AND LIFE-THREATENING.

INTERACTIONS
Drug-drug
Activated charcoal: neutralizes emetic effect. Discourage use together; patient may be given activated charcoal after vomiting.
Antiemetics: may decrease ipecac's therapeutic effectiveness. Advise patient to avoid using together.

Drug-food
Carbonated beverages: may cause abdominal distention. Advise patient to avoid using together.
Milk, milk products: may decrease ipecac's therapeutic effect. Advise patient to avoid using with milk or milk products.
Vegetable oil: delays absorption of drug. Advise patient to avoid using together.

CONTRAINDICATIONS
Contraindicated in semicomatose or unconscious patients and in patients with seizures, severe inebriation, anaphylaxis, severe hypotension, or loss of gag reflex.

OVERDOSE & TREATMENT
Signs and symptoms of overdose include diarrhea, persistent nausea or vomiting (longer than 30 minutes), stomach cramps or pain, arrhythmias, hypotension, myocarditis, difficulty breathing, and unusual fatigue or weakness.

Toxicity from chronic ipecac overdose usually involves use of the concentrated fluid extract in dosage appropriate for the syrup. Signs and symptoms of cardiotoxicity include tachycardia, T-wave depression, atrial fibrillation, depressed myocardial contractility, heart failure, and myocarditis. Other toxic effects include bloody stools and vomitus, hypotension, shock, seizures, and coma. Heart failure is the usual cause of death.

Treatment requires discontinuation of drug followed by symptomatic and supportive care, which may include digitalis and pacemaker therapy to treat cardiotoxic effects. However, no antidote exists for the cardiotoxic effects of ipecac, which may be fatal despite intensive treatment.

NURSING CONSIDERATIONS
• *Alert:* Drug shouldn't be given after ingestion of petroleum products or volatile oils because of potential for dangerous or lethal aspiration.
• *Alert:* Drug shouldn't be given after ingestion of caustic substances such as lye because of potential for additional injury to the esophagus and mediastinum.

• Stomach is usually emptied completely; vomitus also may contain some intestinal material.
• If two doses don't induce vomiting, be prepared for gastric lavage.
• Ipecac syrup usually induces vomiting within 20 to 30 minutes.
• In antiemetic toxicity, ipecac syrup is usually effective if less than 1 hour has elapsed since ingestion of antiemetic.
• No systemic toxicity occurs with doses of 1 oz (30 ml) or less.
• Ipecac syrup is administered before giving activated charcoal, not after.
• Ipecac syrup is commonly abused by bulimics, who binge, then purge.
• Ipecac syrup may be used in small amounts as an expectorant in cough preparations; however, this use has doubtful therapeutic benefit.

PATIENT TEACHING
• Advise parent to keep poison control and doctor's phone numbers readily available.
• Advise patient or parent to consult doctor or poison control center in case of accidental ingestion, before taking or administering ipecac syrup.
• Stress to parents that there are some cases in which ipecac isn't indicated and when it can actually cause more harm than help.
• Remind parent not to give ipecac with milk, milk products, carbonated vegetables, or foods containing vegetable oil.
• Recommend to parents that 1 oz (30 ml) of syrup be available in the home after child's first birthday for immediate use in case of emergency.
• Show parents how to administer drug and tell them what to do in case of accidental poisoning.
• Warn parents not to let child sleep on his back after taking drug. Use a pillow to prop child on his side.
• Advise breast-feeding patient to consult doctor before using this drug, as safety in breast-feeding infants hasn't been established.

---

kaolin and pectin
Kao-Spen, Kapectolin

Pregnancy Risk Category NR

HOW SUPPLIED
Suspension: 5.2 g kaolin, 260 mg pectin/30 ml, 90 g kaolin, 2 g pectin/30 ml

ACTION
Kaolin is a natural hydrated aluminum silicate that is believed to adsorb large numbers

---

of bacteria and toxins and reduce water loss.

Route	Onset	Peak	Duration
P.O.	6-8 hr	Within 48 hr	Unknown

INDICATIONS & DOSAGES
*Adjunct to rest, fluids, and an
appropriate diet in the symptomatic treatment of mild to moderate diarrhea—*
Adults: 60 to 120 ml after each
loose bowel movement.
Children ages 6 to 12: 30 to 60
ml P.O. (Kapectolin) after each
loose bowel movement.
Children ages 3 to 6: 15 to 30
ml P.O. (Kapectolin) after each
loose bowel movement.

ADVERSE REACTIONS
GI: constipation, bloating, fullness.

INTERACTIONS
Drug-drug
*Anticholinergics, clindamycin,
digitalis glycosides, lincomycin,
loxapine, tetracycline, thiothix-
ene:* prolonged use of kaolin
and pectin may interfere with
absorption of these drugs. Advise patient to separate doses by
at least 3 to 4 hours.
Other oral drugs: prolonged
use of kaolin and pectin may interfere with absorption of other
oral drugs. Advise patient to
separate doses by at least 3 to 4
hours.

Drug-herb
Herbal preparations: prolonged
use of kaolin and pectin may interfere with absorption of herbs.
Advise patient to separate doses
by at least 3 to 4 hours.

CONTRAINDICATIONS
Contraindicated if diarrhea is
accompanied by fever or if
there's blood or mucus in stool.

OVERDOSE & TREATMENT
When taken in excessive doses,
kaolin and pectin can lead to
severe constipation and possibly fecal impaction.
  Treatment is symptomatic
and supportive.

NURSING CONSIDERATIONS
• Use cautiously in elderly patient with diarrhea because of
potential for fluid and electrolyte loss.
• Use is recommended in chronic diarrhea only as temporary
treatment until the etiology is
determined. If no relief is seen
within 48 hours, therapy should
be discontinued.
• Because data are lacking,
these products shouldn't be
used by patients who are pregnant or breast-feeding.
• Oral rehydration therapy is
recommended in children with
diarrhea to prevent fluid and
electrolyte loss.

*Liquid contains alcohol.   **May contain tartrazine.   †Canada   ‡Australia   §U.K.

• Store in a well-closed container and protect from freezing.

PATIENT TEACHING
• Instruct patient to shake suspension well before using.
• Inform patient that constipation may occur with this product.
• Advise parent or caregiver that this drug shouldn't be given to children ages 2 or younger.
• Instruct patient to check with doctor if diarrhea isn't controlled within 48 hours.
• Instruct patient to immediately contact doctor if blood or mucus should appear in the stool.
• Inform patient of importance of maintaining adequate hydration and proper diet while taking this product.
• Instruct elderly, pregnant, and breast-feeding patient to contact doctor before taking this drug because safety isn't proven.

---

lactase enzyme
Dairy Ease, LactAid, Lactrase, SureLac

Pregnancy Risk Category NR

HOW SUPPLIED
Caplets: 3,000 FCC U, lactase units, 4,500 FCC U, lactase units, 9,000 FCC U, lactase units
Capsules: 250 mg, lactase units

Drops: 1,250 neutral lactase U/5 drops, lactase units
Tablets (chewable): 3,000 FCC U, lactase units, 9,000 FCC U, lactase units

ACTION
Lactase enzyme hydrolyzes lactose, a complex sugar, into its simple sugar components, glucose and galactose.

Route	Onset	Peak	Duration
P.O.	Immediate	Minutes	Duration of meal

INDICATIONS & DOSAGES
To aid in dairy food digestion in patients with lactose intolerance—
Adults: 1 to 3 tablets, capsules, or caplets with the first bite of dairy food. For chewable tablets, chew, and swallow. Number of tablets will need to be adjusted up or down based on signs and symptoms. Don't exceed more than 6 tablets at a time; or, add 5 to 7 drops per quart of milk, shake gently, and refrigerate for 24 hours. If signs and symptoms (gas, bloating, cramps, or diarrhea) continue, 10 to 15 drops per quart of milk may be added.

ADVERSE REACTIONS
GI: bloating, fullness, GI discomfort.

Reactions may be *common*, uncommon, *life-threatening*, or COMMON AND LIFE-THREATENING.

INTERACTIONS
None reported.

CONTRAINDICATIONS
Because of insufficient data, these products shouldn't be used in patients who are breast-feeding or pregnant.

OVERDOSE & TREATMENT
Although not reported, an overdose of lactase enzyme would be handled with supportive care.

NURSING CONSIDERATIONS
• *Alert:* Use cautiously in patients who may be allergic to molds because Lactaid products are derived from molds.
• These products shouldn't be used in patients who are breast-feeding or pregnant because of insufficient data.
• For the liquid preparations, store at or below room temperature—77° F (25° C)—and refrigerate after opening.
• For capsules and tablets, store at or below room temperature—77° F (25° C)—but don't refrigerate. Keep away from heat.
• Discuss dietary habits with patient.
• Obtain thorough allergy history from patient.

PATIENT TEACHING
• Instruct patient to contact doctor if he experiences any signs and symptoms that are unusual or seem unrelated to the condition for which he took this product.
• Inform patient that the number of tablets or drops will need to be adjusted up or down based on signs and symptoms (gas, bloating, cramps, or diarrhea).
• Inform patient that Lactaid Drops are certified kosher from the Orthodox Union.
• Inform patient that drops may be used with whole, 1%, 2%, nonfat, skim, powdered, or chocolate milk.
• Because of lack of safety information, instruct pregnant and breast-feeding patient not to use this product.

---

loperamide
Imodium A-D, Kaopectate II Caplets, Maalox Anti-Diarrheal Caplets, Pepto Diarrhea Control

Pregnancy Risk Category B

HOW SUPPLIED
Caplets: 2 mg
Capsules: 2 mg
Oral liquid: 1 mg/5 ml

ACTION
Inhibits peristaltic activity, prolonging transit of intestinal contents.

Route	Onset	Peak	Duration
P.O.	Unknown	2.5-5 hr	24 hr

INDICATIONS & DOSAGES

Acute, nonspecific diarrhea—
Adults: initially, 4 mg P.O.;
then 2 mg after each unformed
stool. Maximum dose is 8 mg
daily.
Children ages 8 to 12: 10 ml
(2 mg) t.i.d. P.O. on first day.
Subsequent doses of 5 ml
(1 mg)/10 kg of body weight
may be administered after each
unformed stool. Maximum
dose is 6 mg daily.
Children ages 6 to 8: 10 ml
(2 mg) P.O. b.i.d. on first day. If
diarrhea persists, consult a doctor. Don't exceed 4 mg daily.
Children ages 2 to 5: 5 ml P.O.
t.i.d. on first day. If diarrhea
persists, consult a doctor.

Chronic diarrhea—
Adults: initially, 4 mg P.O.;
then 2 mg after each unformed
stool until diarrhea subsides.
Dosage adjusted to individual
response.

ADVERSE REACTIONS

CNS: drowsiness, fatigue,
dizziness.
GI: dry mouth; abdominal
pain, distention, or discomfort;
constipation; nausea; vomiting.
Skin: rash.
Other: *hypersensitivity reactions.*

INTERACTIONS
Drug-drug
Opioid analgesics: may cause
severe constipation. Advise patient to avoid using together.

CONTRAINDICATIONS
Contraindicated in patients who
are hypersensitive to drug and
when constipation must be
avoided. Also contraindicated
in children younger than age 2.

OVERDOSE & TREATMENT
Clinical effects of overdose
may include constipation, GI irritation, and CNS depression.
    Treatment is with activated
charcoal if ingestion was recent. If patient is vomiting, activated charcoal may be given as
a slurry when patient can retain
fluids. Or, gastric lavage may
be performed, followed by administration of activated charcoal slurry. Monitor for CNS
depression; treat respiratory depression with naloxone.

NURSING CONSIDERATIONS
• Use cautiously in patients with
hepatic disease.
• Drug produces antidiarrheal
action similar to diphenoxylate
but without as many adverse
CNS effects.
• ***Alert:*** Monitor children closely
for CNS effects; they may be
more sensitive than adults to
these effects.

Reactions may be *common*, uncommon, *life-threatening*, or COMMON AND LIFE-THREATENING.

• Ensure adequate fluid intake as tolerated to help prevent dehydration.

• *Alert:* Don't confuse Imodium with Ionamin.

PATIENT TEACHING
• Advise patient not to exceed recommended dosage.
• Tell patient with acute diarrhea to discontinue drug and seek medical attention if no improvement occurs within 48 hours; in chronic diarrhea, tell him to notify doctor and discontinue drug if no improvement occurs after taking 16 mg daily for at least 10 days.
• Advise patient with acute colitis to stop drug immediately if abdominal distention or other signs and symptoms develop, and to notify doctor.
• Warn patient to avoid activities that require mental alertness until CNS effects of drug are known.
• Tell patient to report nausea, abdominal pain, or abdominal discomfort to doctor.
• Advise patient to relieve dry mouth with ice chips or sugarless gum.
• Instruct parent that drug is contraindicated in children younger than age 2.
• Advise breast-feeding patient to consult doctor before using this drug, as safety in breast-feeding infants hasn't been established.

---

magaldrate (aluminum magnesium hydroxide sulfate)
Lowsium, Riopan

Pregnancy Risk Category NR

HOW SUPPLIED
Oral suspension: 540 mg/5 ml

ACTION
Antacid that reduces total acid load in the GI tract, elevates gastric pH to reduce pepsin activity, strengthens the gastric mucosal barrier, and increases esophageal sphincter tone.

Route	Onset	Peak	Duration
P.O.	20 min	Unknown	20-180 min

INDICATIONS & DOSAGES
Antacid—
Adults: 540 to 1,080 mg (5 to 10 ml) of suspension P.O. with water between meals and h.s.

ADVERSE REACTIONS
GI: mild constipation, diarrhea.
GU: increased urine pH levels.
Metabolic: hypokalemia, increased serum gastrin levels.

INTERACTIONS
Drug-drug
Allopurinol, antibiotics (including quinolones, tetracyclines), diflunisal, digoxin, iron salts, isoniazid, penicillamine, phenothiazines, quinidine, salicylates, ticlopidine: decreases pharmacologic effect because of possible impaired absorption. Advise patient to separate administration times by 1 to 2 hours.
Enteric-coated drugs: may release prematurely in stomach. Advise patient to separate doses by at least 1 hour.
Levodopa: when administered together, magaldrate may increase levodopa absorption, increasing risk of toxicity. Advise patient to avoid using together; separate administration times.

Drug-herb
Melatonin: increases inhibitory effects on the *N*-methyl-D-aspartate receptor. Advise patient to avoid using together.

CONTRAINDICATIONS
Contraindicated in patients with severe renal disease.

OVERDOSE & TREATMENT
No information available.

NURSING CONSIDERATIONS
• Use cautiously in patients with mild kidney impairment.

• When giving through NG tube, make sure tube is placed properly and is patent. After instilling, flush tube with water to ensure passage to stomach and to clear tube.
• Monitor serum magnesium level in patients with mild kidney impairment. Symptomatic hypermagnesemia usually occurs only in severe renal failure.
• ***Alert:*** Drug isn't typically used in patients with renal failure to help control hypophosphatemia because it contains magnesium, which may accumulate.
• Drug has a low sodium content and is a good choice for patients on restricted sodium intake.
• Drug may antagonize pentagastrin during gastric acid secretion tests.

PATIENT TEACHING
• Instruct patient to shake suspension well and to follow with water.
• Tell patient taking chewable tablets to chew thoroughly and to follow with a glass of water.
• Advise patient not to take magaldrate indiscriminately or to switch antacids without medical advice.
• Instruct patient to report signs and symptoms of bleeding, tarry stools, or coffee-ground vomitus.

Reactions may be *common*, uncommon, *life-threatening*, or COMMON AND LIFE-THREATENING.

• Drug usually isn't prescribed as an antacid to children younger than age 6 because they typically give vague descriptions of symptoms.

• Although no problems have been reported, aluminum and magnesium may be excreted in breast milk. Instruct breast-feeding patient to contact doctor before using this or any drug.

---

magnesium citrate
(citrate of magnesia)
Citroma, Citro-Mag†

Pregnancy Risk Category NR

HOW SUPPLIED
Oral solution: about 168 mEq magnesium/240 ml

ACTION
Saline laxative that produces an osmotic effect in the small intestine by drawing water into the intestinal lumen.

Route	Onset	Peak	Duration
P.O.	0.5-3 hr	Variable	Variable

INDICATIONS & DOSAGES
Constipation, to evacuate bowel before surgery—
Adults and children ages 12 and older: 11 to 25 g P.O. daily as a single dose or divided.

Children ages 6 to 12: 5.5 to 12.5 g P.O. daily as a single dose or divided.
Children ages 2 to 6: 2.7 to 6.25 g P.O. daily as a single dose or divided.

ADVERSE REACTIONS
GI: abdominal cramping, nausea, diarrhea, laxative dependence with long-term or excessive use.
Metabolic: fluid and electrolyte disturbances with daily use.

INTERACTIONS
Drug-drug
Oral drugs: impairs absorption. Advise patient to separate administration times.

CONTRAINDICATIONS
Contraindicated in patients with abdominal pain, nausea, vomiting, or other signs and symptoms of appendicitis or acute surgical abdomen; myocardial damage; heart block; fecal impaction; rectal fissures; intestinal obstruction or perforation; or renal disease. Also contraindicated in pregnant patients about to deliver.

OVERDOSE & TREATMENT
Long-term use or overdose may cause life-threatening electrolyte disorders. Hypermagnesemia may cause muscle weak-

ness, ECG changes, sedation, confusion, depressed deep tendon reflexes, and respiratory paralysis.

Treatment with diuretics such as furosemide, ethacrynic acid, and ammonium chloride may increase urinary excretion of magnesium.

NURSING CONSIDERATIONS
• *Alert:* Use cautiously in patients with rectal bleeding.
• Time drug administration so that it doesn't interfere with scheduled activities or sleep. Drug produces watery stools in 30 minutes to 6 hours.
• Before giving for constipation, determine if patient has adequate fluid intake, exercise, and diet.
• Chill magnesium citrate before use to make it more palatable.
• Shake suspension well; give with large amount of water when used as laxative. When administering through NG tube, make sure tube is placed properly and is patent. After instilling, flush tube with water to ensure passage to stomach and maintain tube patency.
• *Alert:* Monitor serum electrolyte levels, as ordered, during prolonged use. Magnesium may accumulate in patient with renal insufficiency.

• Drug is for short-term therapy only.

PATIENT TEACHING
• Instruct patient on drug administration.
• Teach patient about dietary sources of bulk, including bran and other cereals, fresh fruit, and vegetables.
• Tell patient not to use for longer than 1 week.
• Tell patient with renal disease or those on a low sodium diet not to use drug without medical advice.
• Advise patient to avoid use with nausea, vomiting, or abdominal pain.
• Warn patient that frequent or prolonged use as a laxative may cause dependence.
• Instruct patient to report adverse effects promptly to doctor.

---

magnesium hydroxide (milk of magnesia)
Milk of Magnesia, Phillips'
Milk of Magnesia, Phillips'
Milk of Magnesia
Concentrated

Pregnancy Risk Category NR

HOW SUPPLIED
Oral suspension: 400 mg/5 ml, 800 mg/5 ml
Chewable tablets: 311 mg

Reactions may be *common*, uncommon, *life-threatening*, or COMMON AND LIFE-THREATENING.

ACTION
Saline laxative that produces an osmotic effect in the small intestine by drawing water into the intestinal lumen.

Route	Onset	Peak	Duration
P.O.	0.5-3 hr	Variable	Variable

INDICATIONS & DOSAGES
Constipation, to evacuate bowel before surgery—
Adults and children ages 12 and older: 2.4 to 4.8 g (30 to 60 ml) P.O. daily as a single dose or divided; 15 to 30 ml (800 mg/5 ml) P.O.
Children ages 6 to 11: 1.2 to 2.4 g (15 to 30 ml) P.O. daily as a single dose or divided; 7.5 to 15 ml (800 mg/5 ml) P.O.
Children ages 2 to 5: 0.4 to 1.2 g (5 to 15 ml) P.O. daily as a single dose or divided; 2.5 to 7.5 ml (800 mg/5 ml) P.O.

Antacid—
Adults and children older than age 12: 5 to 15 ml (liquid) P.O. up to q.i.d. with water; 2.5 to 7.5 ml (liquid, concentrate) P.O. up to q.i.d. with water; 622 mg to 1,244 mg (tablets) P.O. up to q.i.d.

ADVERSE REACTIONS
GI: abdominal cramping, nausea, diarrhea, laxative dependence with long-term or excessive use.

Metabolic: fluid and electrolyte disturbances with daily use.

INTERACTIONS
Drug-drug
Enteric-coated drugs: when used together, magnesium hydroxide may cause premature release of enteric-coated drugs. Advise patient to avoid using together.
Oral drugs: impairs absorption. Advise patient to separate administration times.

CONTRAINDICATIONS
Contraindicated in patients with abdominal pain, nausea, vomiting, or other signs and symptoms of appendicitis or acute surgical abdomen; myocardial damage; heart block; fecal impaction; rectal fissures; intestinal obstruction or perforation; or renal disease. Also contraindicated in pregnant patients about to deliver.

OVERDOSE & TREATMENT
Long-term use or overdose may cause life-threatening electrolyte disorders. Hypermagnesemia may cause muscle weakness, ECG changes, sedation, confusion, depressed deep tendon reflexes, and respiratory paralysis.
Treatment with diuretics such as furosemide, ethacrynic acid, and ammonium chloride may

---

increase urinary excretion of magnesium.

NURSING CONSIDERATIONS
●Drug should be taken 1 hour before or after enteric-coated drug.
●*Alert:* Use cautiously in patients with rectal bleeding.
●Time drug administration so that it doesn't interfere with scheduled activities or sleep. Drug produces watery stools in 30 minutes to 6 hours.
●Patient should have adequate fluid intake, exercise, and diet before taking this drug.
●Suspension should be shaken well and taken with large amount of water when used as laxative. When giving through NG tube, make sure tube is placed properly and is patent. After instilling, flush tube with water to ensure passage to stomach and maintain tube patency.
●*Alert:* Monitor serum electrolyte levels, as ordered, during prolonged use. Magnesium may accumulate in patient with renal insufficiency.
●Drug is for short-term treatment only.

PATIENT TEACHING
●Instruct patient on drug administration.
●Tell patient not to use with kidney disease, abdominal pain, nausea, or vomiting unless directed by doctor.
●Advise patient to report rectal bleeding or lack of effect and to avoid use for longer than 1 week.
●Teach patient about dietary sources of bulk, including bran and other cereals, fresh fruit, and vegetables.
●Warn patient that frequent or prolonged use as a laxative may cause dependence.
●Instruct patient to consult doctor regarding use as an antacid before administering drug to children younger than age 6.
●Inform patient that some magnesium may be excreted in breast milk, although no problems have been reported. Patient should consult doctor before using this drug if breast-feeding.

---

magnesium oxide
Mag-Ox 400, Maox 420, Uro-Mag

Pregnancy Risk Category NR

HOW SUPPLIED
Tablets: 400 mg, 420 mg, 500 mg
Capsules: 140 mg

ACTION
Reduces total acid load in the GI tract, elevates gastric pH, strengthens the gastric mucosal

barrier, and increases esophageal sphincter tone.

Route	Onset	Peak	Duration
P.O.	20 min	Unknown	20-180 min

INDICATIONS & DOSAGES
Antacid—
Adults: 140 mg P.O. with water or milk after meals and h.s.

Laxative—
Adults: 4 g P.O. with water or milk, usually h.s.

Oral replacement therapy in mild hypomagnesemia—
Adults: 400 to 840 mg P.O. daily. Monitor serum magnesium level.

ADVERSE REACTIONS
GI: diarrhea, nausea, abdominal pain.
Metabolic: hypermagnesemia.

INTERACTIONS
Drug-drug
Allopurinol, antibiotics, digoxin, iron salts, penicillamine, phenothiazines: decreases effect because of possible impaired absorption. Advise patient to separate administration times by 1 to 2 hours.
Enteric-coated drugs: may release prematurely in stomach. Advise patient to separate doses by at least 1 hour.

CONTRAINDICATIONS
Contraindicated in patients with severe renal disease.

OVERDOSE & TREATMENT
None reported.

NURSING CONSIDERATIONS
• Use cautiously in patients with mild renal impairment.
• When used as laxative, drug shouldn't be taken within 1 to 2 hours of other oral drugs.
• *Alert:* Monitor serum magnesium levels. With prolonged use and renal impairment, watch for signs and symptoms of hypermagnesemia (hypotension, nausea, vomiting, depressed reflexes, respiratory depression, and coma).
• If diarrhea occurs, be prepared to suggest alternative preparation.

PATIENT TEACHING
• Advise patient not to take magnesium oxide indiscriminately or to switch antacids without doctor's advice.
• Instruct patient to report bleeding, tarry stools, or coffee-ground vomitus.

magnesium sulfate (epsom salts)

Pregnancy Risk Category NR

HOW SUPPLIED
Granules: about 40 mEq magnesium/5 g

ACTION
Saline laxative that produces an osmotic effect in the small intestine by drawing water into the intestinal lumen.

Route	Onset	Peak	Duration
P.O.	0.5-3 hr	Variable	Variable

INDICATIONS & DOSAGES
Constipation, to evacuate bowel before surgery—
Adults and children ages 12 and older: 10 to 30 g P.O. daily as a single dose or divided.
Children ages 6 to 11: 5 to 10 g P.O. daily as a single dose or divided.
Children ages 2 to 5: 2.5 to 5 g P.O. daily as a single dose or divided.

ADVERSE REACTIONS
GI: abdominal cramping, nausea, diarrhea, laxative dependence with long-term or excessive use.
Metabolic: fluid and electrolyte disturbances with daily use.

INTERACTIONS
Drug-drug
Enteric-coated drugs: when used together, magnesium hydroxide may cause premature release of enteric-coated drugs. Advise patient to avoid using together.
Oral drugs: impairs absorption. Advise patient to separate administration times.

CONTRAINDICATIONS
Contraindicated in patients with abdominal pain, nausea, vomiting, or other signs and symptoms of appendicitis or acute surgical abdomen; myocardial damage; heart block; fecal impaction; rectal fissures; intestinal obstruction or perforation; or renal disease. Also contraindicated in pregnant patients about to deliver.

OVERDOSE & TREATMENT
Long-term use or overdose may cause life-threatening electrolyte disorders. Hypermagnesemia may cause muscle weakness, ECG changes, sedation, confusion, depressed deep tendon reflexes, and respiratory paralysis.
  Treatment with diuretics such as furosemide, ethacrynic acid, and ammonium chloride may increase urinary excretion of magnesium.

Reactions may be *common*, uncommon, *life-threatening*, or COMMON AND LIFE-THREATENING.

NURSING CONSIDERATIONS
• Give drug 1 hour before or after enteric-coated drugs.
• **Alert:** Use cautiously in patients with rectal bleeding.
• Time drug administration so that it doesn't interfere with scheduled activities or sleep. Drug produces watery stools in 30 minutes to 6 hours.
• Before giving for constipation, determine if patient has adequate fluid intake, exercise, and diet.
• Shake suspension well; give with large amount of water when used as laxative. When administering through NG tube, make sure tube is placed properly and is patent. After instilling, flush tube with water to ensure passage to stomach and maintain tube patency.
• **Alert:** Monitor serum electrolyte levels, as ordered, during prolonged use. Magnesium may accumulate in patient with renal insufficiency.
• Drug is for short-term therapy only.

PATIENT TEACHING
• Instruct patient on drug administration.
• Tell patient not to use if he has kidney disease, abdominal pain, nausea, or vomiting unless directed by doctor.
• Advise patient to report rectal bleeding or lack of effect and to avoid using for longer than 1 week.
• Teach patient about dietary sources of bulk, including bran and other cereals, fresh fruit, and vegetables.
• Warn patient that frequent or prolonged use as a laxative may cause dependence.
• Instruct patient to consult doctor regarding use as an antacid before administering drug to children younger than age 6.
• Inform patient that some magnesium may be excreted in breast milk, although no problems have been reported. Patient should consult doctor before using this drug if breast-feeding.

---

malt soup extract
Maltsupex, Syllamalt

Pregnancy Risk Category NR

HOW SUPPLIED
Tablets: 750 mg
Powder: 8 g/scoop
Liquid: 16 g/tbs

ACTION
Malt soup extract is a bulk-forming laxative that swells in the intestinal fluid, forming an emollient gel that facilitates passage of intestinal contents and stimulates peristalsis. The extract has been proposed to re-

duce fecal pH, which may contribute to its laxative effect.

Route	Onset	Peak	Duration
P.O.	12-72 hr	2-4 days	Unknown

INDICATIONS & DOSAGES
Powder form—
Adults: up to 4 scoops (32 g) or 2 tbs (32 g) b.i.d. for 3 to 4 days. Maintenance dose is 2 to 4 scoops (16 to 32 g) or 1 to 2 tbs (16 to 32 g) h.s.; or initially, 4 tablets q.i.d. (12 g/day). Maintenance dose is 12 to 36 g/day.
Children ages 6 to 12: up to 2 scoops or 1 tbs (16 g) b.i.d. for 3 to 4 days.
Children ages 2 to 6: 1 scoop or ½ tbs (8 g) b.i.d. for 3 to 4 days.

ADVERSE REACTIONS
GI: esophageal obstruction characterized by chest pain, vomiting, excessive salivation, and inhibited swallowing reflex or choking; diarrhea; bloating; flatulence; fecal impaction.

INTERACTIONS
Drug-drug
Oral drugs: may interfere with the absorption of drugs. Advise patient to avoid using malt soup extract within 2 hours of using other drugs.

Drug-herb
Aloe vera (Aloe barbadensis), *Cascara sagrada* (Rhamnus purshianus), *Chinese rhubarb* (Rheum officinale), *Frangula* (Rhamnus frangula) *Senna* (Cassia senna, Cassia angustifolia), *Yellow dock* (Rumex crispus): may lead to an increased laxative effect. Warn patient against using together.
Other herbs: may interfere with the absorption of herbs. Patient should avoid malt soup extract within 2 hours of taking herbs.

CONTRAINDICATIONS
Contraindicated in patients with acute abdominal pain, nausea, vomiting, signs and symptoms of appendicitis, undiagnosed abdominal pain, bowel obstruction, or dysphagia. Avoid malt soup extract in patients with a history of intestinal ulcerations, stenosis, disabling adhesions, or allergy to barley.

OVERDOSE & TREATMENT
Overdose may led to fecal impaction (especially if not taken with adequate fluid) and abdominal cramping and discomfort.

Treatment is symptomatic and supportive.

NURSING CONSIDERATIONS
• Because bulk-forming laxatives must be taken with sufficient fluids, these drugs may not be warranted in patients with strict fluid requirements

(those with renal dysfunction or heart failure).

• The drug should be used cautiously by diabetic patients or patients who have esophageal strictures, renal disease, or a carbohydrate-restricted diet.

• The powdered form of malt soup extract should be mixed in enough water, milk, or juice to dissolve. Mixing is easier if added to warm milk or warm water.

• The liquid form of malt soup extract should be dissolved in 1 to 2 oz of warm water, stirred, and then added to enough milk, water, or juice.

• Regardless of the preparation, each dose should be followed with at least 8 oz of water. Otherwise, the patient may experience therapeutic failure or fecal impaction.

• The full corrective dose should be used for 3 to 4 days or until relief is noted. The maintenance dose should then be used as needed.

• Store at controlled room temperatures 68° to 77° F (20° to 25° C). Protect powder and tablets from moisture.

• Maltsupex tablets contain tartrazine dye, which may cause allergic reactions, including bronchial asthma in susceptible patients. Although the incidence of tartrazine sensitivity is low, it frequently occurs in individuals who are sensitive to aspirin.

PATIENT TEACHING

• Instruct patient not to use laxative products when abdominal pain, nausea, or vomiting is present unless directed by doctor.

• Instruct patient on a sodium-restricted diet to consult doctor before using this product because of its sodium content.

• Instruct patient to consult doctor if constipation persists.

• If a sudden change in bowel habits that persists for a period of 2 weeks occurs, instruct patient to consult a doctor before using a laxative.

• Advise patient that laxative products shouldn't be used for a period longer than 1 week unless directed by a doctor.

• Advise patient that rectal bleeding or failure to have a bowel movement after use of a laxative may indicate a serious condition. Patient should discontinue use and consult doctor.

• Instruct pregnant or breast-feeding patient to consult a doctor before using this product.

• Advise patient that each dose should be followed with at least 8 oz of water.

meclizine hydrochloride
Bonamine†, Bonine

Pregnancy Risk Category B

HOW SUPPLIED
Tablets (chewable): 25 mg

ACTION
Unknown. Antihistamine that may affect neural pathways originating in the labyrinth to inhibit nausea and vomiting.

Route	Onset	Peak	Duration
P.O.	1 hr	Unknown	8-24 hr

INDICATIONS & DOSAGES
Motion sickness—
Adults and children ages 12 and older: 25 to 50 mg P.O. 1 hour before travel. May repeat dose every 24 hours for the duration of trip.

ADVERSE REACTIONS
CNS: drowsiness, restlessness, excitation, nervousness, auditory and visual hallucinations.
CV: hypotension, palpitations, tachycardia.
EENT: blurred vision, diplopia, tinnitus, dry nose and throat.
GI: dry mouth, constipation, anorexia, nausea, vomiting, diarrhea.
GU: urine retention, urinary frequency.
Skin: urticaria, rash.

INTERACTIONS
Drug-drug
CNS depressants: increases drowsiness. Advise patient to use together cautiously.

CONTRAINDICATIONS
Contraindicated in patients who are hypersensitive to drug.

OVERDOSE & TREATMENT
Signs and symptoms of moderate overdose may include hyperexcitability alternating with drowsiness. Seizures, hallucinations, and respiratory paralysis may occur in profound overdose. Anticholinergic signs and symptoms, such as dry mouth, flushed skin, fixed and dilated pupils, and GI symptoms, are common, especially in children.

Treat overdose by administering gastric lavage to empty stomach contents; emesis with ipecac syrup may be ineffective. Treat hypotension with vasopressors and control seizures with diazepam or phenytoin. Don't give stimulants.

NURSING CONSIDERATIONS
• Use cautiously in patients with asthma, glaucoma, or prostatic hyperplasia.
• Drug may mask signs and symptoms of ototoxicity, brain tumor, or intestinal obstruction.
• Discontinue drug 4 days before diagnostic skin tests to

Reactions may be *common*, uncommon, *life-threatening*, or COMMON AND LIFE-THREATENING.

avoid interference with test response.
• Patient shouldn't take OTC meclizine before skin testing.

PATIENT TEACHING
• Advise patient to avoid hazardous activities that require alertness until CNS effects of drug are known.
• Instruct patient to report persistent or serious adverse reactions promptly.

---

methylcellulose
Citrucel, Citrucel Orange Flavor, Citrucel Sugar-Free Orange Flavor

Pregnancy Risk Category NR

HOW SUPPLIED
Powder: 2 g/tbs (heaping)

ACTION
Bulk-forming laxative that absorbs water and expands to increase bulk and moisture content of stools. The increased bulk encourages peristalsis and bowel movement.

Route	Onset	Peak	Duration
P.O.	12-24 hr	< 3 days	Variable

INDICATIONS & DOSAGES
Chronic constipation—
Adults and children ages 12 and older: 1 tbs (heaping) in 8 oz (240 ml) of cold water daily to t.i.d.
Children ages 6 to 12: ½ the adult dose in 8 oz (240 ml) of cold water daily.

ADVERSE REACTIONS
GI: nausea, vomiting, diarrhea with excessive use; esophageal, gastric, small intestinal or colonic strictures when drug is chewed or taken in dry form; abdominal cramps, especially in severe constipation; laxative dependence with long-term or excessive use.

INTERACTIONS
None significant.

CONTRAINDICATIONS
Contraindicated in patients with abdominal pain, nausea, vomiting, or other signs and symptoms of appendicitis or acute surgical abdomen and in those with intestinal obstruction or ulceration, disabling adhesions, or difficulty swallowing.

OVERDOSE & TREATMENT
No information available.

NURSING CONSIDERATIONS
• Before giving for constipation, determine if patient has adequate fluid intake, exercise, and diet.
• Each adult dose contains approximately 3 mg of sodium,

---

105 mg of potassium, and contributes 60 calories from sucrose.

• Drug is especially useful in debilitated patients and in those with postpartum constipation, irritable bowel syndrome, diverticulitis, and colostomies. It's also used to treat laxative abuse and to empty colon before barium enema examinations.

• Drug isn't absorbed systemically and is nontoxic.

• **Alert:** Don't confuse Citrucel with Citracal.

PATIENT TEACHING

• Tell patient to take drug with at least 8 oz (240 ml) of liquid to mask grittiness.

• Teach patient about dietary sources of bulk, including bran and other cereals, fresh fruit, and vegetables.

• Tell patient to increase fluid intake.

---

mineral oil (liquid petrolatum)

Fleet Enema Mineral Oil, Kondremul, Kondremul Plain, Lansoÿl†, Liqui-Doss, Milkinol, Neo-Cultol, Petrogalar Plain

Pregnancy Risk Category C

HOW SUPPLIED

Emulsion: 2.75 ml/5 ml, 4.75 ml/5 ml
Oral liquid: in pints, quarts, gallons
Enema: 120 ml, 133 ml

ACTION

Lubricant laxative that increases water retention in stools by creating a barrier between colon wall and feces that prevents colonic reabsorption of fecal water.

Route	Onset	Peak	Duration
P.O.	6-8 hr	Variable	Variable
P.R.	2-15 min	Unknown	Unknown

INDICATIONS & DOSAGES

Constipation, preparation for bowel studies or surgery—
Adults and children ages 12 and older: 15 to 45 ml P.O. h.s.; or 120 ml P.R. (as enema).
Children ages 6 to 11: 5 to 15 ml P.O. h.s.; or 30 to 60 ml P.R. (as enema).
Children ages 2 to 6: 30 to 60 ml P.R. (as enema).

ADVERSE REACTIONS

GI: nausea; vomiting; diarrhea with excessive use; abdominal cramps, especially in severe constipation; hemorrhoids; decreased absorption of nutrients and fat-soluble vitamins, resulting in deficiency; slowed healing after hemorrhoidectomy;

laxative dependence with long-term or excessive use.
Respiratory: *lipid pneumonia.*
Skin: anal pruritus, anal irritation, perianal discomfort.

INTERACTIONS
Drug-drug
Docusate salts: may increase mineral oil absorption and cause lipid pneumonia. Advise patient to separate administration times.
Fat-soluble vitamins (A, D, E, K): may decrease absorption after prolonged administration. Monitor for vitamin deficiency.

Drug-food
Any food: may delay drug action. Advise patient to take drug 2 hours before or after eating.

CONTRAINDICATIONS
Contraindicated in patients with abdominal pain, nausea, vomiting, or other signs and symptoms of appendicitis or acute surgical abdomen and in those with fecal impaction or intestinal obstruction or perforation.

OVERDOSE & TREATMENT
No information available.

NURSING CONSIDERATIONS
• Use cautiously in young children and in elderly or debilitated patients because of susceptibility to lipid pneumonia

through aspiration, absorption, and transport from intestinal mucosa.
• *Alert:* Use cautiously in patients with rectal bleeding.
• Before taking for constipation, patient should have adequate fluid intake, exercise, and diet.
• Drug should be taken on an empty stomach because it delays passage of food from stomach and is more active on an empty stomach.
• Drug may be taken with fruit juice or carbonated drink to disguise taste.
• Drug may be used when patient needs to ease strain of evacuation.

PATIENT TEACHING
• Advise patient to take drug only at bedtime on an empty stomach and not to take it for longer than 1 week. Tell him to take drug with fruit juice or carbonated drink to disguise taste.
• To avoid soiling clothing, advise patient of possible rectal leakage from excessive dosages.
• Teach patient about dietary sources of bulk, including bran and other cereals, fresh fruit, and vegetables.
• Instruct patient to report adverse effects promptly to doctor.

● Elderly patient may be at increased risk for aspiration; advise caution in use.

● Instruct parent or caregiver that mineral oil isn't to be given to children younger than age 6, because of potential for aspiration.

● Instruct parent or caregiver that enema form is contraindicated in children younger than age 2.

---

nizatidine
Axid AR

Pregnancy Risk Category C

HOW SUPPLIED
Tablets: 75 mg

ACTION
Competitively inhibits action of H_2 at receptor sites of the parietal cells, decreasing gastric acid secretion.

Route	Onset	Peak	Duration
P.O.	0.5 hr	0.5-3 hr	12 hr

INDICATIONS & DOSAGES
Prevention of heartburn, acid indigestion, or sour stomach—
Adults and children ages 12 and older: 75 mg P.O. daily or b.i.d. 30 to 60 minutes before meals or beverages that cause heartburn. Maximum 150 mg daily for up to 2 weeks.

ADVERSE REACTIONS
CNS: somnolence.
CV: *arrhythmias.*
Hematologic: eosinophilia.
Hepatic: elevated liver function tests results, hepatocellular injury.
Metabolic: hyperuricemia.
Skin: diaphoresis, rash, urticaria.
Other: fever.

INTERACTIONS
Drug-drug
Aspirin: may elevate serum salicylate levels (with high doses). Monitor closely.

Drug-food
Tomato-based vegetable juices: may decrease potency of drug. Advise patient to avoid using together.

Drug-lifestyle
Smoking: may increase gastric acid secretion and worsen the disease. Advise patient not to smoke.

CONTRAINDICATIONS
Contraindicated in patients hypersensitive to H_2-receptor antagonists.

OVERDOSE & TREATMENT
Signs and symptoms of overdose are cholinergic, including lacrimation, salivation, emesis, miosis, and diarrhea.

Treatment may include use of activated charcoal, emesis, or lavage, with clinical monitoring and supportive therapy.

NURSING CONSIDERATIONS
• False-positive urobilinogen test results may occur during drug therapy.
• Because drug is excreted primarily by the kidneys, reduce dosage in patients with moderate to severe renal insufficiency.
• Drug loses some potency when mixed with tomato-based vegetable juices. Ask pharmacist about compatibility.
• Assess for abdominal pain.
• Note presence of blood in emesis, stool, or gastric aspirate.
• For patient on maintenance therapy, remember that effects of continuous drug therapy for longer than 1 year aren't known.
• In elderly patients, renal function may be reduced; discuss dose modification with patient, if needed.

PATIENT TEACHING
• Urge patient to avoid cigarette smoking because it may increase gastric acid secretion and worsen disease.
• Advise patient to report abdominal pain and blood in stools or emesis.
• Inform parent or caregiver that safety and efficacy haven't been established in children.

• Instruct breast-feeding patient to consult doctor before taking this drug, because nizatidine is secreted and concentrated in breast milk.

---

pancreatin
Hi-Vegi-Lip Tablets, 4X
Pancreatin 600 mg, 8X
Pancreatin 900 mg,
Pancrezyme 4X Tablets

Pregnancy Risk Category C

HOW SUPPLIED
Hi-Vegi-Lip Tablets
Tablets (enteric-coated):
2,400 mg pancreatin, 4,800 U lipase, 60,000 U protease, and 60,000 U amylase

4X Pancreatin 600 mg
Tablets (enteric-coated):
2,400 mg pancreatin, 12,000 U lipase, 60,000 U protease, and 60,000 U amylase

8X Pancreatin 900 mg
Tablets (enteric-coated):
7,200 mg pancreatin, 22,500 U lipase, 180,000 U protease, and 180,000 U amylase

Pancrezyme 4X Tablets
Tablets (enteric-coated):
2,400 mg pancreatin, 12,000 U lipase, 60,000 U protease, and 60,000 U amylase

---

ACTION
Replaces endogenous exocrine pancreatic enzymes and aids digestion of starches, fats, and proteins.

Route	Onset	Peak	Duration
P.O.	Unknown	Unknown	1-2 hr

INDICATIONS & DOSAGES
Exocrine pancreatic secretion insufficiency; digestive aid in diseases associated with deficiency of pancreatic enzymes, such as cystic fibrosis—
Adults and children: dosage varies with condition being treated. Usual initial dose is 8,000 to 24,000 U of lipase activity P.O. before or with each meal or snack. Total daily dose may also be given in divided doses at 1- to 2-hour intervals throughout day.

ADVERSE REACTIONS
GI: nausea, diarrhea with high doses.
Metabolic: hyperuricemia.
Skin: perianal irritation.
Other: allergic reactions.

INTERACTIONS
Drug-drug
Antacids: may negate pancreatin's beneficial effect. Advise patient to avoid using together.
Iron-containing products: decreases the absorption of these products. Advise patient to avoid using together.

CONTRAINDICATIONS
Contraindicated in patients who are hypersensitive to drug, pork protein, or enzymes and in those with acute pancreatitis or acute exacerbations of chronic pancreatitis.

OVERDOSE & TREATMENT
Signs and symptoms of overdose include hyperuricosuria, hyperuricemia, diarrhea, abdominal cramps, and transient intestinal upset.
    Treatment is symptomatic and supportive.

NURSING CONSIDERATIONS
●Use with caution in pregnant or breast-feeding patients.
●Minimal USP standards dictate that each milligram of bovine or porcine pancreatin contains lipase 2 U, protease 25 U, and amylase 25 U.
●To avoid indigestion, monitor patient's dietary intake to ensure a proper balance of fat, protein, and starch intake. Dosage varies according to degree of maldigestion and malabsorption, amount of fat in diet, and enzyme activity of individual preparations.
●Fewer bowel movements and improved stool consistency indicate effective therapy.

• Drug isn't effective in GI disorders unrelated to pancreatic enzyme deficiency.

• Enteric coating on some products may reduce available enzyme in upper portion of jejunum.

PATIENT TEACHING

• Instruct patient to take before or with meals and snacks.

• Tell patient not to crush or chew enteric-coated forms. Capsules containing enteric-coated microspheres may be opened and sprinkled on a small quantity of cooled, soft food. Stress importance of swallowing immediately without chewing and following with glass of water or juice.

• Warn patient not to inhale powder form or powder from capsules; may irritate skin or mucous membranes.

• Tell patient to store in airtight containers at room temperature.

• Instruct patient not to change brands without medical advice.

• Instruct patient to report adverse effects promptly to doctor.

---

phosphorated carbohydrate solution
Emetrol, Nausea Relief, Nausetrol

Pregnancy Risk Category C

HOW SUPPLIED
Solution: 1.87 g dextrose, 1.87 g fructose, and 21.5 mg phosphoric acid/5 ml

ACTION
Hyperosmolar solutions of carbohydrates when combined with phosphoric acid relieve nausea and vomiting by acting in a direct fashion on the wall of the gastrointestinal tract. This action reduces smooth muscled contractions.

Route	Onset	Peak	Duration
P.O.	Rapid	Unknown	Unknown

INDICATIONS & DOSAGES
Nausea—
Adults: 15 or 30 ml (1 to 2 tbs) P.O. every 15 minutes until nausea and vomiting decreases. Don't take for longer than 1 hour or more than five doses.
Children ages 2 to 12: 5 or 10 ml (1 to 2 tsp) P.O. every 15 minutes until nausea and vomiting decrease. Don't take for longer than 1 hour or more than five doses.

ADVERSE REACTIONS
GI: abdominal pain, diarrhea.

INTERACTIONS
Drug-lifestyle
Alcohol use: possible additive effects. Advise patient to avoid

alcohol consumption while taking this drug.

CONTRAINDICATIONS
These solutions contain fructose and shouldn't be given to patients with hereditary fructose intolerance. Also, diabetic patients should avoid such drugs because they contain a significant amount of sugar. Patients with asthma, glaucoma, or enlargement of the prostate gland shouldn't take this drug unless advised to by a doctor.

OVERDOSE & TREATMENT
Ingestion of large amounts of phosphoric acid may irritate the oropharynx, esophagus, or GI tract. Signs and symptoms include nausea, vomiting, hematemesis, bloody diarrhea, abdominal pain, perforation, and GI bleeding.

If patient hasn't vomited, emesis shouldn't be induced because of the possibility of severe irritation to the GI tract. Instead, gastric lavage is recommended.

NURSING CONSIDERATIONS
• A patient taking sedatives or tranquilizers shouldn't take this drug without first consulting his doctor.
• Use with caution in diabetic patient if ordered; closely monitor blood glucose levels.

• Nausea and vomiting that are refractory to treatment may signify a serious underlying condition.
• Drug shouldn't be diluted with fluids. Patient shouldn't drink anything for at least 15 minutes after administration.

PATIENT TEACHING
• Instruct patient not to dilute drug with liquid.
• Instruct patient not to ingest fluids orally before or after (at least 15 minutes) taking a dose.
• Have diabetic patient monitor blood glucose levels closely if taking this drug.
• Instruct patient to report adverse effects promptly to his doctor.

---

psyllium
Effer-Syllium Instant Mix, Fiberall, Genfiber, Hydrocil Instant, Konsyl, Konsyl-D, Maalox Daily Fiber Therapy, Metamucil, Metamucil Sugar Free, Modane Bulk, Mylanta Natural Fiber Supplement, Perdiem Fiber, Prodiem Plain†, Reguloid Natural, Restore, Serutan, Syllact, Unilax, V-Lax

Pregnancy Risk Category NR

HOW SUPPLIED
Chewable pieces: 1.7 g/piece, 3.4 g/piece
Effervescent powder: 3.4 g/packet, 3.7 g/packet
Granules: 2.5 g/tsp, 4.03 g/tsp
Powder: 3.3 g/tsp, 3.4 g/tsp, 3.5 g/tsp, 4.94 g/tsp
Wafers: 3.4 g/wafer

ACTION
Bulk-forming laxative that absorbs water and expands to increase bulk and moisture content of stool, thus encouraging peristalsis and bowel movement.

Route	Onset	Peak	Duration
P.O.	12-24 hr	3 days	Variable

INDICATIONS & DOSAGES
Constipation, bowel management—
Adults and children ages 12 and older: 2.5 to 7 g P.O. per dose. Up to 30 g daily in divided doses.
Children ages 6 to 11: 2.5 to 3.75 g P.O. per dose. Up to 15 g daily given in divided doses.

ADVERSE REACTIONS
GI: nausea, vomiting, diarrhea with excessive use; esophageal, gastric, small intestine, and rectal obstruction when drug is taken in dry form; abdominal cramps, especially in severe constipation.

INTERACTIONS
Drug-drug
Anticoagulants, digoxin, salicylates: may bind or absorb these drugs, leading to a decrease in their effect. Advise patient to separate administration times by at least 2 hours.
Potassium-sparing diuretics, potassium supplements: may promote loss of potassium and interfere with the effects of these drugs. Advise patient to avoid using together.

CONTRAINDICATIONS
Contraindicated in patients who are hypersensitive to drug and in those with abdominal pain, nausea, vomiting, or other symptoms of appendicitis; intestinal obstruction or ulceration; fecal obstruction; disabling adhesions; or difficulty swallowing.

OVERDOSE & TREATMENT
Although no cases of overdose have been reported, signs and symptoms would probably include abdominal pain and diarrhea.
    If overdose should occur, treatment would be symptomatic and supportive.

NURSING CONSIDERATIONS
• Before giving for constipation, determine if patient has ade-

---

quate fluid intake, exercise, and diet.

• Mix with at least 8 oz (240 ml) of cold, pleasant-tasting liquid such as orange juice, to mask grittiness and stir only a few seconds. Have patient drink mixture immediately so it doesn't congeal. Follow with additional glass of liquid.

• For dosages in children younger than age 6, consult a doctor.

• Drug may reduce appetite if taken before meals.

• Drug isn't absorbed systemically and is nontoxic. It's especially useful in debilitated patients and in those with postpartum constipation, irritable bowel syndrome, or diverticular disease. It's also used to treat chronic laxative abuse and with other laxatives to empty colon before barium enema examinations.

PATIENT TEACHING

• Teach patient how to properly mix and take drug. Tell him to take drug with at least 8 oz of water.

• Tell patient to report chest pain, vomiting, or difficulty breathing or swallowing.

• Advise patient that inhaling powder may cause allergic reactions, especially in those with psyllium sensitivity or respiratory disorders.

• Tell patient that laxative effect usually occurs in 12 to 24 hours but may be delayed 3 days.

• Advise diabetic patient to check label and use a sugar-free psyllium product.

• Teach patient about dietary sources of bulk, including bran and other cereals, fresh fruit, and vegetables.

pyrantel pamoate
Antiminth, Combantrin†, Pin-Rid, Pin-X, Reese's Pinworm Medicine

Pregnancy Risk Category C

HOW SUPPLIED
Tablets: 62.5 mg
Capsules (soft-gel): 180 mg
Oral suspension: 50 mg/ml

ACTION
Blocks neuromuscular action, paralyzing the worm and causing its expulsion by normal peristalsis.

Route	Onset	Peak	Duration
P.O.	Variable	1-3 hr	Variable

INDICATIONS & DOSAGES
Roundworm, pinworm—
Adults and children ages 2 and older: 11 mg/kg P.O. as a single dose. Maximum dose is 1 g. For pinworm, dose should be repeated in 2 weeks.

ADVERSE REACTIONS
CNS: headache, dizziness, drowsiness, insomnia, weakness.
GI: anorexia, nausea, vomiting, gastralgia, abdominal cramps, diarrhea, tenesmus.
Hepatic: transient elevation of AST.
Skin: rash.
Other: fever.

INTERACTIONS
Drug-drug
Piperazine salts: possible antagonism. Advise patient to avoid using together.

CONTRAINDICATIONS
Contraindicated in patients who are hypersensitive to drug.

OVERDOSE & TREATMENT
Signs and symptoms of overdose are unlikely but may include vomiting and diarrhea.

Treatment of overdose is largely supportive, particularly of CV and respiratory functions. After recent ingestion (within 4 hours), empty stomach by induced emesis or gastric lavage. Follow with activated charcoal to decrease absorption. Osmotic cathartics may be helpful.

NURSING CONSIDERATIONS
• Use cautiously in patients with severe malnutrition or anemia or in patients with hepatic dysfunction.
• Dietary restrictions, laxatives, or enemas aren't necessary.
• Drug should be given to all family members for pinworm infections.
• Drug may reduce appetite if taken before meals.
• Drug should be protected from light.

PATIENT TEACHING
• Inform patient that pyrantel may be taken with food, milk, or fruit juices; however, it may decrease appetite if taken before meals.
• Instruct patient to shake suspension well.
• Teach patient about personal hygiene, especially good handwashing technique. To avoid reinfection, teach patient to wash perianal area daily, to change undergarments and bedclothes daily, and to wash hands and clean fingernails before meals and after bowel movements.
• Advise patient to refrain from preparing food for others.
• Tell patient to take entire dose as prescribed.
• Inform parent or caregiver that safety and efficacy haven't been established for children younger than age 2.
• Instruct breast-feeding patient that safety hasn't been estab-

lished; advise her to consult a doctor before taking this drug.

---

ranitidine hydrochloride
Zantac 75

Pregnancy Risk Category B

HOW SUPPLIED
Tablets: 75 mg

ACTION
Competitively inhibits action of H_2 at receptor sites of the parietal cells, decreasing gastric acid secretion.

Route	Onset	Peak	Duration
P.O.	1 hr	1-3 hr	13 hr

INDICATIONS & DOSAGES
Relief from heartburn—
Adults: 75 mg P.O. daily or b.i.d. Don't exceed 150 mg daily.

Prevention of heartburn—
Adults: 75 mg, 30 to 60 minutes before meals. Don't exceed 150 mg daily.

ADVERSE REACTIONS
CNS: vertigo, malaise, headache.
EENT: blurred vision.
GU: increased serum creatinine levels.
Hematologic: *reversible leukopenia, pancytopenia.*

Hepatic: elevated liver enzymes, jaundice.
Skin: rash.
Other: *anaphylaxis, angioedema.*

INTERACTIONS
Drug-drug
Antacids: may interfere with ranitidine absorption. Advise patient to separate doses, if possible.
Diazepam: decreases absorption of diazepam. Monitor patient closely.
Glipizide: may increase hypoglycemic effect. Adjust glipizide dosage, as needed.
Procainamide: may decrease renal clearance of procainamide. Monitor patient closely for toxicity.
Warfarin: may interfere with warfarin clearance. Monitor patient closely.

Drug-lifestyle
Smoking: may increase gastric secretion and worsen disease. Advise patient to avoid smoking.

CONTRAINDICATIONS
Contraindicated in patients who are hypersensitive to drug.

OVERDOSE & TREATMENT
No cases of overdose have been reported. However, treatment would involve emesis or gastric

---

Reactions may be *common*, uncommon, *life-threatening*, or COMMON AND LIFE-THREATENING.

lavage and supportive measures, as needed. Drug is removed by hemodialysis.

NURSING CONSIDERATIONS
- Use cautiously in patients with hepatic dysfunction and impaired renal function.
- Adjust dosage in patients with impaired hepatic or renal function, as ordered.
- Assess patient for abdominal pain. Note presence of blood in emesis, stool, or gastric aspirate.
- Drug may cause false-positive results in urine protein tests using Multistix.
- *Alert:* Don't confuse ranitidine with ritodrine or rimantadine; or Zantac with Xanax.

PATIENT TEACHING
- Instruct patient on proper use of preparation. If patient is taking a single dose, advise him to do so at bedtime.
- Instruct patient not to take product for longer than 2 weeks without medical supervision.
- Instruct patient to take without regard to meals because absorption isn't affected by food.
- Instruct patient not to take other acid-reducing drugs along with ranitidine.
- Advise patient to swallow tablet whole, instead of chewing it.

- Urge patient to avoid cigarette smoking because it may increase gastric acid secretion and worsen disease.
- Advise patient to report abdominal pain and blood in stool or emesis.
- Inform elderly patient of increased risk for adverse effects; emphasize importance of regular follow-up visits with the doctor.
- Inform breast-feeding patient that drug is excreted in breast milk; she should contact the doctor before taking this drug.

---

senna
Agoral, Black-Draught, Ex-lax, Fletcher's Castoria, Nature's Way, Senexon, Senna-Gen, Senokot, Senokotxtra, X-Prep Liquid*

Pregnancy Risk Category C

HOW SUPPLIED
Capsules: 10 mg
Tablets: 6 mg, 8.6 mg, 15 mg, 17 mg, 25 mg
Granules: 15 mg/5 ml, 20 mg/5 ml
Liquid: 25 mg/15 ml, 33 mg/ml
Syrup: 8.8 mg/5 ml
Suppositories: 30 mg

ACTION
Unknown. Stimulant laxative that increases peristalsis, proba-

bly by direct effect on smooth muscle of the intestine. It's thought to either irritate the musculature or stimulate the colonic intramural plexus. Drug also promotes fluid accumulation in colon and small intestine.

Route	Onset	Peak	Duration
P.O.	6-10 hr	Variable	Variable

INDICATIONS & DOSAGES
For use as a laxative—
Adults and children ages 12 and older: 12 to 50 mg of sennosides once daily or b.i.d.; 30 mg P.R. once daily or b.i.d.
Children ages 6 to 11: 50% of adult dosage.
Children ages 1 to 5: 33% of adult dosage.

For use as a bowel evacuative—
Adults: a standardized dose of senna fruit extract or concentrate to provide 105 to 157.5 mg of sennosides given 12 to 14 hours before the procedure.

ADVERSE REACTIONS
GI: nausea; vomiting; diarrhea; loss of normal bowel function with excessive use; abdominal cramps, especially in severe constipation; malabsorption of nutrients; cathartic colon (syndrome radiologically resembling ulcerative colitis) with long-term misuse; possible constipation after catharsis; yellow or yellow-green cast to feces; diarrhea in breast-feeding infants of mothers receiving senna; darkened pigmentation of rectal mucosa with long-term use (usually reversible 4 to 12 months after stopping drug); protein-losing enteropathy; laxative dependence with excessive use.
GU: red-pink discoloration in alkaline urine; yellow-brown discoloration in acidic urine.
Metabolic: electrolyte imbalance, such as hypokalemia.

INTERACTIONS
None significant.

CONTRAINDICATIONS
Contraindicated in patients with ulcerative bowel lesions; nausea, vomiting, abdominal pain, or other symptoms of appendicitis or acute surgical abdomen; fecal impaction; or intestinal obstruction or perforation. Also contraindicated in patients who are hypersensitive to the drug.

OVERDOSE & TREATMENT
Long-term use or overdose may cause diarrhea, hypokalemia, loss of essential nutrients and dehydration.

Treatment is symptomatic.

NURSING CONSIDERATIONS
- Before taking for constipation, patient should have adequate fluid intake, exercise, and diet.
- Limit diet to clear liquids after X-Prep Liquid is taken.
- Product shouldn't be exposed to excessive heat or light.
- Drug is used for short-term therapy.
- Senna is one of the most effective laxatives for counteracting constipation caused by narcotic analgesics.
- In phenolsulfonphthalein excretion test, senna may turn urine pink to red, red to violet, or red to brown.
- Infant of breast-feeding patient using senna may develop diarrhea.
- Elderly patient may be more prone to laxative dependency than younger patient.

PATIENT TEACHING
- Tell patient to follow instructions provided with product, because dosages vary depending on product used.
- Teach patient about dietary sources of bulk, including bran and other cereals, fresh fruit, and vegetables.
- Tell patient to take drug with plenty of water.
- Tell patient to report persistent or severe reactions.
- Warn patient that drug may turn urine pink, red, violet, or brown, depending on urinary pH.
- Instruct patient that laxative use shouldn't exceed 1 week. Excessive use may result in dependence or electrolyte imbalance.
- Tell patient that bowel movement may have a yellow or yellow-green cast.
- Advise elderly patient that he may be more prone to laxative dependency than younger patient.
- Inform parents or caregiver that these products aren't usually given to children.

---

simethicone
Alka-Seltzer Gas Relief, Flatulex, GasAid, Gas-X, Gas-X Extra Strength, Gerber Gas Drops, Infant's Mylicon Drops, Maalox Anti-Gas Tablets, Mylanta Gas, Mylanta Gas Maximum Strength, Ovol†, Ovol-40†, Ovol-80†, Phazyme, Phazyme 95, Phazyme 125 Maximum Strength

Pregnancy Risk Category C

HOW SUPPLIED
Tablets: 40 mg, 55 mg , 60 mg, 80 mg, 95 mg, 125 mg
Capsules: 125 mg
Capsules (softgel): 125 mg
Drops: 40 mg/0.6 ml

ACTION
By its defoaming action, drug disperses or prevents formation of mucus-surrounded gas pockets in the GI tract.

Route	Onset	Peak	Duration
P.O.	Immediate	Immediate	Unknown

INDICATIONS & DOSAGES
Flatulence, functional gastric bloating—
Adults and children older than age 12: 40 to 125 mg P.O. after each meal and h.s., up to 500 mg daily.
Adults (drops): 40 to 80 mg P.O. after each meal and h.s., up to 500 mg daily.
Children ages 2 to 12 (drops): 40 mg (0.6 ml) after each meal and h.s. Maximum 12 doses daily.
Children younger than age 2 (drops): 20 mg (0.3 ml) after each meal and h.s. Maximum 12 doses daily.

ADVERSE REACTIONS
GI: expulsion of excessive liberated gas as belching, rectal flatus.

INTERACTIONS
Drug-drug
Alginic acid: may decrease the effectiveness of this drug. Advise patient to avoid using together.

CONTRAINDICATIONS
Contraindicated in patients who are hypersensitive to drug.

OVERDOSE & TREATMENT
No information available.

NURSING CONSIDERATIONS
• Drug isn't recommended for treating infant colic because of limited information on safety in children.
• Drug doesn't prevent formation of gas.
• ***Alert:*** Don't confuse simethicone with cimetidine.

PATIENT TEACHING
• Tell patient taking chewable tablet form to chew tablet thoroughly before swallowing.
• Advise patient to change position often and ambulate to aid flatus passage.
• Instruct parent to consult doctor before giving drug to child.
• Instruct patient or parent to inform a doctor promptly of adverse effects.
• Tell parent that infant drops can be mixed with 1 oz of cool water, infant formula, or other liquid.

---

sodium citrate (citrate salts)
Citra pH

Pregnancy Risk Category C

HOW SUPPLIED
Solution: 450 mg sodium citrate (105 mg sodium/5 ml)

ACTION
Antacids neutralize gastric acid, thereby leading to an increase in the pH of the stomach and duodenal bulb. Antacids also increase the tone of the lower esophagus and may have astringent properties.

Route	Onset	Peak	Duration
P.O.	Rapid	Unknown	20 min-3 hr

INDICATIONS & DOSAGES
Symptomatic relief of upset stomach associated with hyperacidity (heartburn, gastroesophageal reflux, acid indigestion, sour stomach)—
Adults: 30 ml P.O. daily (dilute with 30 to 90 ml water).

ADVERSE REACTIONS
Other: milk-alkali syndrome (headache, nausea, irritability, and weakness).

INTERACTIONS
Drug-drug
Oral drugs: antacids may alter the absorption of other drugs when given together. Antacids should be given 2 hours before or after the administration of other drugs.

CONTRAINDICATIONS
Contraindicated in patients on a sodium-restricted diet and in patients with severe renal dysfunction.

OVERDOSE & TREATMENT
Large doses of antacids may result in metabolic alkalosis. Supportive care involves respiratory control. Rebreathing of the patient's expired air may be helpful initially. Calcium gluconate may be needed to control tetany if severe alkalosis occurs.

NURSING CONSIDERATIONS
• Use cautiously in patients with renal dysfunction, heart failure, hypertension, peripheral or pulmonary edema, or toxemia of pregnancy.
• Assess renal function before starting drug.
• The sodium content may be significant for patients with high blood pressure.
• Dilute with 30 to 90 ml of water before administering orally.
• Wait 2 hours before or after regularly scheduled prescription drugs before administering antacids.
• Notify doctor if relief isn't obtained or if signs and symptoms of GI bleeding occur.

---

*Liquid contains alcohol.   **May contain tartrazine.   †Canada   ‡Australia   §U.K.

PATIENT TEACHING

- Tell patient not to take prescription drugs within 2 hours of antacids.
- Tell patient to notify doctor immediately if patient experiences black, tarry stools or vomit that resembles coffee grounds.
- If patient has high blood pressure, advise patient to monitor blood pressure closely because of the high sodium content in sodium citrate preparations.
- Have patient notify doctor if signs and symptoms of milk alkali syndrome appear (headache, nausea, irritability, weakness).
- Inform patient that taking excessive amounts of antacids may cause the stomach to eventually produce larger amounts of gastric acid. Tell patient not to use the maximum dose of antacids for longer than 2 weeks.

---

sodium phosphates
Fleet Enema, Fleet Pediatric Enema, Fleet Phospho-Soda

Pregnancy Risk Category NR

HOW SUPPLIED
Liquid: 2.4 g/5 ml sodium phosphate and 900 mg sodium biphosphate/5 ml
Enema: 160 mg/ml sodium phosphate and 60 mg/ml sodium biphosphate

ACTION
Saline laxative that produces an osmotic effect in the small intestine by drawing water into the intestinal lumen.

Route	Onset	Peak	Duration
P.O.	0.5-3 hr	Variable	Variable
P.R.	5-10 min	Variable	Variable

INDICATIONS & DOSAGES
Constipation; preparation for surgery or endoscopic exam; P.R. as enema—
Adults and children ages 12 and older: 1 adult bottle (133 ml) P.R. as enema.
Children ages 5 to 11: 1 children's bottle (66 ml) P.R. as enema.
Children ages 2 to 5: Prepare ½ children's bottle by unscrewing cap and removing 2 tbs of liquid with measuring spoon. Replace cap and give remaining liquid in bottle P.R. as enema.

Constipation; preparation for surgery or endoscopic exam; P.O.—
Adults and children ages 12 and older: 20 to 45 ml (4 to 9 tsp) P.O. diluted in 4 oz water. Follow with 8 oz water.
Children ages 10 to 11: 10 to 20 ml (2 to 4 tsp) P.O. diluted in 4 oz water. Follow with 8 oz water.
Children ages 5 to 9: 5 to 10 ml (1 to 2 tsp) P.O. diluted in

4 oz water. Follow with 8 oz water.

ADVERSE REACTIONS
GI: abdominal cramping, laxative dependence with long-term or excessive use.
GU: rectal irritation (bleeding, itching, burning) with enema preparations.
Metabolic: fluid and electrolyte disturbances, such as hypernatremia and hyperphosphatemia, with daily use; hypocalcemia.

INTERACTIONS
None significant.

CONTRAINDICATIONS
Contraindicated in patients with abdominal pain, nausea, vomiting, or other symptoms of appendicitis or acute surgical abdomen; intestinal obstruction or perforation; edema; heart failure; megacolon; or impaired renal function; also contraindicated in patients on sodium-restricted diets.

OVERDOSE & TREATMENT
Overdose, or retention of enema, may cause hypocalcemia, hyperphosphatemia, hypernatremia, dehydration, and acidosis.

To treat, monitor electrolyte levels, correct imbalance, and give fluids for dehydration.

NURSING CONSIDERATIONS
• Use cautiously in patients with large hemorrhoids or anal excoriations, in patients with impaired renal function, electrolyte disturbances, colostomy, or in patients on diuretics or other drugs that may affect electrolyte levels.
• Before giving for constipation, determine if patient has adequate fluid intake, exercise, and diet.
• *Alert:* Up to 10% of sodium content of drug may be absorbed.
• *Alert:* Severe electrolyte imbalances may occur if recommended dosage is exceeded.
• Patient shouldn't use adult-size enema in children younger than age 12 or full child-size enema in children younger than age 5.
• The enema for adults contains 191 mEq sodium and 95.5 mEq for children's enema.

PATIENT TEACHING
• Tell patient to follow closely directions provided with enema to reduce risk of injury.
• Tell patient to take oral form on empty stomach, upon rising, at least 30 minutes before eating, or at bedtime.
• Teach patient about dietary sources of bulk, including bran and other cereals, fresh fruit, and vegetables.

• Warn patient about adverse reactions and stress importance of using drug only for short-term therapy.

• Instruct patient to report adverse reactions promptly to doctor.

• Tell patient to notify doctor if there's no return of liquid after enema.

• Tell patient not to use with nausea, vomiting, abdominal pain, or a sudden change in bowel movements lasting for longer than 2 weeks.

• Advise patient to notify the doctor if rectal bleeding occurs, or if bowel movement doesn't occur.

---

witch hazel (hamamelis water)*
A•E•R, Preparation H Medicated Wipes, Tucks Hemorrhoidal*, Witch Hazel*

Pregnancy Risk Category NR

HOW SUPPLIED
Liquid (various strengths)
Cream: 50%
Premoistened pads: 50%

ACTION
Witch hazel is a mild astringent made from the twigs and branches of *Hamamelis virginiana*. Astringents cause contraction and wrinkling of tissues and work to decrease local edema, inflammation, and exudation.

Route	Onset	Peak	Duration
Topical	Unknown	Unknown	Unknown

INDICATIONS & DOSAGES
Temporary relief of anal irritation or itching, hemorrhoids, or posthemorrhoidectomy discomfort, vaginal infection, postepisiotomy discomfort—
Adults and children ages 12 and older: apply up to six times daily—in the morning, evening, and after each bowel movement.

ADVERSE REACTIONS
Other: itching, burning.

INTERACTIONS
Drug-drug
MAO inhibitors, tricyclic antidepressants: combination products containing vasoconstrictors (phenylephrine) interact with these drugs. Advise patient to avoid using together, if possible; if drugs must be used together, monitor patient closely.

CONTRAINDICATIONS
Patients taking MAO inhibitors shouldn't take combination products containing phenylephrine.

Reactions may be *common*, uncommon, *life-threatening*, or COMMON AND LIFE-THREATENING.

OVERDOSE & TREATMENT
Little information is available on the signs and symptoms of overdoses of witch hazel.

Because the product contains alcohol, treatment would involve respiratory and cardiac support. Gastric lavage may be useful in certain patients. Emesis or activated charcoal isn't recommended.

NURSING CONSIDERATIONS
• If patient is taking prescription drugs for high blood pressure or depression, consult doctor before using combination products containing phenylephrine or other vasoconstrictors.
• Patient should be taught proper use of drug.
• If condition doesn't improve or worsens within 7 days, patient should consult doctor.
• If bleeding occurs, patient should contact doctor immediately.
• Product is for external use only; patient should avoid contact with the eyes.
• Safety in pregnant and breast-feeding patients hasn't been established; patient should consult a doctor before taking this drug.

PATIENT TEACHING
• Tell patient to clean the affected area with mild soap and warm water, rinse thoroughly, and dry gently by patting or blotting with toilet tissue or soft cloth before using product. Instruct him to apply drug by patting affected area.
• Tell patient that this product is for external use only; he should avoid drug contact with eyes.
• Tell patient to contact doctor immediately if bleeding, protrusion, or seepage occurs.
• Tell patient to consult a doctor if condition doesn't improve or worsens within 7 days, or if moderate to severe pain occurs or continues.

Combination products

Brand name and active ingredients	Indications and dosages	Nursing considerations
Alka-Seltzer Antacid Gold • citric acid 832 mg • potassium bicarbonate 312 mg • sodium bicarbonate 958 mg	*Heartburn, acid indigestion, and sour stomach* **Adults:** 2 tablets P.O. every 4 hours p.r.n. Maximum 8 tablets daily. Maximum 6 tablets daily in adults ages 60 and older. **Children:** ½ of adult dose. Maximum 4 tablets daily.	• Have patient dissolve in 4-oz glass of water before taking. • Tell patient not to take if he is taking prescription drugs, unless directed by a doctor. • Tell patient not to use maximum dose for longer than 2 weeks. • Advise patient not to use if he's on a sodium-restricted diet.
Alka-Seltzer Tablets • aspirin 325 mg • citric acid 1,000 mg • sodium bicarbonate 1,700 mg **Alka-Seltzer Original** • aspirin 325 mg • citric acid 1,000 mg • sodium bicarbonate 1,916 mg **Alka-Seltzer–Extra Strength** • aspirin 500 mg • citric acid 1,000 mg • sodium bicarbonate 1,916 mg	*Heartburn, acid indigestion, sour stomach with headache or body aches and pains; upset stomach with headache from overindulgence in food or drink* **Adults:** dissolve 2 tablets in 4 oz water and drink every 4 hours p.r.n. Maximum 8 doses daily. Maximum 4 doses daily in adults ages 60 and older.	• Tell patient not to take if also taking prescription drugs unless directed by a doctor, especially drugs for thinning of the blood, diabetes, gout, or arthritis. • Tell patients to avoid using to treat chickenpox or flu symptoms in children or adolescents. • Advise patients not to use during the last 3 months of pregnancy. • Tell patient not to use maximum dose for longer than 10 days. • Patient who is allergic to aspirin, who has asthma or bleeding problems, who's on a sodium-restricted diet or consumes more than 3 alcoholic drinks per day should avoid use unless directed by a doctor.

Combination products (continued)

Brand name and active ingredients	Indications and dosages	Nursing considerations
Alka-Seltzer Tablets (continued)		• Tell patient to discontinue use and notify a doctor if ringing in ears or hearing loss, persistent or worsening pain, new symptoms, or redness or swelling occurs. • Drug contains phenylalanine.
Anusol • mineral oil • pramoxine hydrochloride 1% • zinc oxide 12.5%	*Pain, soreness, burning, and itching from hemorrhoids and other anorectal disorders; forms protective coating over inflamed tissues to help prevent drying* **Adults:** apply to affected area up to 5 times daily (morning, evening, and after bowel movements).	• Teach patient to clean affected area with soap and water and blot or pat dry before use. • Have patient report symptoms that are new or worsening or that persist for longer than 1 week and to report any bleeding, redness, irritation, swelling, or pain. • Tell patient not to exceed recommended dose. • Tell patient not to put product into rectum.
Di-Gel • calcium carbonate 280 mg • magnesium hydroxide 128 mg • simethicone 20 mg	*Indigestion, heartburn, sour stomach, and gas* **Adults:** 2 to 4 tablets P.O. every 2 hours after or between meals and h.s. Maximum 24 tablets daily.	• Have patient consult a doctor before taking, if also taking prescription drugs. • Tell patient not to use maximum dose for longer than 2 weeks. • Alert patient with kidney disease to avoid this product unless directed by a doctor. • May cause constipation or diarrhea.

(continued)

Combination products *(continued)*

Brand name and active ingredients	Indications and dosages	Nursing considerations
Fleet Medicated Pre-Moistened Rectal/Vaginal Pads • alcohol 7% • glycerin 10% • witch hazel 50%	*External itching, burning, and irritation from hemorrhoids and other anorectal disorders* **Adults and children ages 12 and older:** apply to affected area up to 6 times daily.	• Teach patient to clean affected area with soap and water and to blot or pat dry before use. • Tell patient not to exceed recommended dose. • Tell patient not to put product into rectum. • Tell patient to report symptoms that worsen or persist for longer than 1 week, and any bleeding.
Fleet Pain Relief Pads • glycerin 12% • pramoxine hydrochloride 1%	*Pain, soreness, and burning from hemorrhoids and other anorectal irritations; protects inflamed skin* **Adults:** apply to affected area up to 5 times daily (morning, evening, and after bowel movements).	• Teach patient to clean affected area with soap and water and to blot or pat dry before use. • Tell patient to report new or worsening symptoms; symptoms persisting for longer than 1 week; and bleeding, redness, irritation, swelling, or pain. • Tell patient not to exceed recommended dose. • Tell patient not to put product into rectum.
Gaviscon Extra Strength Liquid Antacid • aluminum hydroxide 508 mg/ 10 ml • magnesium carbonate 475 mg/ 10 ml	*Heartburn, sour stomach, acid indigestion, and upset stomach* **Adults and children ages 12 and older:** 2 to 4 tsp q.i.d., or as directed by a doctor.	• Advise patient to take drug after meals or at bedtime, followed by ½ glass of water. • Tell patient not to take more than 16 tsp in 24 hours or 16 tsp daily for longer than 2 weeks, unless otherwise directed by a doctor. • Warn patient with kidney disease not to use. • Tell patient that this product may have a laxative effect. • Tell patient on sodium restriction not to use this product ex-

Combination products (continued)

Brand name and active ingredients	Indications and dosages	Nursing considerations
Gaviscon Extra Strength Liquid Antacid *(continued)*		cept under the advice and supervision of a doctor. Each tsp contains 0.9 mEq sodium. • Antacids may interact with certain prescription drugs. Tell patient not to take with prescription drugs unless directed by a doctor. • Tell patient on sodium restriction not to use this product except under the advice and supervision of a doctor. Each tbs contains 1.7 mEq sodium.
Gaviscon Regular Strength Liquid Antacid • aluminum hydroxide 95 mg/15 ml • magnesium carbonate 358 mg/ 15 ml	*Heartburn, sour stomach, acid indigestion, and upset stomach* **Adults and children ages 12 and older:** 1 or 2 tbs q.i.d. or as directed by a doctor.	• Instruct patient to take after meals or h.s., followed by 1½ glasses of water. • Tell patient not to take more than 8 tbs in 24 hours or 8 tbs daily for longer than 2 weeks. • Tell patient with kidney disease not to use this drug unless directed by a doctor. • Tell patient that this drug may have a laxative effect. • Antacids may interact with certain prescription drugs. Tell patient not to take with prescription drugs unless directed by a doctor.
Gaviscon Regular Strength Tablets • aluminum hydroxide 80 mg • magnesium trisilicate 20 mg	*Heartburn, sour stomach, acid indigestion, and upset stomach associated with these conditions*	• Inform patient that each regular-strength tablet contains 0.8 mEq sodium. Each extra-strength tablet contains approximately 1.3 mEq sodium. • Tell patient on sodium restriction not to use this product unless directed by a doctor. • Tell patient to take drug after meals and at bedtime, or p.r.n.

(continued)

Combination products *(continued)*

Brand name and active ingredients	Indications and dosages	Nursing considerations
Gaviscon Extra Strength Tablets *(continued)* • aluminum hydroxide 160 mg • magnesium carbonate 105 mg	**Adults and children ages 12 and older:** chew 2 to 4 tablets q.i.d., or as directed by a doctor.	• Tell patient to follow tablet with ½ glass of water or other liquid. • Tell patient not to swallow tablet whole. • Antacids may interact with certain prescription drugs. Tell patient not to take with prescription drugs unless directed by a doctor. • Tell patient not to take more than 16 tablets in a 24-hr period or 16 tablets daily for longer than 2 weeks, unless directed by a doctor.
Gelusil • aluminum hydroxide 200 mg • magnesium hydroxide 200 mg • simethicone 20 mg	*Heartburn, sour stomach, acid indigestion, and gas* **Adults:** 2 to 4 tablets P.O. 1 hour after meals and h.s. Maximum 12 tablets daily.	• Tell patient not to take with prescription drugs unless directed by a doctor. • Tell patient not to use maximum dose for longer than 2 weeks. • Tell patient with kidney disease not to use drug unless directed by a doctor.
Hemorrhoid Cream • phenylephrine 0.25% • pramoxine hydrochloride 1% • mineral oil 20% • white petrolatum 30% **Hemorrhoid Ointment** • light mineral oil 12.5% • phenylephrine 0.25% • pramoxine hydrochloride 1%	*Shrinkage of swollen tissue; relief from pain, burning, itching, and discomfort from hemorrhoids and anorectal irritation* **Adults and children ages 12 and older:** apply to affected area up to 5 times daily (morning, eve-	• Teach patient to clean affected area with soap and water and to blot or pat dry before use. • Tell patient not to take with prescription drugs for hypertension or depression, unless directed by a doctor. • Tell patient to report new or worsening symptoms or symptoms that persist for longer than 1 week and also to report any bleeding, redness, irritation, swelling, or pain. • Tell patient not to exceed recommended dose.

Combination products *(continued)*

Brand name and active ingredients	Indications and dosages	Nursing considerations
Hemorrhoid Ointment *(continued)* • white petrolatum 82.15%	ning, and after bowel movements).	• Tell patient not to put product into rectum. • Tell patient with heart disease, hypertension, thyroid disease, diabetes, or difficulty urinating because of enlarged prostate not to use drug unless directed by a doctor.
Imodium Advanced • loperamide 2 mg • simethicone 125 mg	*Controls symptoms of diarrhea, bloating, pressure, and cramps* **Adults and children ages 12 and older:** 2 tablets P.O. after first loose stool, then 1 tablet after next loose stool. Maximum 4 tablets daily. **Children ages 9 to 11 (60 to 95 lb):** 1 tablet P.O. after first loose stool, then ½ tablet P.O. after next loose stool. Maximum 3 tablets daily. **Children ages 6 to 8 (48 to 59 lb):** 1 tableP.O. after first loose stool, then ½ tablet P.O. after next loose stool.	• Tell patient to take each dose with water. • Inform patient that drug may cause drowsiness or dizziness. • Tell patient to use caution when driving or performing tasks that require mental alertness until effects are known. • Tell patient to drink plenty of clear fluids to prevent dehydration. • Have patient notify doctor if diarrhea is persistent or if abdominal pain, distention, or fever occurs. • Tell patient not to exceed recommended dose. • Tell patient not to take drug if he has a fever over 101° F (38.3° C), blood or mucus in stool, or history of rash or other allergic reaction to loperamide. • Tell patient not to use for longer than 2 days if he's taking an antibiotic or has a history of liver disease, unless directed by a doctor.

(continued)

Combination products *(continued)*

Brand name and active ingredients	Indications and dosages	Nursing considerations
Imodium Advanced *(continued)*	Maximum 2 tablets daily.	
Maalox • aluminum hydroxide 225 mg/5 ml • magnesium hydroxide 200 mg/5 ml	*Acid indigestion, heartburn, sour stomach, and upset stomach* **Adults:** 4 tsp P.O. q.i.d. Maximum 12 tsp daily.	• Tell patient not to take with prescription drugs unless directed by a doctor. • Tell patient not to use maximum dose for longer than 2 weeks. • Tell patient with kidney disease not to use drug unless directed by a doctor.
Maalox Anti-Gas • aluminum hydroxide 500 mg/5 ml • magnesium hydroxide 450 mg/5 ml • simethicone 40 mg/5 ml	*Heartburn, sour stomach, acid indigestion, gas, and upset stomach* **Adults:** 2 to 4 tsp P.O. q.i.d. Maximum 12 tsp daily.	
Mylanta Gelcaps • calcium carbonate 550 mg • magnesium hydroxide 125 mg	*Indigestion, heartburn, sour stomach, upset stomach, or symptoms of overindulgence in food or drink* **Adults:** 2 to 4 gelcaps P.O. p.r.n. Maximum 24 gelcaps daily.	• Tell patient not to take with prescription drugs unless directed by a doctor. • Tell patient with kidney disease not to use drug unless directed by a doctor.
Mylanta Supreme • calcium carbonate 400 mg/5 ml • magnesium hydroxide 135 mg/5 ml	*Indigestion, heartburn, sour stomach, upset stomach, or symptoms of overindulgence in food or drink*	• Inform patient that refrigeration of drug may improve flavor. • Tell patient not to take with prescription drugs unless directed by a doctor. • Tell patient not to use maximum dose for longer than 2 weeks.

Combination products *(continued)*

Brand name and active ingredients	Indications and dosages	Nursing considerations
Mylanta Supreme *(continued)*	**Adults:** 2 to 4 tsp P.O. between meals and h.s. Maximum 18 tsp daily.	• Tell patient with kidney disease not to use drug unless directed by a doctor.
Mylanta Tablets • calcium carbonate 350 mg • magnesium hydroxide 150 mg **Mylanta Maximum Strength Tablets** • calcium carbonate 700 mg • magnesium hydroxide 300 mg	*Indigestion, heartburn, sour stomach, upset stomach, or symptoms of overindulgence in food or drink* **Adults:** 2 to 4 tablets P.O. between meals and h.s. Maximum 20 regular-strength or 10 maximum-strength tablets daily.	• Tell patient not to take with prescription drugs unless directed by a doctor. • Tell patient not to use maximum dose for longer than 2 weeks. • Tell patient with kidney disease not to use drug unless directed by a doctor.
Pepcid Complete • calcium carbonate 800 mg • famotidine 10 mg • magnesium hydroxide 165 mg	*Heartburn from acid indigestion and sour stomach* **Adults and children ages 12 and older:** 1 tablet P.O. when symptoms occur. Maximum 2 tablets daily.	• Tell patient not to use drug if he's allergic to famotidine or other acid reducers or if he has difficulty swallowing. • Instruct patient to avoid use with other products containing famotidine or other acid reducers. • Tell patient not to take with prescription drugs unless directed by a doctor. • Have patient discontinue use and notify a doctor if pain continues or symptoms last for longer than 2 weeks. • Tell patient to chew tablets completely and not to swallow tablets whole.

(continued)

Combination products *(continued)*

Brand name and active ingredients	Indications and dosages	Nursing considerations
Perdiem Overnight Relief • psyllium 3.25 g/tsp • senna 0.74 g/tsp	*Constipation* **Adults and children ages 12 and older:** 1 to 2 tsp P.O. daily to b.i.d. **Children ages 7 to 11:** 1 tsp P.O. daily to b.i.d. *Severe constipation* **Adults and children ages 12 and older:** 2 tsp P.O. every 6 hours. Maximum 5 tsp daily.	• Tell patient to take with 8-oz glass of water or other liquid, to decrease risk of choking. • Tell patient not to chew tablet. • Tell patient not to use drug if he has difficulty swallowing or esophageal narrowing. • Tell patient to discontinue use and notify doctor if he has chest pain, vomiting, difficulty swallowing, or difficulty breathing after taking drug; if symptoms are no better in 1 week; or if rectal bleeding occurs. • Tell patient not to use drug if he's allergic to psyllium.
Preparation H Cooling Gel • phenylephrine 0.25% • witch hazel 50%	*Local itching and discomfort from hemorrhoids; shrinks hemorrhoidal tissue; protects irritated anorectal areas* **Adults and children ages 12 and older:** apply externally to the affected area up to q.i.d., usually in morning, evening, and after each bowel movement.	• Teach patient to clean affected area with soap and water and to blot or pat dry before use. • Tell patient not to exceed recommended dose. • Tell patient not to put product into rectum. • Tell patient not to take with prescription drugs for hypertension or depression unless directed by a doctor. • Tell patient not to use drug if he has heart disease, hypertension, thyroid disease, diabetes, or difficulty urinating because of enlarged prostate, unless directed by a doctor.

Combination products *(continued)*

Brand name and active ingredients	Indications and dosages	Nursing considerations
Riopan Plus • magaldrate 540 mg/5 ml • simethicone 40 mg/5 ml **Riopan Plus Double Strength** • magaldrate 1080 mg/5 ml • simethicone 40 mg/5 ml	*Heartburn, sour stomach, acid indigestion, upset stomach from overindulgence in food and drink, and gas* **Adults:** 1 to 2 tsp P.O. between meals and h.s. Maximum 12 tsp daily.	• Tell patient that refrigeration improves drug's taste. • Tell patient not to take with prescription drugs unless directed by a doctor. • Tell patient not to use maximum dose for longer than 2 weeks. • Tell patient with kidney disease not to use drug unless directed by a doctor.
Rolaids • calcium carbonate 550 mg • magnesium hydroxide 110 mg **Rolaids Extra Strength** • calcium carbonate 675 mg • magnesium hydroxide 135 mg	*Heartburn, sour stomach, acid indigestion, and upset stomach* **Adults:** 1 to 4 regular-strength tablets or 2 to 4 extra-strength tablets P.O. as symptoms occur. Repeat hourly p.r.n. Maximum 10 extra-strength or 12 regular-strength tablets daily.	• Tell patient not to take with prescription drugs unless directed by a doctor. • Tell patient not to use maximum dose for longer than 2 weeks.
Senokot-S • docusate sodium 50 mg • sennosides 8.6 mg	*Constipation* **Adults and children ages 12 and older:** 2 tablets P.O. daily. Maximum 4 tablets b.i.d. **Children ages**	• Tell patient to take at bedtime. • Tell patient not to take with abdominal pain, nausea, or vomiting unless directed by a doctor. • Have patient discontinue use and notify a doctor if symptoms are no better in 1 week or if rectal bleeding occurs. *(continued)*

Combination products *(continued)*

Brand name and active ingredients	Indications and dosages	Nursing considerations
Senokot-S *(continued)*	**6 to 11:** 1 tablet P.O. daily. Maximum 2 tablets b.i.d. **Children ages 2 to 5:** ½ tablet P.O. daily. Maximum 1 tablet b.i.d.	
Tempo • aluminum hydroxide 200 mg • magnesium hydroxide 200 mg • simethicone 25 mg	*Heartburn, sour stomach, acid indigestion, gas, and upset stomach* **Adults:** 1 to 4 tablets P.O. q.i.d. Maximum 16 tablets daily.	• Tell patient not to take with prescription drugs unless directed by a doctor. • Tell patient not to use maximum dose for longer than 2 weeks. • Tell patient with kidney disease not to use drug unless directed by a doctor. • Product contains phenylalanine.
Titralac Plus • calcium carbonate 420 mg • simethicone 21 mg	*Heartburn, sour stomach, acid indigestion, and symptoms associated with gas* **Adults:** 2 tablets P.O. every 2 to 3 hours as symptoms occur. Maximum 19 tablets daily.	• Tell patient not to take with prescription drugs unless directed by a doctor. • Tell patient not to use maximum dose for longer than 2 weeks. • Tell patient to chew, swallow, or allow tablet to dissolve in mouth.

6

Genitourinary system

The genitourinary (GU) system consists of the reproductive and urinary systems and serves two independent functions: reproduction and elimination of renal filtrates (urine). Except for the male urethra, the normal internal reproductive and urinary systems are associated only by proximity. The external portions of the two systems are associated by the location of the urethral meatus in the external genitalia. This logistical association leaves both systems vulnerable to some of the same pathogens and conditions.

The male and female reproductive systems each supply half of what is needed for conception, and the female provides an environment for gestation with a mechanism for delivery.

The external female reproductive system is made up of the labia majora and labia minora, clitoris, fourchette, fossa navicularis, vestibule, vestibular bulb, Skene's glands, Bartholin's glands, hymen (temporary structure), and vaginal introitus. The internal female reproductive system includes bilateral ovaries (gonads) and fallopian tubes, uterus, and vagina.

Externally, the male reproductive system is made up of the penis, including glans penis, prepuce, and foreskin. Bilateral testicles (gonads), with associated epididymis in the scrotum; bilateral vas deferens, seminal vesicles, and ejaculatory ducts; bilateral Cowper's (bulbourethral) glands; a prostate gland; and a urethra compose the internal male reproductive system.

The normal urinary system includes bilateral kidneys and ureters and a urinary bladder, bladder sphincter, urethra, and urethral meatus. The structure of the urinary system protects the kidneys from invasive pathogens by creating a series of barriers. Urine flows immediately from the kidneys through the ureter and into the bladder. The bladder empties voluntarily through the urethra at intervals.

Treating GU disorders
Patients tend to use OTC drugs to maintain reproductive health, prevent conception, and treat reproductive system and

urinary tract disorders. User privacy, easy access, and reduced expense add to the appeal of OTC drugs for these kinds of disorders. Patients using OTC drugs are usually treating signs and symptoms that are easy to treat at home. By asking during the routine patient assessment what GU conditions the patient is treating with OTC drugs, you can gain critical information about previously unreported or underreported conditions and about chronic GU system problems. A patient with a recurring GU disorder, such as vaginal candidiasis, is more likely to recognize the underlying cause of her signs and symptoms than is a patient having these signs and symptoms for the first time.

When you tell the patient which signs and symptoms he needs to report, you enable him to make informed and appropriate decisions about OTC drug treatment. Although many GU disorders can be successfully treated with OTC drugs, it's wise to give patients guidelines because of the dangers associated with serious GU disorders left untreated or that receive insufficient or delayed treatment.

Signs and symptoms

Signs and symptoms of GU conditions can include lower abdominal pain, back pain, and localized pain. Other signs and symptoms are abnormal urine color or odor, changes of voiding patterns, urinary frequency and urgency, incontinence, abnormal vaginal discharge, menstrual changes, abnormal ejaculation or ejaculatory changes, urethral meatus discharge, swelling, tenderness, and itching, rash, and lesions possibly involving the entire peritoneal area. The sources of these signs and symptoms can range from transient irritation to life-threatening pathogenic disorders.

Common disorders

Pathogenic GU system disorders include urinary tract infection (UTI), inflammation, and obstruction; urethral spasm, kidney stones, neoplasms, trauma-induced changes, fertility problems, coital disorders, impotence, sexually transmitted diseases (STDs), prostate disorders, testicular disorders, menstrual irregularities, uterine disorders, vaginal infections, ovarian conditions, fallopian tube disorders, and disorders of the external genitalia.

Disorders of the GU system are the topic of many popular

advertising campaigns for personal products. Advertisements of some products, such as those for incontinence, can lead patients to believe that some signs and symptoms are unavoidable and to be taken in stride.

Patient teaching
Effective patient teaching during patient assessment promotes the best outcome for patient self-assessment. Encourage patients to investigate OTC products, including herbs and dietary supplements, before use. Inform patients that reactions can occur with the use of OTC products. Local irritation, especially involving mucosal tissue, can leave the patient vulnerable to invasive pathogens. Encourage the patient to read all instructions and product information and to report any adverse reactions.

Contraception
Foam, cream, jelly, and suppository spermicides (nonoxynol 9, octoxynol 9) are used to prevent conception and have a reported failure rate of 2% to 30%. These chemical barrier products also provide limited virucidal and bactericidal activity. Both a mechanical barrier (diaphragm, cervical cap, or condom) and a chemical barri-

er (spermicide) should be used by patients who rely on OTC contraception. Spermicides can be used as back-up contraception during episodes when efficacy of a prescription contraceptive is temporarily compromised (concurrent oral contraceptive and antibiotic therapies, following missed oral contraceptive doses).

Spermicides, which are administered vaginally, create a hostile environment for sperm, reducing the potential for viable sperm to travel past the uterine cervix.

Signs and symptoms
Not applicable.

Serious conditions
Not applicable.

Complications
Vaginal bacterial flora may be altered, allowing for invasive infections and increasing the risk of bacteriuria.

Local irritation caused by product sensitivity can be experienced by either partner.

Nursing considerations
• Sexually active patients at risk for STDs should receive regular testing and evaluation.
• Sexually active patients wishing to prevent conception, and for whom prescription contra-

ceptives are contraindicated, may require additional encouragement to use mechanical and chemical barrier methods.

• Patient assessment should include questions regarding use of OTC contraceptives and the occurrence of any adverse reactions.

Patient teaching

• Make sure the patient understands that contraceptive use reduces but doesn't eliminate the potential for pregnancy and that she should use chemical and mechanical methods concurrently.

• Inform the patient that spermicides should be used in conjunction with a barrier method of contraception and that spermicides don't prevent STDs.

• Instruct the patient to read carefully and adhere to administration and storage instructions. Effectiveness of individual spermicides can vary and depends strongly on a high level of patient compliance.

• Tell patient that vaginally administered products may cause local irritation in either partner. If irritation occurs, patient should stop using the product. If irritation persists, the patient should contact her doctor.

• Inform the patient that vaginal lubricants aren't spermicides.

Vaginal discharge

Abnormal vaginal discharge is produced in the vagina or higher in the reproductive tract. It can result from pregnancy, infection, mechanical irritation (from a tampon), chemical irritation (from a douche), product sensitivity (systemic or vaginally administered drugs), altered vaginal pH, neoplasms, and cervical disorders.

Signs and symptoms

Normal vaginal secretions are part of the self-cleaning properties of the vagina. Consistency and amount of secretions can fluctuate during times of stress or the normal monthly hormonal changes. Large amounts of vaginal discharge with an appearance, consistency, and odor that is different from normal vaginal secretions should alert the patient to signs of trouble. Opacity can range from clear to purulent; color can include white, blood-tinged, yellow, or greenish. Consistency can range from watery to thick and curdlike. Vulvar and perineal irritation may occur as a result of contact with the discharge.

Serious conditions

Untreated or delayed treatment of STDs can result in sterility, cancer of the GU tract, or death. The infected patient's own health, as well as that of anyone who has had sexual contact with the patient, is at risk. Many perinatal infections can also be transmitted to the fetus or newborn.

Abnormal vaginal discharge coupled with postcoital pain and bleeding may be related to cellular invasion and erosion of the cervical epithelium. Self-treatment delays appropriate medical evaluation and intervention.

Complications

Most cleansing preparations make cosmetic claims to soothe, deodorize, or refresh. Overuse of these products can disrupt the normal physiology of the vagina and external genitalia. Some products contain chemicals that irritate the mucosa. Inappropriate use may lead to irritation, burning, swelling, and infection. Douching is also linked to pelvic inflammatory disease (PID) and ectopic pregnancy.

Nursing considerations

- Obtain a thorough history including medical conditions, sexual history, any use of feminine deodorants and frequency of use, as well as any other associated signs and symptoms accompanying the discharge.

- Appropriate feminine hygiene practices, including daily cleansing, preferably with unscented soap, is usually adequate.
- A patient with a history of multiple vaginal yeast infections should contact her doctor for further evaluation.

Patient teaching

- Inform the patient that she should report any change in vaginal discharge and all episodes of self-treatment.
- Untreated STDs in sexually active individuals may expose other individuals to the infection.
- Advise the patient to follow the manufacturer's recommendations for proper use of feminine hygiene products.
- Tell the pregnant patient not to douche unless her doctor advises it.
- Warn the patient with thyroid disorder or iodine allergy that some douche products contain povidone-iodine, which can be absorbed from the vagina.

Itching

Vaginal, pubic, and perineal itching may result from local irritation (urinary incontinence, vaginal discharge), product sensitivity (soaps, personal hygiene products), systemic disorders, parasites, mycotic infection, and drug reactions.

Signs and symptoms

Patients may complain of itchiness in the pubic area, including the vulva and perineum.

Serious conditions

Untreated itchiness in these areas can be caused by pubic lice, STDs, neoplasms, and the disease process.

Complications

Delayed medical evaluation and treatment of STDs, neoplasms, mycotic infection, urinary tract disorders, or other diseases places the patient at risk for greater morbidity and, in some cases, mortality.

Local trauma from scratching makes the patient susceptible to invasive pathogens. Proliferation of pubic lice increases the potential of spreading this infestation to other individuals.

Nursing considerations

• Patients may be reluctant to report both pubic area itchiness and use of OTC drug treatments.
• Obtain a detailed history, including onset, duration, and treatments used.
• Patient assessment should include questions about incontinence and any other urinary tract signs and symptoms.
• Physical examination should include visual check for pubic lice.

Patient teaching

• Inform patient that persistent itching signals an underlying condition that needs treatment; and that, although relief measures can be taken during treatment, the itching will resolve when the underlying condition has resolved.
• Instruct patient to report prolonged episodes of itching to the doctor for further evaluation and treatment.

Dysmenorrhea

Uterine cramps normally occur immediately before and during menses and are often treated successfully with OTC drugs. The increase in oxygen demand of the uterus, caused in part by an increase in frequency of uterine contractions and dysrhythmia of the contractions, produces uterine hypoxia and pain.

Signs and symptoms

Dysmenorrhea may involve sharp, intermittent pain or dull, aching pain. It's usually characterized by mild to severe cramping or colicky pain in the pelvis or lower abdomen that may radiate to the thighs and lower sacrum.

Serious conditions

Any pain should always be thoroughly assessed. Dysmenorrhea may accompany a serious medical condition, one that cannot be treated successfully with OTC drugs. Endometriosis typically produces steady, aching pain that begins before menses and peaks at the height of menstrual flow. Associated signs and symptoms may include premenstrual spotting, dyspareunia, infertility, nausea and vomiting, painful defecation, and rectal bleeding and hematuria with menses. Pelvic inflammatory disease produces dysmenorrhea accompanied by fever; malaise; foul-smelling, purulent vaginal discharge; severe abdominal pain; nausea and vomiting; and diarrhea. Tumors may cause lower abdominal pain that worsens with menses. The pain may be constant or intermittent. Associated signs and symptoms may include backache, constipation, menorrhagia, and if the tumor is large, ureteral obstruction.

Complications

A patient with persistent pain that is unrelieved by the recommended maximum daily dose of OTC pain reliever shouldn't attempt self-treatment, unless advised to do so by the doctor. High doses or unsupervised long-term use of acetaminophen may cause liver damage. NSAIDs can cause GI bleeding, especially when used inappropriately. Some OTC combination products may contain an NSAID or acetaminophen, so the milligram content of all products needs to be considered when calculating the total daily dose consumed.

Nursing considerations

• Obtain a menstrual and sexual history.
• Have the patient describe the pain fully, including quality, location, duration, and relief measures.
• Explore associated signs and symptoms, such as nausea and vomiting, altered bowel or urinary habits, bloating, pelvic or rectal pressure, and unusual fatigue, irritability, or depression.
• Ask about the patient's method of contraception. An intrauterine device may cause severe cramping and heavy menstrual flow.

Patient teaching

• Teach pain relief exercises such relaxation and distraction.
• Encourage the use of a heating pad. Heat reduces abdomi-

nal muscle tension and increases blood flow.

• Inform the patient that a regular schedule of exercise may reduce the level of discomfort.

Urinary tract infection

Urinary tract infections (UTIs) can affect either the lower urinary tract (the urinary bladder and urethra) or the upper urinary tract (the kidney). Inflammation caused by microorganisms usually travels up the urethra, but a UTI could also come from an organism in the bloodstream or lymphatic system that travels directly to the kidney. No OTC cure exists for UTIs, but OTC drugs can relieve bothersome signs and symptoms of this condition.

Signs and symptoms

The classic symptom experienced by patients with a lower UTI is painful, frequent urination with small voids and urgency. Upper UTIs typically cause severe flank pain and tenderness over the costovertebral angle. Malaise, fever, chills, nausea, vomiting, and signs and symptoms of a lower UTI may also be present.

Serious conditions

Fortunately, a patient suffering from the unmistakable and bothersome signs and symptoms of a UTI will most certainly seek medical evaluation. Urinary frequency, and sometimes urinary hesitancy and urgency, can accompany bladder calculus, prostatic cancer (at an advanced stage), prostatitis, a tumor in the female reproductive tract, or urethral stricture.

Complications

Phenazopyridine is the generic name for the OTC drug that can relieve UTI signs and symptoms. Once excreted into the urine, it exerts a topical analgesic effect on the mucosa and relieves the discomforts of a UTI, while the patient awaits the cure brought about by antibiotic therapy. Phenazopyridine isn't meant to be used for longer than 2 days, nor should it be used to treat pain that hasn't been medically evaluated. Doing so delays appropriate diagnosis and treatment.

Nursing considerations

• Assess the patient's normal pattern of voiding.

• Ask about the onset and duration of the abnormal urinary signs and symptoms.

• Explore the patient's medical history for UTIs, other urologic problems, recent urologic procedures, and neurologic disorders.

• Obtain culture and sensitivity tests, as appropriate.

Patient teaching
• Instruct the patient to report immediately recurrence or worsening of signs and symptoms.
• If the patient is prone to UTIs, advise against douching. This may cause a change in the pH of the vagina and natural flora.
• Inform the patient that phenazopyridine can turn the urine dark orange and the drug has been known to stain contact lenses.
• Advise the patient to discontinue using phenazopyridine if he starts to appear jaundiced. This may indicate impaired renal excretion.
• Emphasize that phenazopyridine treats only the pain associated with the infection but not the *cause* of the infection.
• Tell the patient to take phenazopyridine after meals.

butoconazole nitrate
clotrimazole
miconazole nitrate
nonoxynol 9
octoxynol
octoxynol 9
phenazopyridine
  hydrochloride
tioconazole

---

butoconazole nitrate
Femstat 3, Mycelex 3

Pregnancy Risk Category C

HOW SUPPLIED
Vaginal cream: 2% with applicators supplied

ACTION
Unknown. Thought to control or destroy fungus by disrupting cell membrane permeability, thereby causing osmotic instability.

Route	Onset	Peak	Duration
Vaginal	Unknown	Unknown	Unknown

INDICATIONS & DOSAGES
Vulvovaginal mycotic infections caused by Candida *species—*
Nonpregnant women: one applicatorful vaginally h.s. for 3 days. If needed, treat for another 3 days.
Pregnant women during second or third trimester: one applicatorful vaginally h.s. for 6 days.

ADVERSE REACTIONS
GU: vulvovaginal burning and itching, soreness, discharge, swelling.
Skin: finger itching.

INTERACTIONS
None significant.

CONTRAINDICATIONS
Contraindicated in patients who are hypersensitive to drug and in patients in the first trimester of pregnancy.

OVERDOSE & TREATMENT
No information available.

NURSING CONSIDERATIONS
• Breast-feeding women should use cautiously.
• Confirm diagnosis by smears or cultures.
• Drug may be used with oral contraceptive and antibiotic therapy.
• Ascertain that patient understands directions for use and length of therapy.
• Use of drug in pregnant women is restricted to second and third trimesters and only when potential benefits outweigh possible risks to fetus.

PATIENT TEACHING
- Teach patient how to apply drug, and tell her not to use tampons during treatment.
- Instruct patient to contact doctor if infection persists for longer than 3 days.
- Advise patient to keep affected area cool and dry, wear loose-fitting cotton clothing, avoid feminine hygiene sprays, wash area daily with unscented soap and dry thoroughly with clean towel, and prevent reinfection by wiping perineum from front to back.
- Instruct patient to clean applicator with soap and water after each use.
- Advise patient to use drug for prescribed length of time, even during menses.
- Tell patient that drug should be placed high in the vagina, except during pregnancy.
- Advise patient to refrain from sexual intercourse until treatment is complete. Patient's sexual partner should consult doctor if penile itching, redness, or discomfort occurs.
- Alert patient that drug base may weaken latex products (such as condom or diaphragm); their use within 3 days of drug administration isn't recommended as method of birth control.
- Tell patient not to store drug in temperatures above 104° F

(40° C) and to avoid freezing the drug.
- Inform breast-feeding patient that it's unclear if drug is excreted in breast milk. Tell her to consult doctor before using this drug.

---

clotrimazole
Femizol 7, Gyne-Lotrimin, Gyne-Lotrimin 3, Gyne-Lotrimin 3 Combination Pack, Gyne-Lotrimin 7, Mycelex-7

Pregnancy Risk Category B

HOW SUPPLIED
Vaginal cream: 1%
Vaginal tablets: 100 mg, 200 mg
Combination pack: vaginal tablets 100 mg, and topical cream 1%

ACTION
Fungistatic, but may be fungicidal, depending on level. Alters fungal cell-wall permeability and produces osmotic instability.

Route	Onset	Peak	Duration
Vaginal-	Unknown	Unknown	Unknown

INDICATIONS & DOSAGES
Vulvovaginal candidiasis—
Adults and children ages 12 and older: one 100-mg vaginal tablet inserted daily h.s. for 7

consecutive days; or one applicatorful of vaginal cream daily h.s. for 7 days. Apply topical cream to affected areas in the morning and evening for 7 days.

ADVERSE REACTIONS
GI: lower abdominal cramps.
GU: mild vaginal burning or irritation, cramping, urinary frequency.

INTERACTIONS
None reported.

CONTRAINDICATIONS
Contraindicated in patients who are hypersensitive to drug. Also contraindicated for ophthalmic use.

OVERDOSE & TREATMENT
No information available.

NURSING CONSIDERATIONS
• Breast-feeding patients should use cautiously because it's unknown if drug is excreted in breast milk.
• *Alert:* Don't confuse clotrimazole with co-trimoxazole.
• Because small amounts of this drug may be absorbed from the vagina, patient should use only when deemed medically essential during the first trimester of pregnancy, and only after consulting the doctor.

PATIENT TEACHING
• Inform breast-feeding patient that it's unclear if drug is excreted in breast milk. Tell her to consult doctor before using this drug.
• Warn patient not to let drug come in contact with eyes.
• Caution patient that frequent or persistent yeast infections may be symptomatic of a more serious medical problem such as AIDS.
• Tell patient to refrain from sexual intercourse during vaginal treatment.
• Warn patient that topical preparation may stain clothing.
• Emphasize need to continue treatment for full course and to notify doctor if no improvement occurs after 3 days for vulvovaginal candidiasis, or if vulvovaginal candidiasis recurs within 2 months.
• Tell patient to avoid use with abdominal pain, fever, or malodorous vaginal discharge.
• Tell patient to discontinue use and notify doctor if vaginal pruritus or discomfort occurs after use.
• Tell patient to stop treatment if vaginal itching or discomfort occurs after use.

---

miconazole nitrate
Femizol-M, Monistat 3, Monistat 3 Combination Pack, Monistat 7, Monistat 7 Combination Pack, M-Zole 7 Dual Pack

Pregnancy Risk Category B (vaginal)

HOW SUPPLIED
Vaginal cream: 2%
Vaginal suppositories: 100 mg

ACTION
A fungicidal imidazole that disrupts fungal cell membrane permeability.

Route	Onset	Peak	Duration
Vaginal	Unknown	Unknown	Unknown

INDICATIONS & DOSAGES
Vulvovaginal candidiasis—
Adults and children ages 12 and older: one applicatorful or one 100-mg suppository (Monistat 7) vaginally h.s. for 7 days; course may be repeated if needed.

ADVERSE REACTIONS
CNS: headache.
GU: pelvic cramps; vulvovaginal burning, pruritus, and irritation with vaginal cream.

INTERACTIONS
None significant.

CONTRAINDICATIONS
Contraindicated in patients who are hypersensitive to drug or its components.

OVERDOSE & TREATMENT
No information available.

NURSING CONSIDERATIONS
• Use should be avoided within 72 hours of vaginal forms and certain latex products, such as condoms or vaginal contraceptive diaphragms because of possible interaction.

PATIENT TEACHING
• Advise patient that drug is for perineal or vaginal use only and to keep drug out of eyes.
• Caution patient that frequent or persistent yeast infections may be a symptom of a more serious medical problem, such as AIDS.
• Tell patient to cautiously insert vaginal form high into the vagina, using the applicator provided.
• Tell patient that drug may stain clothing.
• Warn patient to discontinue drug if sensitivity or chemical irritation occurs.
• Tell patient to use drug for full treatment period prescribed and to notify doctor if signs and symptoms persist or worsen at end of therapy.

*Liquid contains alcohol.   **May contain tartrazine.   †Canada   ‡Australia   §U.K.

- Advise patient to avoid tampons and sexual intercourse during vaginal treatment.
- Emphasize need to continue treatment for full course and to notify doctor if no improvement occurs after 3 days for vulvovaginal candidiasis, or if vulvovaginal candidiasis recurs within 2 months.
- Tell patient to avoid use with abdominal pain, fever, or malodorous vaginal discharge.
- Tell patient to discontinue use and notify doctor if vaginal pruritus or discomfort occurs after use.
- Tell patient to store vaginal product between 59° and 86° F (15° and 30° C).
- Inform parent or caregiver that safety for use in children younger than age 2 hasn't been established. Parent or caregiver should consult doctor before administering this drug.
- Inform breast-feeding patient that safety hasn't been established for use. Tell her to use drug with caution.

---

nonoxynol 9
Advantage 24, Because, Beyond Seven, Conceptrol, Delfen, Durex, Emko, Encare Semicid, Gynol II Contraceptive, Gynol II Extra Strength Contraceptive Jelly, Kimono, Koromex, Koromex Crystal Clear Gel, K-Y Plus, LifeStyles, Ramses, Shur-Seal, Trojan, VCF

octoxynol
Koromex

octoxynol 9
Ortho-Gynol Contraceptive

Pregnancy Risk Category C

HOW SUPPLIED
nonoxynol 9
Jelly: 3%, 5%, 8%, 15%
Foam: 8%, 12.5%
Gel: 2%, 2.2%, 3.5%, 4%
Film: 28%; 2-inch squares
Vaginal suppository: 2.27%; 100 mg, 150 mg
octoxynol
Cream: 3%
octoxynol 9
Gel: 1%

ACTION
Spermicide that immobilizes and kills sperm combined with a medium that creates a mechanical barrier over the cervical opening.

Route	Onset	Peak	Duration
Vaginal	5-15 min	Unknown	Unknownl

INDICATIONS & DOSAGES
Contraception—
Adults: Vaginal use according to the manufacturer's recommendations at least 10 minutes (but no more than 60 minutes) before sexual intercourse. Condom use according to manufacturer's instructions.

ADVERSE REACTIONS
GU: penile or vaginal discomfort, irritation, soreness, itching.
Skin: dermatitis, erythema, irritation.

INTERACTIONS
None reported.

CONTRAINDICATIONS
Contraindicated in patients who are hypersensitive to active ingredient and in patients with history of toxic shock syndrome.

OVERDOSE & TREATMENT
No information available.

NURSING CONSIDERATIONS
•Efficacy of contraceptive foam is higher than that of other forms.
•Vaginal contraceptive suppositories have low contraceptive efficacy.
•Douching sooner than 6 to 8 hours after intercourse diminishes or eliminates spermicide action and may propel viable sperm into the uterus.

PATIENT TEACHING
•Advise the patient to use products with concentrations of 8% or higher, if tolerated.
•Instruct patient to use mechanical contraceptive along with chemical contraceptive for highest efficacy.
•Advise against pretesting condoms, which increases the risk of product failure.
•Advise patient that chemical contraceptive products don't prevent the transmission of sexually transmitted diseases (STDs); mechanical contraceptive methods shouldn't be relied on to prevent exposure to STDs.
•Instruct patient to carefully read and follow product instruction.
•Advise patient that use of this drug more than 60 minutes before intercourse requires reapplication of a full dose.
•Advise patient that douching should be delayed at least 6 to 8 hours after intercourse.
•Instruct patient to report adverse effects promptly to doctor.
•Advise parent or caregiver that this drug isn't to be used by children.

phenazopyridine hydrochloride (phenylazo diamino pyridine hydrochloride)
AZO-Standard, Baridium, Prodium

Pregnancy Risk Category B

HOW SUPPLIED
Tablets: 95 mg

ACTION
Exerts local anesthetic action on urinary mucosa through unknown mechanism.

Route	Onset	Peak	Duration
P.O.	Unknown	Unknown	Unknown

INDICATIONS & DOSAGES
Pain with urinary tract irritation or infection—
Adults and children ages 12 and older: 190 mg P.O. t.i.d. after meals for 2 days.

ADVERSE REACTIONS
CNS: headache.
EENT: staining of contact lenses.
GI: nausea, GI disturbances.
Hematologic: hemolytic anemia, methemoglobinemia.
Skin: rash, pruritus.
Other: *anaphylactoid reactions*.

INTERACTIONS
None significant.

CONTRAINDICATIONS
Contraindicated in patients who are hypersensitive to drug and in patients with glomerulonephritis, severe hepatitis, uremia, renal insufficiency, or pyelonephritis during pregnancy.

OVERDOSE & TREATMENT
Symptoms of overdose include methemoglobinemia (most obvious as cyanosis), along with renal and hepatic impairment and failure.

To treat overdose of phenazopyridine, empty stomach immediately by inducing emesis with ipecac syrup or by gastric lavage. Administer methylene blue, 1 to 2 mg/kg I.V., or 100 to 200 mg ascorbic acid P.O. to reverse methemoglobinemia. Provide symptomatic and supportive measures (respiratory support and correction of fluid and electrolyte imbalances). Monitor laboratory parameters and vital signs closely. Contact local or regional poison control center for specific instructions.

NURSING CONSIDERATIONS
• When drug is combined with an antibacterial, to treat UTIs, therapy shouldn't extend beyond 2 days.

Reactions may be *common*, uncommon, ***life-threatening***, or COMMON AND LIFE-THREATENING.

- Drug should be used only as an analgesic.
- Drug colors urine red or orange, and it may stain certain materials.
- Use with caution in elderly patients because of possible decreased renal function.
- Drug may alter results of Diastix or Chemstrip uG, Acetest, and Ketostix.
- Drug may interfere with Ehrlich's test for urine urobilinogen, phenolsulfonphthalein excretion tests of kidney function, sulfobromophthalein excretion tests of liver function, and urine tests for protein, corticosteroids, or bilirubin levels.

PATIENT TEACHING

- Teach patient ways to prevent UTIs.
- Advise patient that taking drug with meals may minimize GI distress.
- Caution patient to stop drug and seek medical advice immediately if skin or sclera becomes yellow-tinged, which may indicate drug accumulation because of impaired renal excretion.
- Inform patient that drug colors urine red or orange; it may stain fabrics or contact lenses.
- Tell diabetic patient that drug may alter Diastix or Chemstrip uG results. Patient should use Clinitest for accurate urine glucose test results. Also tell pa-

tient that drug may interfere with urinary ketone tests (Acetest or Ketostix).
- Advise patient to seek medical advice if urinary tract pain persists. Tell patient that drug shouldn't be used for long-term treatment.
- Inform breast-feeding patient that safety of drug hasn't been established.

tioconazole
Vagistat-1

Pregnancy Risk Category C

HOW SUPPLIED
Vaginal ointment: 6.5%

ACTION
A fungicidal imidazole that alters cell-wall permeability.

Route	Onset	Peak	Duration
Vaginal	Unknown	Unknown	Unknown

INDICATIONS & DOSAGES
Vulvovaginal candidiasis—
Adults and children ages 12 and older: 1 applicatorful (about 4.6 g) vaginally one time only, h.s.

ADVERSE REACTIONS
CNS: headache.
GI: abdominal pain.
GU: burning, discharge, vaginal pain, genital pruritus, dys-

uria, dyspareunia, vulvar edema, irritation.

INTERACTIONS
None reported.

CONTRAINDICATIONS
Contraindicated in patients who are hypersensitive to this drug or to other imidazole antifungal drugs (ketoconazole, miconazole). Also contraindicated in pregnant patients and in patients with diabetes mellitus, HIV infection, or AIDS.

OVERDOSE & TREATMENT
None reported.

NURSING CONSIDERATIONS
• Pregnant women and patients with diabetes mellitus, HIV infection, or AIDS should use only under direction of doctor.
• Breast-feeding patients should stop breast-feeding while taking drug because it isn't known if drug is excreted in breast milk.
• Notify doctor if patient reports irritation or sensitivity.
• *Alert:* Don't confuse tioconazole with terconazole.

PATIENT TEACHING
• If patient is pregnant, tell her not to use this product unless directed by doctor.
• Inform breast-feeding patient that it's unknown if drug is excreted in breast milk. Tell her to stop breast-feeding and consult doctor before using this drug.
• Review proper use of drug with patient. Written instructions for patient are available with product.
• Tell patient to insert drug high into vagina.
• Tell patient not to use with abdominal pain, high fever, malodorous vaginal discharge, vomiting, or diarrhea unless directed by doctor.
• To avoid contamination of ointment, tell patient to open applicator just before use.
• Tell patient to use sanitary napkins, instead of tampons, to avoid staining clothing.
• Advise patient to avoid sexual intercourse on night after insertion.
• Tell patient that drug may be used during her menstrual period.
• Tell patient that drug base may react with latex, causing decreased effectiveness of condoms and diaphragms (for up to 72 hours after treatment is completed).
• Advise patient to seek medical advice if signs and symptoms don't improve within 3 days, persist for longer than 1 week, or return within 2 months.

Combination products

Brand name and active ingredients	Indications and dosages	Nursing considerations
Diurex PMS • acetaminophen 1,000 mg • pamabrom 50 mg • pyrilamine maleate 30 mg	*Premenstrual symptoms* **Adults and children ages 12 and older:** 2 caplets P.O. with water q 6 hours p.r.n. Maximum 8 caplets in 24 hours.	• Tell patient not to take drug for longer than 10 days. • Inform patient that drug may turn urine a golden color. • Tell patient not to exceed recommended dose. • If patient is taking other drugs, she should consult doctor before taking this drug. • Warn patient that drug may cause drowsiness. • Tell patient to use caution when driving or operating machinery.
Midol Maximum Strength PMS Formula • acetaminophen 500 mg • pamabrom 25 mg • pyrilamine maleate 15 mg	*Premenstrual symptoms* **Adults and children ages 12 and older:** 2 caplets or gelcaps P.O. with water q 4 hours p.r.n. Maximum 8 caplets or gelcaps in 24 hours.	• Tell patient not to take drug for longer than 10 days. • Tell patient to notify doctor if pain lasts longer than 10 days. • Warn patient that drug may cause drowsiness. • Tell patient to avoid alcohol, sedatives, and tranquilizers, unless directed by doctor. • Tell patient to use caution when driving or operating machinery. • Tell parent that drug may cause excitability in children. • Drug dose contains caffeine equal to 1 cup of coffee. • Tell patient to limit use of drugs, food, or beverages that contain caffeine. • Tell patient with emphysema, chronic bronchitis, or glaucoma not to take this drug, unless directed by doctor. • Tell patient who drinks more than 3 alcoholic beverages per

(continued)

Combination products (continued)

Brand name and active ingredients	Indications and dosages	Nursing considerations
Midol Maximum Strength Teen Formula • acetaminophen 500 mg • pamabrom 25 mg	*Premenstrual symptoms* **Adults and children ages 12 and older:** 2 caplets P.O. with water q 4 hours p.r.n. Maximum 8 caplets in 24 hours.	day to consult doctor before taking this drug. • Tell patient not to take drug for longer than 10 days. • Tell patient to notify doctor if pain lasts longer than 10 days. • Tell patient who drinks more than 3 alcoholic beverages per day to consult doctor before taking this drug.
Pamprin Maximum Strength • acetaminophen 250 mg • magnesium salicylate 250 mg • pamabrom 25 mg	*Premenstrual symptoms* **Adults and children ages 12 and older:** 2 caplets P.O. with water q 4 to 6 hours p.r.n. Maximum 8 caplets in 24 hours.	• Tell patient not to take drug for longer than 10 days. • Tell patient not to take for fever for longer than 3 days. • Tell patient to notify doctor for ringing in ears, hearing loss, persistent or worsening pain or fever, new symptoms, redness, or swelling. • Tell patient not to take with nticoagulants, or if she has diabetes, gout, arthritis, or allergies to salicylates, unless directed. • Tell pregnant patient not to take during the last 3 months of pregnancy.
Pamprin Maximum Strength Multi-Symptom Menstrual Relief • acetaminophen 500 mg • pamabrom 25 mg • pyrilamine maleate 15 mg	*Premenstrual symptoms* **Adults and children ages 12 and older:** 2 tablets or caplets P.O. with water q 4 to 6 hours p.r.n. Maximum 8 tablets or caplets in 24 hours.	• Tell patient not to take drug for longer than 10 days. • Warn patient that drug may cause drowsiness. • Tell patient to avoid alcohol, sedatives, and tranquilizers unless directed by doctor. • Tell patient to use caution when driving or operating machinery. • Warn parent that drug may cause excitability in children.

Combination products *(continued)*

Brand name and active ingredients	Indications and dosages	Nursing considerations
Pamprin Maximum Strength Multi-Symptom Menstrual Relief *(continued)*		• Tell patient with emphysema, chronic bronchitis, or glaucoma not to take this drug, unless directed by doctor. • Tell patient who drinks more than 3 alcoholic beverages per day to consult doctor before taking this drug.
Premsyn PMS • acetaminophen 500 mg • pamabrom 25 mg • pyrilamine maleate 15 mg	*Premenstrual symptoms* **Adults and children ages 12 and older:** 2 caplets P.O. with water q 4 to 6 hours p.r.n. Maximum 8 caplets in 24 hours.	• Tell patient to continue use throughout menstrual cycle, if needed. • Tell patient not to take drug for longer than 10 days. • Warn patient that drug may cause drowsiness. • Tell patient to avoid alcohol, sedatives, and tranquilizers, unless directed by doctor. • Tell patient to use caution when driving or operating machinery. • Warn parent that drug may cause excitability in children. • Tell patient with emphysema, chronic bronchitis, or glaucoma not to take this drug, unless directed by doctor. • Tell patient who drinks more than 3 alcoholic beverages per day to consult doctor before taking this drug.
Tylenol Menstrual Relief • acetaminophen 500 mg • pamabrom 25 mg	*Premenstrual symptoms* **Adults and children ages 12 and older:** 2 caplets P.O. with water q 4 to 6 hours p.r.n. Maximum 8 caplets in 24 hours.	• Tell patient not to use with other products containing acetaminophen. • Tell patient to notify doctor if she experiences new symptoms, redness or swelling, or worsening or persistence of symptoms.

7

Integumentary system

The skin, hair, nails, sweat glands, and subcutaneous tissue make up the integumentary system. Because it has a complex structure, and important functions, the skin is classified as an organ. Seven distinct functions have been attributed to the skin: protection (its primary function), maintenance of homeostasis, excretion, temperature regulation, vitamin synthesis, sensory perception, wound healing, and visual appeal.

Anatomy

The skin has two distinct layers, the epidermis and the dermis, which are above a layer of subcutaneous fatty tissue. The epidermis is the outermost structure of the skin. Structurally, it's avascular and about 0.1 mm thick (depending on the site). It consists of five layers: horny cell, stratum lucidum, granular cell, prickle cell, and basal cell. The epidermis rejuvenates itself through the process of keratinization. New cells originate in the basal layer of the epidermis and migrate up through the various epidermal layers, undergoing mor-

phologic and biochemical changes as they are pushed upward. When they reach the horny cell layer at the top of the epidermis, they have become anucleated cells called keratinocytes.

Directly under the epidermis is the dermis. The dermis is the principal mass of the skin, 1 to 4 mm thick and composed of collagen and reticular and elastin bundles. It encloses the appendages of the epidermis (hair, nails, and glands) and supports the nerve and vascular network of the skin. The dermis protects the underlying tissues from mechanical trauma and maintains homeostasis. It's also a water-storage organ and, as such, influences thermoregulation, sensory innervation, and wound healing.

An intact integument provides a physical barrier against foreign substances and microorganisms. Intercellular bonding in the epidermis, and the collagen, elastin, and ground substance in the dermis, provide mechanical strength.

Disorders of the skin may localize in one area of the skin or involve all layers simultaneously. Common skin conditions include inflammation (generally noninfectious), benign or malignant cellular proliferation, pigment abnormalities, infections, and infestations.

Because the skin is a large, visible organ, and our culture is obsessed with perfection and beauty, skin disorders are often self-diagnosed and self-treated. Common skin disorders that are treated with OTC drugs include acne, xerosis, superficial infections, psoriasis, insect bites and stings, infestations, hair loss, dermatitis, scrapes and abrasions, and superficial burns.

Acne

Acne is an inflammatory disorder of the pilosebaceous unit (hair follicle and its oil gland). Inflammation and plugging of the follicular ducts lead to formation of comedones (open blackheads and closed whiteheads), papules, pustules, and in severe cases, cysts. Acne is caused by a complex of interrelated factors, and the exact cause is unknown. Abnormally adherent keratinocytes and accumulation of sebum and keratinous debris are the main cellular factors in the presentation of acne. Factors that contribute to its development include bacteria *(Propionibacterium acnes)* in the pilosebaceous units, drugs (such as exogenous androgens, ACTH, glucocorticoids, hydantoins, isoniazid), friction (football helmets, headbands, hats), and oil-based cosmetics and hair products (pomade acne).

Signs and symptoms
Characteristically, acne occurs during adolescence at the onset of puberty, but it may occur as late as the seventh decade of life. It may cause an array of lesions, including primary lesions, comedones, erythematous papules, pustules, and cysts. Although they contain purulent material, pustules typically aren't infected. The purulent material is an accumulation of leukocytes that's a response to inflammation. Cystic lesions form when closed comedones rupture, releasing contents into the dermis. Fever, malaise, pain, and prostration may accompany extensive cystic acne. Because acne occurs on the face, the social stigma may lead patients to use many OTC drugs and cover-ups in an attempt to hide the disorder.

Serious conditions
Acnelike lesions on the face and trunk may actually be *Staphylococcus aureus* folli-

culitis. Inappropriate treatment can lead to deeper follicular and perifollicular infection, resulting in the formation of an abscess. If the infection invades numerous contiguous follicles, a carbuncle will form. These infections require systemic antibiotics.

Complications

Inappropriate treatment or manipulation of the lesions in an attempt to express contents can cause secondary infection or scarring. Less serious, but nonetheless important, problems can arise from overzealous efforts at cleansing. Overuse of exfoliating brushes or sponges may disrupt the integrity of the skin surface and set the stage for secondary infections. The wide range of OTC acne preparations includes scrubs, soaps, facial masks, and washes. Although these items have a place in the treatment of mild to moderate acne, some contain ingredients that may be sensitizing or too harsh for certain skin types.

Nursing considerations

• Products should be used as directed on the package. If irritation occurs, the patient should stop the drug and, after irritation subsides, use the medication every other day.

• If irritation persists, the product should be discontinued and a dermatologist consulted.
• Observe for signs and symptoms of manipulation (squeezing) of lesions in an attempt to express contents; this may cause rupture, secondary infection, cyst formation, or scarring.

Patient teaching

• Teach the patient about the causes and course of the disorder; dispel misconceptions about the effects of hygiene or diet.
• Discuss ways to avoid factors known to exacerbate the disorder.
• Advise the patient that use of heavy makeup or cover-ups to mask lesions actually adds oil and increases follicular plugging.
• Teach the patient to use gentle skin cleansing techniques and never to squeeze lesions.
• Advise the patient that harsh abrasives, brushes, or sponges irritate the skin, intensify inflammatory phase of acne, and increase risk of infection.
• Explain the possible adverse effects of any drug being used.

Xerosis

Xerosis is dry skin that reflects dehydration of the stratum corneum by intrinsic or extrinsic factors. A decrease in epidermal free fatty acids, an intrinsic change seen with aging, leads to dry skin in elderly patients. Xerosis may affect any area of the body but usually affects the lower legs and feet. Generalized dryness may occur in some disease states, such as ichthyosis, thyroid disorders, or atopic dermatitis. Other factors that may affect hydration of the skin may include low ambient humidity, particularly during the winter months.

Signs and symptoms

Dryness may appear as irregular areas, measuring from 1 mm to a few centimeters. Dryness caused by an underlying disease may be more generalized. Sensitivity and pruritus may accompany the dryness, and patients with atopic dermatitis may experience scaling or flaking accompanied by erythema.

Serious conditions

Generalized scaling, dryness, and pruritus unresponsive to bland emollients may suggest an underlying disorder such as diabetes, thyroid dysfunction, psoriasis, or exfoliative erythroderma. The patient should see a doctor for evaluation. Dryness of the feet that doesn't respond to bland emollients suggests a fungal infection—common in

elderly, diabetic, and immunocompromised patients.

Complications

Untreated fungal infections, particularly in diabetic or immunocompromised patients, may spread and become debilitating. Uncontrolled systemic disease of any category can have serious adverse effects. Patients who have been self-treating and have no relief from signs or symptoms should see a doctor.

Nursing considerations

• Identify the moisturizer or emollient that the patient is using.
• Some products may be sensitizers, particularly in elderly patients; perfumes and additives can irritate sensitive skin.
• Observe the patient for signs and symptoms of continued pruritus in the absence of dry skin; look for excoriations or purpura caused by scratching.
• Ask the patient about bathing habits and use of bath additives and soap; hot baths and excessive use of soap exacerbate xerosis.
• Be alert to possible tinea infections in high-risk populations.

Patient teaching

• Advise the patient to take tepid, rather than hot, baths or showers.

• Advise the patient to avoid use of harsh soaps, which increase dryness.

• Inform the patient that soap is necessary only in axillae, groin, and feet—the only areas of the body that produce odor.

• If xerosis is severe, tell the patient to limit bathing to every other day.

• Teach the patient gentle drying techniques: don't rub skin with a towel; pat skin gently, leaving some moisture on the skin; immediately apply a bland emollient after patting dry.

• Advise the patient to maintain high humidity level in the home with humidifiers or cool mist vaporizers.

• Suggest that the patient avoid wearing rough or constricting clothing, which can traumatize dry skin.

• If the condition doesn't improve, advise the patient to consult a doctor.

Superficial infections

Infection is the presence and growth of a microorganism that produces tissue damage. Microorganisms may be bacteria, viruses, or fungi. The pathogens may be resident flora that proliferate because of an underlying disease (such as diabetes, cancer, or immunosuppression) or acquired through impaired defense mechanisms that protect against the proliferation or invasion of microorganisms. These mechanisms include an intact integument (first line of defense), the mononuclear phagocyte system (MPS), the inflammatory response, and the immune system.

The MPS, also referred to as the reticuloendothelial system (RES), recognizes and phagocytoses microorganisms. Cell injury initiates inflammation to neutralize the inflammatory agent, remove necrotic material, and establish an environment for healing and repair. Components of inflammation include a vascular response, a cellular response, formation of exudate, and healing.

Bacterial infections of the skin are most commonly caused by *Staphylococcus aureus* or *Streptococcus pyogenes.* Most are superficial, arising from minor, superficial breaks in the skin or secondary infection in preexisting dermatitis (impetiginization).

Viral infections of the skin are usually caused by human papillomavirus (HPV), varicella zoster, herpes zoster, or herpes simplex. Common warts, plantar warts, and flat warts are symptoms of cutaneous infection of keratinized skin with HPV; they are spread by direct skin-to-skin contact. In contrast, varicella zoster (chickenpox) is transmitted through airborne droplets as well as direct contact. Herpes zoster (shingles) is reactivation of varicella zoster infection. Herpes simplex virus is transmitted by skin-to-skin or mucosa-to-skin contact. Immunocompromise, irradiation, and systemic corticosteroids can facilitate the infection.

Fungal infections of the skin are usually caused by dermatophytes: *Trichophyton, Microsporum, Epidermophyton*, or *Candida*. This unique group of dermatophytes can infect nonviable keratinized cutaneous tissues—stratum corneum, nails, and hair. Fungal infections may be acquired from contaminated earth, animals, or other people. Dermatophytes synthesize keratinases, which digest keratin and, therefore, provide nutrients for the invading fungi. Atopy, topical and systemic corticosteroids, ichthyosis, and collagen vascular disease are host factors that facilitate the fungal infection. Sweating, occlusive clothing, occupational exposure, and ge-

ographic location (areas of high humidity) are local factors favoring fungal infections.

Signs and symptoms

Signs and symptoms of infection depend on the invading organism and the patient's underlying health status and immune competency. Inflammation usually accompanies infection, but it isn't always indicative of infection. The signs of inflammation include redness (rubor), heat (calor), pain (dolor), and swelling (tumor).

Bacterial infections caused by *Staphylococcus aureus* and *Streptococcus pyogenes* are superficial and usually involve the epidermis (impetigo) or extend into the dermis (ecthyma). These infections are characterized by crusting, erosions, and ulcers.

Viral infection signs and symptoms depend on the type of virus. Human papillomavirus causes common warts, plantar warts, or flat warts. Common warts are firm, hyperkeratotic papules (rarely larger than 10 mm) having a cleft surface and vegetations. Plantar warts are small, shiny, sharply marginated papules that evolve into a plaque with a rough hyperkeratotic surface and brown-black dots.

Superficial infections 255

Varicella zoster is characterized by successive crops of pruritic vesicles that evolve to papules, crusting, and in some cases, scars. The primary lesions are vesicles on an erythematous base, described as a "dewdrop on a rose petal." Mild constitutional signs and symptoms—low-grade fever, malaise, headache, general aches and pains, severe backache—usually appear 2 or 3 days before the skin lesions. Lesions appear on the face and scalp and spread rapidly to the trunk and limbs.

Herpes zoster (shingles) begins with a prodrome of nerve pain or paresthesia, usually appearing 3 to 5 days, but possibly up to 14 days, before lesions appear. Heightened sensitivity to mild stimuli (allodynia) may be seen in some cases. Constitutional signs and symptoms that may also appear are headache, malaise, and fever. The lesions evolve from the primary lesion, a papule, to vesicles and bullae and then to pustules and crusting. The lesions are grouped and are distributed unilaterally along a dermatome. Dermatomes of predilection are (in order of highest to lowest occurrence) thoracic, trigeminal, lumbosacral, and cervical. The clear or hemorrhagic vesicles occur on an erythematous base.

Herpes simplex virus (cold sore, fever blister, herpetic whitlow) is characterized by primary or recurrent grouped vesicles on an erythematous base in keratinized skin or on mucous membranes. The incubation period is 2 to 20 days after infection. The primary herpes lesion may be symptomatic or accompanied by trivial symptoms. The herpes virus resides in the basal nerve ganglion, and vesicles form at the site of inoculation. Regional lymphadenopathy and low-grade fever may be present; headache, malaise, and myalgia may appear 3 to 4 days after the appearance of lesions. Recurrence is secondary to precipitating factors such as trauma, excessive sun exposure, illness, or immunosuppression.

Fungal infections of the epidermis (tinea pedis, tinea corporis, tinea cruris, tinea manuum) are characterized by erythema, chronic diffuse desquamation, or bulla formation. Burning and stinging are the most common symptoms that prompt a patient to seek medical intervention. Fungal infections of the nails (onychomycosis) and hair (trichomycosis) also occur.

Serious conditions

Bacterial infections of the skin in otherwise healthy individuals are usually localized. In patients who are immunocompromised (by disease or drug), have diabetes, are debilitated, or have other underlying conditions, bacterial infections of the skin can have systemic ramifications. Patients with a clinical cutaneous infection accompanied by fever and constitutional signs and symptoms should be evaluated by a doctor. Unresponsive, nonhealing cutaneous infections in patients with diabetes may be secondary to underlying osteomyelitis, particularly when the infection is over a bony prominence.

Cutaneous viral infections also may evolve to systemic infection in compromised hosts. Warts that are proliferating can reflect a depressed or compromised immune system and should be evaluated by a doctor. Varicella zoster in adults can be life-threatening and always mandates referral to a doctor. Herpes zoster appears in a unilateral dermatomal pattern. Lesions that cross the midline could indicate an underlying malignancy. Herpes simplex virus, if disseminated, could also be a symptom of immunocompromise or malignancy.

Complications

Prolonged self-treatment of any type of infection without resolution can lead to systemic complications. In the case of herpes zoster infections, postherpetic neuralgia can be a debilitating complication when treatment is inadequate.

Nursing considerations

• Assess lesions for characteristics, inflammation, pain, and possible progression of infection.
• Assess the patient's overall medical status.
• Assess the patient's hygiene and living conditions.
• Review all the patient's OTC and prescription drugs.

Patient teaching

• Teach the patient and family about how infection is spread.
• Teach the patient good hygiene skills.
• Instruct the patient and family about signs and symptoms of progressing infection and the need to seek medical attention for appropriate treatment.
• Teach the patient how to avoid precipitating or aggravating factors.

Psoriasis

Psoriasis is a chronic, genetic, inflammatory disease of unknown cause. It is proliferation of normal skin cells caused by an increased cell turnover rate. Normally, a cell takes about 28 days to move from the site of mitosis, the basal cell layer, to the stratum corneum. In psoriasis, this rate may be 4 to 5 days, so that immature cells arrive at the surface, and the normal sloughing of epidermal cells is impeded. Large areas of scale (hyperkeratosis) accumulate on the skin surface. Onset can be at any age, but the disease tends to be more severe if the onset is in childhood. Remissions and exacerbations mark the course of psoriasis. Aggravating factors include streptococcal pharyngitis, emotional upset, stress, hormonal changes, and certain drugs.

Signs and symptoms

Signs and symptoms vary with the type of psoriasis and the patient. The characteristic lesions of psoriasis are red papules that coalesce to form plaques that are covered with silvery scales. Pruritus may or may not occur and there may be pain when fissuring or psoriatic arthritis is present. Commonly affected areas include the elbows, knees, scalp, umbilicus, and perineum. Other signs and symptoms may include nail pitting, intergluteal pinking, and dry or brittle hair.

Serious conditions

Many skin diseases have similar signs and symptoms. Psoriasis that fails to respond to OTC drugs suggests the presence of other diseases, such as seborrheic dermatitis, lichen simplex chronicus, candidiasis, psoriasiform drug eruptions, or glucagonoma syndrome.

A potentially fatal condition that can mimic psoriasis in its early stages is mycosis fungoides (cutaneous T-cell lymphoma). This disease is often misdiagnosed as psoriasis but won't respond to conventional treatments.

Complications

A severe flare of disease may evolve into exfoliative erythroderma. This condition is characterized by problems involving thermoregulation, iron, electrolyte imbalance, and high-output cardiac failure, which can be fatal. The patient with generalized psoriasis is at high risk for infection. Finally, psoriatic arthritis can be crippling.

Nursing considerations

• Evaluate the patient for signs and symptoms of infection, particularly if he's in a high-risk population.
• Over-the-counter topical corticosteroids may be help treat mild psoriasis.

• Cool, moist compresses on trigger points, lubricating baths, and continuous use of bland emollients may relieve pruritus.

• Lack of response to treatment or the spread of lesions should be evaluated by a doctor to verify diagnosis and prescribe appropriate interventions.

Patient teaching

• Teach the patient about the disease and possible complications.

• Instruct the patient on use of bland emollients and importance of keeping the skin moist at all times.

• Suggest that the patient use a cool mist vaporizer to help increase humidity in the environment.

• Encourage tepid baths with additives, such as colloidal oatmeal to help hydrate the skin, add lubrication, and help ease pruritus (if present).

• Explain the importance of applying bland emollients immediately after bathing and patting, not rubbing, dry.

• Instruct the patient on signs and symptoms of infection.

• Emphasize the importance of seeking medical care if condition doesn't clear or worsens.

Insect bites and stings

Bees, wasps, spiders, fleas, mosquitoes, chiggers, and ticks commonly cause bites and stings. Reactions to bites and stings are classified as local reactions (type I), systemic reactions (type II), and delayed, or serum sickness reactions (type III).

A local reaction starts with the release of histamine. Systemic reactions are also mediated by the release of histamine but may become more severe, leading to a life-threatening situation. It may include profound hypotension, MI, brain damage, or renal failure. These severe reactions are immediate and mediated by immunoglobulin E antibodies. A delayed or serum sickness reaction may occur hours or weeks after the bite or sting. Immune complexes formed between allergens and specific immunoglobulin G antibodies may mediate this type of reaction.

Signs and symptoms

Type I reactions cause immediate, sharp pain, edema, and pruritus, which usually subside within a few hours. If the bite or sting is on the head or in the mouth, the reaction will be more severe. If a local reaction involves an entire extremity, the patient will be at higher risk of a future systemic reaction to the same type of bite or sting.

Type II reactions vary in severity. A mild type II reaction includes diffuse pruritus, urticaria, distant edema, and flushing. A more severe type II reaction may cause such life-threatening signs and symptoms as laryngeal edema or bronchospasm, resulting in respiratory compromise.

Type III reactions appear days to weeks after the original bite or sting and may cause flu-like signs and symptoms such as fever, myalgia, or chills. Guillain-Barré syndrome has occurred in some patients.

Serious conditions

Tick bites may cause Lyme disease or Rocky Mountain spotted fever; these conditions require systemic treatment.

Bites from black widow or brown recluse spiders can have devastating neurologic, respiratory, and cardiac consequences. Brown recluse spider bites may also cause necrosis resulting in large defects and possible tissue loss.

Complications

Glomerulonephritis or myocarditis may complicate a delayed, or serum sickness reaction to a bite or sting. Patients with atopic dermatitis have more severe local reactions than patients with healthy skin. Elderly, pediatric, and debilitated patients are at particular risk of complications from envenomation.

Nursing considerations

• Altered skin integrity in elderly, pediatric, or debilitated patients increases the risk of infection.
• Evaluate the area around bite or sting for evidence of spread or necrosis.
• Be alert to complications secondary to allergic response.

Patient teaching

• If a wound is present, explain appropriate wound care.
• If reaction, no matter how minor, doesn't resolve, refer the patient to a doctor.
• Instruct the patient on signs and symptoms of delayed reaction.

Infestations

The two most common ectoparasites in human infestations are mites (scabies) and lice (pediculosis). Transmission is through person-to-person contact. The female scabies mite burrows into the skin by secreting a substance that lyses the stratum corneum; there she lays one or two eggs a day during her 30-day life span. The mite feeds on intracellular, lymphlike fluid in the stratum granulosum. The saliva, body secretions, and feces of the mite cause severe pruritus.

In contrast, the louse needs human blood to survive. It attaches itself to the skin and injects saliva into the site of attachment. The saliva prevents the blood from clotting and causes an allergic reaction. The body louse can lay eggs on fabric or in the seams of clothing. Eradication requires treatment of the person and the environment.

Signs and symptoms
Irregular, linear, gray-brown, or pearly mite burrows are generally prominent in the web spaces of the hands, on the flexor surfaces of the wrists, in the axillary folds, and on the buttocks. The lesions may be vesicular or papular. Pruritus is the most significant symptom, and excoriations are usually evident.

Small, erythematous papules and wheals characterize lice infestation. Nits can be seen attached to the hair shafts. Cervical adenopathy may accompany severe infestation of the head.

Serious conditions
Atopic dermatitis, neurodermatitis, contact dermatitis, dermatitis herpetiformis, lichen planus, or psoriasis should be considered.

Complications
Excoriations secondary to severe pruritus compromise the barrier function of the skin and increase the risk of secondary infection. In immunocompromised persons, the result may be bacteremia, sepsis, or even death.

Lice infestation can lead to keratoconjunctivitis, photophobia, and secondary pyoderma. Eczema, nodular granulomas, urticaria, and a severe psychological reaction known as delusions of parasitosis also may occur. Certain species of lice also serve as vectors for epidemic typhus fever, relapsing fever, or trench fever.

Nursing considerations
• Crowded living conditions enhance transmission of both scabies and lice.
• Some patients have a severe psychological response to the condition called delusions of parasitosis.
• Itching from scabies may persist for up to 2 weeks after treatment.

• Severe, generalized excoriations can increase the risk of secondary infection.

• The debilitated or immuno-compromised patient has a more severe response.

Patient teaching

• Instruct the patient, family, and significant other on appropriate application of drug.

• Instruct the patient on the appropriate handling of linens, clothing, brushes, and combs.

• Explain that significant pruritus may last up to 2 weeks after treatment.

Hair loss

Hair loss, or alopecia, may be nonscarring or scarring.

Alopecia areata, androgenetic alopecia, telogen effluvium, and anagen effluvium are the nonscarring alopecias. The cause of alopecia areata is unknown. The effect of androgen on genetically predisposed hair follicles causes androgenetic alopecia (male-pattern baldness). Telogen effluvium can be caused by pregnancy, switching oral contraceptives, major medical procedures, major trauma, and significant illness. Anagen effluvium is usually caused by drugs, alcohol intoxication, or chemotherapy.

Scarring (cicatricial) alopecia is caused by damage or destruction of the hair follicles by inflammation (infectious or noninfectious) or other pathologic processes.

Signs and symptoms

Alopecia areata occurs in sharply defined normal-appearing skin with visible hair follicles and no scarring or atrophy. Occasionally, broken-off, stubby hairs (called exclamation point hairs) remain. The hair loss may be scattered; there may be a total loss of scalp hair or a generalized loss of body hair (alopecia areata universalis).

Androgenetic alopecia is a gradual thinning of the hair in men and women. A receding hairline may be the first indication of alopecia.

Diffuse shedding of the scalp hair is the main symptom of telogen effluvium; hair comes out easily if the fingers or a comb are run through the hair. Anagen effluvium has the same symptoms as telogen effluvium, but it occurs more quickly and is more pronounced.

Scarring (cicatricial) alopecia appears as areas of hair loss with obvious scarring. Atrophy and complete loss of hair follicles are seen.

Serious conditions

Nonscarring alopecia that appears in a patchy (moth-eaten) pattern can be a sign of secondary syphilis. Other diseases that can produce alopecia include white-patch tinea capitis, traction alopecia, and early chronic cutaneous lupus erythematosus.

Significant weight loss within a short period of time, significant illness, certain drugs (lithium, bromocriptine, cimetidine, clofibrate, retinoids), heavy metal poisoning with mercury or lead, and pesticides can also induce hair loss.

Basal cell epithelioma, squamous cell carcinoma, metastatic tumors, lymphomas, and adnexal tumors can cause scarring alopecia. Systemic diseases that can induce scarring alopecia include scleroderma and dermatomyositis. It can be associated with autoimmune disorders such as vitiligo, thyroid disease (Hashimoto's thyroiditis), and familial autoimmune polyendocrinopathy syndrome (hypoparathyroidism, Addison's disease, and mucocutaneous candidiasis).

Complications

Although alopecia has few complications, hair loss may be a sign of an underlying health problem.

Nursing considerations

• Hair loss for any reason causes anxiety in patients.
• Not all hair loss is genetic; it may be a sign of an underlying medical condition.
• Stress can be a factor in hair loss.

Patient teaching

• Advise a patient with patchy hair or scarring alopecia to consult a doctor.
• Advise the patient that inflammation associated with hair loss can be a sign of a more serious condition.
• Reassure the patient that in most cases of alopecia without scarring, hair will grow back.

Dermatitis

Atopic, contact, and seborrheic dermatitis are skin inflammations characterized by itching, erythema, and skin lesions with a variety of borders and patterns of distribution. Atopic dermatitis is hereditary; contact dermatitis is caused by exposure to allergens or irritants; and the cause of seborrheic dermatitis isn't known.

Signs and symptoms

Contact dermatitis can be acute, subacute, or chronic. Acute dermatitis appears as well-demarcated plaques of erythema, edema, and vesiculation; oozing erosions may also occur. Subacute dermatitis appears as plaques of erythema with small, dry scales or superficial desquamation. Small, firm papules may also be present. Chronic dermatitis appears as plaques with lichenification, exaggerated skin lines, and excoriations caused by scratching of chronic, intensely itchy lesions. Small, firm, rounded, or flat-topped papules may be present.

Patients with acute atopic dermatitis have poorly defined erythematous patches, papules, and plaques; widespread edema, erosion, crusting, and excoriations; and possibly scales. Patients with chronic atopic dermatitis have lichenification, fissuring, alopecia, and periorbital pigmentation. Skin hyperexcitability and intense itching are hallmark signs and symptoms.

Yellowish, red, often greasy, or white dry scaling macules or papules characterize seborrheic dermatitis. Commonly affected areas include the external ear, scalp (dandruff, cradle cap), nasolabial folds and cheeks, axillae, groin, and submammary areas.

Serious conditions

Conditions that mimic dermatitis include psoriasis, dermatophytosis, and early stages of mycosis fungoides (cutaneous T-cell lymphoma). Rare disorders that mimic atopic dermatitis include acrodermatitis enteropathica, gluten-sensitive enteropathy, glucagonoma syndrome, phenylketonuria, some immunologic disorders, and selective immunoglobulin A deficiency.

Complications

Secondary infection by *Staphylococcus aureus* can cause extensive erosions and crusting, and herpes simplex infection (eczema herpeticum) may be life-threatening. Problems with thermoregulation may be a concern when large areas of the body are involved. Protein and iron losses are common.

Nursing considerations

• Assess the patient for secondary infection.
• Counsel the patient on avoidance of aggravating factors.

Patient teaching

• Instruct the patient about strategies to keep skin lubricated.
• Teach the patient to avoid aggravating and precipitating factors.
• Teach the patient how to reduce inflammation by using

cool compresses and emollients.

• Advise the patient to limit exposure to known external irritants.

Scrapes and abrasions

Scrapes and abrasions are usually caused by trauma, which disrupts the integrity of the skin and alters its barrier function, permitting invasion of infecting microorganisms.

Signs and symptoms

Erosion, pain, exudate, and crusting may be the only signs and symptoms. Erythema is usually evident but doesn't necessarily indicate infection. In superficial scrapes and abrasions, acute erythema reflects inflammation, which is a normal part of the healing process.

Serious conditions

The most serious condition resulting from superficial skin disruptions is secondary infection, especially in debilitated or immunocompromised patients.

Complications

Few complications of superficial infections occur. However, a lesion that doesn't heal should be evaluated by a doctor. Skin cancers can develop in nonhealing wounds, and prolonged healing may indicate a disorder such as diabetes.

Nursing considerations

• Be alert to signs of secondary infection.

• Inquire which drugs the patient may be using; some topical antibiotics are sensitizers.

Patient teaching

• Teach the patient the signs and symptoms of infection.

• Encourage the patient to seek medical care if a lesion doesn't heal in a timely manner.

Superficial burns

Burns can be caused by thermal, chemical, electrical, or UV radiation. Factors that influence the extent of the burn injury are the energy source, duration of exposure to that source, and conductance of the tissue exposed. At the time of the burn, blood flow to the local burn area increases, vessels dilate, and histamine release increases capillary permeability. Superficial, or partial-thickness, damage affects the top two or three layers of the epidermis.

Signs and symptoms

The signs and symptoms of burns include erythema, swelling, blisters, sloughing of the epidermis, and pain.

Serious conditions
Sunburn may cause a photo-toxic reaction. Systemic lupus erythematosus can cause a sunburnlike erythema. Erythropoietic protoporphyria can also cause erythema, vesicles, edema, and purpura.

Complications
Repeated serious, blistering sunburns can lead to development of basal cell epithelioma, squamous cell carcinoma, or malignant melanoma later in life. Secondary infection is also a consideration when blisters or erosions appear.

Nursing considerations
• Be alert to the development of unusual skin lesions; some skin cancers result from sun exposure or burns.
• Evaluate the patient for possible secondary infection.

Patient teaching
• Explain the importance of sunscreen use.
• Teach the patient the signs and symptoms of secondary infection.
• Instruct the patient with burns (other than sunburn) about appropriate wound care.

aluminum acetate
  solution
bacitracin
benzalkonium chloride
benzocaine
benzoyl peroxide
calamine
chlorhexidine gluconate
chlorophyll derivatives,
  chlorophyllin copper
  complex
clotrimazole
coal tar
colloidal oatmeal
dextranomer
dibucaine
diphenhydramine
  hydrochloride, topical
gentian violet
hydroactive dressings
  and granules, flexible
hydrocortisone
hydrocortisone acetate
hydrogen peroxide
hydroquinone
iodine
isopropyl alcohol
ketoconazole
lidocaine hydrochloride,
  topical
miconazole nitrate
minoxidil, topical
neomycin sulfate
permethrin
povidone-iodine
pramoxine hydrochloride
pyrethrins
pyrithione zinc
salicylic acid
selenium sulfide

sodium hypochlorite
sulfur
terbinafine hydrochloride
tetracaine hydrochloride
tetracycline
  hydrochloride,
  chlortetracycline
  hydrochloride
thimerosal
tolnaftate
triclosan, irgasan
undecylenic acid and
  derivatives
urea
vitamins A, D, and E,
  topical
witch hazel
zinc oxide

---

aluminum acetate solution
Buro-Sol

Pregnancy Risk Category NR

HOW SUPPLIED
Solution: 0.23% aluminum
acetate

ACTION
Aluminum acetate solution is
an astringent and helps to con-
strict blood vessels.

Route	Onset	Peak	Duration
Topical	Immediate	Unknown	Unknown

Reactions may be *common*, uncommon, *life-threatening*, or COMMON AND LIFE-THREATENING.

INDICATIONS & DOSAGES
Acute skin inflammation (contact dermatitis, poison ivy, insect bites, jewelry rashes, mild sunburn, athlete's foot), dry skin—
Adults and children: 1:20 to 1:40 solution applied topically via soaked gauze dressing for 15 to 30 minutes, 4 to 6 times daily.

ADVERSE REACTIONS
Skin: irritation.

INTERACTIONS
Drug-drug
Collagenase: diminishes therapeutic effect of collagenase. Thoroughly rinse area with normal saline solution before applying collagenase.

CONTRAINDICATIONS
None reported.

OVERDOSE & TREATMENT
No information available.

NURSING CONSIDERATIONS
• Thoroughly rinse drug from area before applying collagenase.
• Tell patient not to cover wet dressing with impervious cover, such as plastic.
• Hot solution may irritate skin.
• Safety and efficacy of use with fluids other than water haven't been established.

• If dressing is applied to skin and reintroduced into solution, discard the solution.
• Safety and efficacy of use for chickenpox haven't been established.
• Aluminum acetate solution can be safely used as pretreatment for topical antifungals and corticosteroids.

PATIENT TEACHING
• Advise patient to read carefully and follow package instructions.
• Instruct patient to use room temperature tap water when preparing solution.
• Instruct patient to saturate clean white cloth, gently squeeze, and apply to the affected area.
• Caution patient against placing plastic or other impervious cover over wet dressing.
• Instruct patient to discontinue use if extension of inflammation occurs, if increased irritation is experienced, or if symptoms haven't diminished within 1 week.
• Advise patient to avoid contact of solution with eyes.

bacitracin
Baciguent

Pregnancy Risk Category C

HOW SUPPLIED
Ointment: 500 U/g

ACTION
Bactericidal or bacteriostatic, depending on organism and concentration of drug; inhibits bacterial cell-wall synthesis. Effective against gram-positive organisms.

Route	Onset	Peak	Duration
Topical	Unknown	Unknown	Unknown

INDICATIONS & DOSAGES
Topical infections, abrasions, cuts, minor burns, or wounds—
Adults and children: apply thin film q.d. to t.i.d., depending on severity of condition. Drug shouldn't be used for longer than 1 week.

ADVERSE REACTIONS
Skin: allergic contact dermatitis.

INTERACTIONS
None reported.

CONTRAINDICATIONS
Contraindicated in patients who are hypersensitive to drug or its components. Also not to be used in eyes, on mucous membranes, or in external ear canal if eardrum is perforated.

OVERDOSE & TREATMENT
No information available.

NURSING CONSIDERATIONS
• Clean skin before applying drug, especially if skin is crusted or suppurative.
• Anticipate alternative treatment for burns that cover more than 20% of body surface, especially if patient suffers from impaired renal function.
• Prolonged use may result in overgrowth of nonsusceptible organisms, particularly *Candida* species.
• Patients allergic to neomycin may also be sensitive to bacitracin.
• Before applying drug, obtain culture and sensitivity tests, as ordered.
• *Alert:* Don't confuse bacitracin with Bactroban.

PATIENT TEACHING
• Tell patient to stop using drug and to seek medical advice if improvement doesn't occur or if condition worsens.
• Instruct patient to report persistent or severe adverse reactions.
• Tell patient not to use drug for longer than 1 week, except with medical advice.

Reactions may be *common*, uncommon, *life-threatening*, or COMMON AND LIFE-THREATENING.

benzalkonium chloride
Band-Aid Medicated
Bandages, Benza, Clinical
Care Antimicrobial Wound
Cleaner, Dermoplast
Antibacterial Spray, Disintyl,
Formula Magic Antimicrobial/
Antifungal Powder, Humex,
Johnson's Antibacterial
Towelettes, Nexcare
Antibacterial Bandages, Ony-
Clear, Orchid Fresh
Antimicrobial Ostomy
Cleanser

Pregnancy Risk Category NR

HOW SUPPLIED
Ointment: 0.2%
Powder: 0.01%
Solution: 0.0025% to 0.5%,
17%
Spray: 0.0025% to 0.5%, 17%

ACTION
The drug is a cationic surfactant that has antimicrobial effects on gram-positive and
gram-negative bacteria but no
effect on bacterial spores. The
mechanism of bactericidal action isn't known but may result
from enzyme inactivation,
which disrupts cell membranes,
and the denaturation of microbe
lipoprotein. The drug also has
wetting, emulsifying, keratolytic, and detergent actions.

Route	Onset	Peak	Duration
Topical	Immediate	Unknown	Unknown

INDICATIONS & DOSAGES
*First aid antisepsis for skin,
mucous membranes, and
wounds—*
**Adults and children ages 2
and older:** *Topical spray—*
applied from 6 to 12 inches
away; if dressing used, area
must dry first. Not to exceed 3
applications per day. *Topical
application of nonspray form—*
refer to product label for directions.

ADVERSE REACTIONS
Skin: irritation.

INTERACTIONS
None reported.

CONTRAINDICATIONS
Contraindicated for use with
occlusive dressings, casts, and
anal or vaginal packs because
of potential for irritation and
chemical burning.

OVERDOSE & TREATMENT
Ingestion can cause GI tract
irritation, with nausea and vomiting. Systemic toxicity symptoms include restlessness, ap-
prehension, weakness, confusion, dyspnea, cyanosis,
collapse, seizures, and coma.
Respiratory muscle paralysis

can cause death. Alcohol use promotes absorption.

Immediately give several glasses of mild soap solution, milk, or egg whites beaten in water; start gastric lavage, using a mild soap solution. Support respirations, as needed, and give oxygen. Give a short-acting parenteral barbiturate to treat seizure activity.

NURSING CONSIDERATIONS
• *Alert:* Ingestion can cause death.
• Apply antiseptic agents to intact skin surrounding the wound rather than directly on wound bed, to avoid irritating the tissue.
• Drug doesn't achieve complete sterilization because of lack of activity against bacterial spores, infectious hepatitis, and *Mycobacterium tuberculosis*.
• Have patient rinse detergents and soaps from the skin or other areas before use because they reduce the antibacterial activity of benzalkonium chloride.

PATIENT TEACHING
• Advise patient that drug is inactivated by soap and anionic detergents; tell him to rinse area thoroughly before applying drug.
• Advise patient that drug doesn't cause complete sterilization.

• Instruct patient to read carefully and follow instructions on package and to report any adverse reactions to a doctor.
• Advise patient to avoid contact of drug with eyes.

---

benzocaine
Americaine, Boil-Ease, Dermoplast, Outgro

Pregnancy Risk Category C

HOW SUPPLIED
Aerosol: 20%
Ointment: 20%

ACTION
A local anesthetic that inhibits conduction of nerve impulses from sensory nerves, temporarily reducing perception of local discomfort.

Route	Onset	Peak	Duration
Topical	Immediate	Unknown	Unknown

INDICATIONS & DOSAGES
Local pain, itching, or discomfort from sunburn, insect bites, minor cuts, scrapes, and burns, or other minor skin irritations—
Adults and children ages 2 and older: apply to affected area p.r.n.; hold spray 6 to 12 inches from affected area, and spray liberally up to q.i.d.

ADVERSE REACTIONS
Skin: urticaria, edema, contact dermatitis, burning, stinging, tenderness.

INTERACTIONS
Drug-drug
Class I antiarrhythmics: potential for synergistic effect. Use together with caution.

CONTRAINDICATIONS
Contraindicated in patients who are hypersensitive to drug or its components.

OVERDOSE & TREATMENT
None reported.

NURSING CONSIDERATIONS
• Benzocaine topical creams and ointments should be stored in tight containers, protected from light; prolonged exposure to temperatures higher than 86° F (30° C) should be avoided.
• Excessive use may cause methemoglobinemia in infants. Don't use in children younger than age 1.

PATIENT TEACHING
• Advise patient to read carefully and follow package instruction.
• Tell patient to spray product into palm of hand and apply to face, avoiding contact with eyes.

• Instruct patient to discontinue use if symptoms don't subside within 1 week and to contact doctor for evaluation.

---

benzoyl peroxide
Acne-5, Acne-10, Ambi 10, Benoxyl 5 Lotion, Benoxyl 10 Lotion, BlemErase, Clean and Clear, Clearasil, Clear By Design, Dryox, Exact, Fostex, Loroxide, Neutrogena Acne Mask, Neutrogena on the Spot, Oxy Balance, Oxy 5, Oxy 10, PanOxyl, Perfectoderm, Persa-Gel 10, Vanoxide, ZAPZYT

Pregnancy Risk Category C

HOW SUPPLIED
Bar: 5%, 10%
Cleanser: 10%
Cream: 2.5%, 5%, 10%
Facial mask: 5%
Gel: 2.5%, 5%, 10%, 20%
Liquid: 5%, 10%
Lotion: 5%, 7.5%, 10%

ACTION
Antibacterial effect on *Propionibacterium acnes* may result from the generation of free oxygen radicals that bind to and destroy bacterial proteins. Drug may also be a mild keratolytic, causing increased turnover of epithelial cells and enhanced resolution of comedones.

---

*Liquid contains alcohol.   **May contain tartrazine.   †Canada   ‡Australia   §U.K.

Route	Onset	Peak	Duration
Topical	3-4 wk	8-12 wk	Unknown

tives such as cinnamon, benzocaine, and tetracaine.

INDICATIONS & DOSAGES
*Mild to moderate acne vulgaris,
oily skin—*
**Adults and children older
than age 12:** apply a small
amount topically q.d. or b.i.d. to
freshly cleansed and dried affected area. Begin with 2.5%
strength and progress to
stronger strength p.r.n.
Cleanser—Wash q.d. or b.i.d.,
rinse thoroughly, and pat dry.

ADVERSE REACTIONS
Skin: excessive drying with
peeling, erythema, and edema;
allergic contact dermatitis.

INTERACTIONS
Drug-drug
Sunscreens containing PABA:
transient skin discoloration.
Use together cautiously.
Tretinoin: skin irritation. Use
together cautiously.

Drug-lifestyle
Sun exposure: increases skin irritation. Tell patient to use sunscreen and avoid unnecessary
exposure.

CONTRAINDICATIONS
Contraindicated in patients who
are hypersensitive to benzoyl
peroxide. Cross-sensitivity may
occur with benzoic acid deriva-

OVERDOSE & TREATMENT
Symptoms of overdose may include excessive scaling, erythema, and edema.
　Treatment includes discontinuing use and consulting a doctor. Cool compresses, emollients, or topical corticosteroids
may provide symptomatic relief.

NURSING CONSIDERATIONS
● Benzoyl peroxide is for external use only.
● Drug shouldn't come in contact with eyes, eyelids, lips,
other mucous membranes, inflamed skin, or open skin or
wounds. If contact occurs, patient should rinse with water
immediately.
● Some dryness and peeling occur with use. Excessive dryness, peeling, or other skin reaction should be evaluated by a
doctor.
● Symptoms may not improve
before 2 to 6 weeks of benzoyl
peroxide treatment.
● Various concentrations are
available, but few data indicate
that effectiveness is dose-
related.
● Irritation is dose-related; patient should start with the lowest concentration (2.5%), and
increase if it has no effect.

• Gels last longer and release more benzoyl peroxide than lotions or creams; reserve creams for patient with dry or sensitive skin. Recommend liquids, which are the most irritating, only for patients who don't respond to gels or lotions.

• It isn't known if drug appears in breast milk. Breast-feeding women should use it cautiously.

• Some products may contain sulfites.

PATIENT TEACHING

• Advise patient to read carefully and follow package instructions.

• Tell patient to cleanse area thoroughly before applying.

• Inform patient that drug will bleach hair and fabrics.

• Instruct patient to start with lowest concentration (2.5%) and increase exposure time and concentration as needed and tolerated.

• Inform patient that drug may cause temporary warmth or mild stinging. If excessive stinging or burning occurs with any application, patient should rinse skin with soap and water and not reapply drug until the next day.

• Advise patient to expect some dryness and peeling. To avoid irritation, tell patient to start with one application daily and increase as tolerated. If excessive redness or discomfort occurs, patient should decrease dose or discontinue use. If excessive irritation occurs, patient should discontinue use and consult a doctor.

• Tell patient to avoid other sources of skin irritation, such as alcohol-containing topical products, sun lamps, or excessive sun exposure.

• Warn asthmatic patient that product may contain sulfites.

• Tell patient that normal use of water-based cosmetics is allowed.

---

calamine
Calamox, Resinol

Pregnancy Risk Category NR

HOW SUPPLIED
Cream: 8%
Lotion: 8%
Ointment: 6%, 17%

ACTION
Mild astringent and antipruritic properties may help to soothe minor skin irritations.

Route	Onset	Peak	Duration
Topical	Immediate	Unknown	Unknown

INDICATIONS & DOSAGES
Temporary relief from itching, pain, and discomfort caused by insect bites, poison ivy, poison

---

oak, poison sumac, and other minor skin irritations—
Adults and children older than age 2: topical application to affected area t.i.d. or q.i.d.

ADVERSE REACTIONS
Skin: rash, dermatitis.

INTERACTIONS
None reported.

CONTRAINDICATIONS
Contraindicated on open or oozing areas of skin.

OVERDOSE & TREATMENT
No information available.

NURSING CONSIDERATIONS
• Calamine is well tolerated and has no significant adverse effects.
• Calamine should be used for minor skin irritation but shouldn't be applied to open or oozing skin.

PATIENT TEACHING
• Advise patient to read carefully and follow package instructions.
• Instruct patient to avoid allowing drug to come in contact with eyes.
• Advise patient to discontinue use of drug and seek evaluation by doctor if symptoms don't subside or if rash, burning, or irritation occurs.

• Caution patient not to apply drug to open or oozing skin.

---

chlorhexidine gluconate
BactoShield, Bactoshield 2, Betasept, Dina-Hex Skin Cleanser, Dyna-Hex 2 Skin Cleanser, Exidine-2 Scrub, Exedine-4 Scrub, Exedine Skin Cleanser, E-Z Scrub, Hibiclens, Hibistat, Hibistat Towelette

Pregnancy Risk Category B

HOW SUPPLIED
Aerosol, metered: 4%
Foam: 4 %
Liquid: 2%, 4%
Solution: 0.5%, 2%, 4%
Sponge or brush: 4%
Wipes: 0.5%

ACTION
Persistent broad-spectrum antimicrobial (gram-positive and gram-negative bacteria).

Route	Onset	Peak	Duration
Topical	Immediate	Unknown	Several hr

INDICATIONS & DOSAGES
Skin and wound cleanser—
Adults: rinse area thoroughly with water. Apply sufficient amount of drug to cover affected area, and wash gently. Rinse thoroughly.

Germicidal alternative to conventional handwashing—
Adults: apply 5 ml chlorhexidine (or use individual wipe); rub vigorously until dry (about 15 seconds).

ADVERSE REACTIONS
EENT: deafness when instilled into middle ear.
Skin: irritation, dermatitis (especially when applied to genital areas), photosensitivity reactions, urticaria.
Other: *hypersensitivity reactions with anaphylaxis,* bronchospasm, cough, wheezing, dyspnea.

INTERACTIONS
None reported.

CONTRAINDICATIONS
Contraindicated in patients who are hypersensitive to chlorhexidine gluconate; not for use in ears or eyes.

OVERDOSE & TREATMENT
If drug is ingested in large quantities or by children, signs and symptoms of alcohol intoxication may appear.

Treat with gastric lavage using milk, egg white, gelatin, or mild soap.

NURSING CONSIDERATIONS
• Patient shouldn't put in the ear, especially if eardrum is ruptured, because deafness may result.
• Serious and permanent eye injury has occurred when chlorhexidine enters and remains in the eye.
• Patient shouldn't use on wounds involving more than the superficial skin layers.

PATIENT TEACHING
• Caution patient against allowing drug to contact eyes, ears, or mouth and to rinse promptly and thoroughly with water if contact does occur.
• Instruct patient to read carefully and follow drug instructions.
• Advise patient not to use chlorhexidine repeatedly as a general skin cleanser over large body areas unless directed by a doctor.
• Inform patient that drug isn't for use on wounds involving more than superficial skin layers.

chlorophyll derivatives, chlorophyllin copper complex
Chloresium, Derifil, PALS

Pregnancy Risk Category NR

HOW SUPPLIED
Solution: 0.2%
Spray: 0.2%

Tablets (chlorophyll and chlorophyll derivatives): 20 mg, 100 mg
Tablets (chlorophyllin copper complex): 14 mg, 100 mg
Water-soluble ointment: 0.5%

ACTION

The exact mechanism of action is unknown. Chlorophyll derivatives may stimulate protein synthesis or have antimicrobial effects and, when taken orally, may bind to odorous microbial compounds in the GI tract. Chlorophyll derivatives help to produce a clean, granulating wound base for epithelialization or skin grafting, soothe inflamed tissues, and control wound odor. Chlorophyll derivatives are also taken orally to help control ostomy odors. This is characterized as true deodorization rather than odor masking.

Route	Onset	Peak	Duration
Topical	Unknown	Unknown	Unknown
P.O.	1-2 wk	Unknown	Unknown

INDICATIONS & DOSAGES

Wound care, deodorization—
Adults and children older than age 12: use a continuous wet dressing to apply solution, or instill directly into ulcers or cavities (refer to specific product directions). Apply ointment generously to area and cover with dressing.

Control of ostomy odor—
Adults and children older than age 12: 50 to 200 mg per day, P.O., in divided doses, with meals. Doses shouldn't exceed 300 mg daily.

ADVERSE REACTIONS

GI: diarrhea.
Skin: pruritus, mild irritation.

INTERACTIONS

Drug-drug
Laxatives (bisacodyl, docusate, milk of magnesia, senna): enhances laxative effect. Caution against using together.

Drug-herb
Agar, aloe, black hellebore, buckthorn bark, cascara sagrada, rhubarb: enhances laxative effect. Caution against using together.

CONTRAINDICATIONS

None reported.

OVERDOSE & TREATMENT

No information available.

NURSING CONSIDERATIONS

• For best results with ointment, dressings should be changed every 48 to 72 hours.
• Chlorophyll derivatives may be used topically on arterioscle-

rotic ulcers, diabetic ulcers, and other chronic ulcers; malignant skin lesions that need deodorization; skin grafts; and thermal, chemical, or radiation injuries.

- Tablets may be placed in ostomy or taken by mouth.
- Effect of oral tablets may not be apparent for several weeks.

PATIENT TEACHING
- Advise patient to read carefully and follow package instructions.
- Inform patient that if cramping or diarrhea occurs, the oral dose should be reduced.
- Advise patient that the oral tablets will stain the stool dark green.
- Caution patient that solution and ointment are for external use only.
- Advise patient to use the lowest dose that effectively controls odor.

---

clotrimazole
Lotrimin AF Antifungal Jock-Itch Lotion, Lotrimin AF Antifungal Jock-Itch Cream, Lotrimin AF Antifungal Cream, Mycelex

Pregnancy Risk Category B

HOW SUPPLIED
Topical cream: 1%
Topical lotion: 1%
Topical solution: 1%

ACTION
Fungistatic or fungicidal (dose-dependent) drug that alters fungal cell-wall permeability and creates osmotic instability.

Route	Onset	Peak	Duration
Topical	Unknown	Unknown	Unknown

INDICATIONS & DOSAGES
Superficial fungal infections (tinea corporis, tinea cruris, tinea pedis)—
Adults and children ages 3 and older: apply thinly, and massage into affected and surrounding area, morning and evening for 2 to 4 weeks.

ADVERSE REACTIONS
Skin: erythema, stinging, blistering, peeling, edema, pruritus, urticaria, burning, general irritation.

INTERACTIONS
None significant.

CONTRAINDICATIONS
Contraindicated in patients who are hypersensitive to drug or its components. Also contraindicated for ophthalmic use.

OVERDOSE & TREATMENT
No information available.

NURSING CONSIDERATIONS
• Area should be cleaned before applying topical drug.
• Tinea cruris usually responds within 2 weeks; tinea pedis or corporis, 4 weeks.
• If condition doesn't improve, doctor should review the diagnosis.
• It's unknown whether drug appears in breast milk. Breastfeeding patients should use cautiously.
• Drug isn't recommended for use in children younger than age 3.

PATIENT TEACHING
• Advise patient to read carefully and follow package instructions.
• Tell patient to notify doctor if tinea cruris doesn't respond within 2 weeks, or tinea pedis or corporis within 4 weeks.
• Tell patient with tinea pedis to apply drug between toes, to wear well-fitting, ventilated shoes, and to change socks at least once daily.
• Caution patient to watch for and report irritation or sensitivity and to discontinue use if irritation occurs.
• Inform patient of the importance of using drug for the full treatment even though symptoms may have improved.
• Warn patient not to use occlusive wrappings or dressings.
• Warn patient to avoid drug contact with eyes.

---

coal tar
Coal Tar, Carbonis Detergens, Denorex, DHS Tar, Doak Tar, Doak Tar Distillate, Estar, Exorex, Fototar, Ionil T, Medotar, Neutrogena T/Derm, Oxipor VHC, PsoriGel, Taraphilic Ointment, Tegrin, Tegrin for Psoriasis, Tegrin Medicated Soap for Psoriasis

Pregnancy Risk Category C

HOW SUPPLIED
Cream: 2%, 5%
Gel: 5%, 7.5%
Liquid: 40%
Lotion: 5%, 25%
Oil: 5%
Ointment: 1%
Shampoo: 5%, 7%, 9%, 12.5%
Solution: 20%

ACTION
Drug has antieczematous, keratoplastic, and antipruritic properties; it decreases epidermal proliferation and dermal infiltration.

Route	Onset	Peak	Duration
Topical	Unknown	Unknown	Unknown

Reactions may be *common*, uncommon, *life-threatening*, or COMMON AND LIFE-THREATENING.

INDICATIONS & DOSAGES

Seborrheic dermatitis, dandruff—
Adults and children ages 2 and older: apply coal tar shampoos to wet hair and scalp, and rinse; then repeat the application, leave on for 5 minutes, and rinse. Frequency of shampoo use depends on severity of condition. Use at least twice weekly for 2 weeks, and then once weekly. May be used daily, if warranted.

Psoriasis, atopic dermatitis—
Adults and children ages 2 and older: apply to affected area q.d. to q.i.d. Gently massage, and then remove excess after several minutes. Coal tar bath oil emulsions are added to bath water; soak for 10 to 20 minutes, and then pat skin dry. Use q.d. to once every 3 days for 30 to 45 days.

ADVERSE REACTIONS

Skin: rash, burning, photosensitivity reactions, skin discoloration, hair discoloration.

INTERACTIONS

Drug-drug
Other psoriasis therapy: disulfiram (Antabuse) reaction if alcohol-containing coal tar products are used. Patient shouldn't use together unless otherwise directed.

Drug-lifestyle
Sun exposure: photosensitivity. Patient should avoid exposure to sun or sunlamps for 24 hours after treatment.

CONTRAINDICATIONS

Contraindicated in patients who are hypersensitive to drug or its components. Don't use on acutely inflamed or broken skin or on genital and rectal area. Also contraindicated in patients younger than age 2 and in those with lupus erythematosus, polymorphous light eruptions, or other condition characterized by photosensitivity. Patients with psoriasis who are also receiving UV therapy shouldn't use this drug, unless directed by a doctor.

OVERDOSE & TREATMENT

For ingestion, don't induce emesis; encourage patient to drink water.

For ocular exposure, irrigate with water. Contact a poison control center or doctor.

NURSING CONSIDERATIONS

• Use during exacerbation of psoriasis may result in total body exfoliation.
• Coal tar products shouldn't be used with other psoriasis therapies because of risk of photosensitivity.

• Don't use in children younger than age 2.

PATIENT TEACHING
• Caution patient to read carefully and follow package instructions.
• Tell patient that emollients may be used 1 hour after coal tar if dryness occurs.
• Instruct patient to discontinue use and consult a doctor if symptoms don't improve or if they worsen.
• Advise patient not to use coal tar products if photosensitive or hypersensitive to any component.
• Advise patient not to allow coal tar products to come in contact with eyes.
• Instruct patient not to apply to genital or rectal areas or to inflamed, broken, or infected skin.
• Advise patient that product may stain hair, clothing, and bathtub.

---

colloidal oatmeal
Avalon Oat Soak, Aveeno Baby Bath, Aveeno Daily Moisturizing Bath, Aveeno Soothing Bath, Jergens ActiBath, Nutra-Soothe

Pregnancy Risk Category NR

HOW SUPPLIED
Bath tablets: 20%
Powder: 43%, 100%

ACTION
Nonalkaline antipruritic, lubricating, and cleansing agent.

Route	Onset	Peak	Duration
Topical	Unknown	Unknown	Unknown

INDICATIONS & DOSAGES
Chronic or acute skin irritation or dryness—
Adults and children: 1 to 2 baths daily for 10 to 20 minutes each. Prepare bath before entering tub; sprinkle powder into full-force stream of warm water and stir thoroughly; or, drop 1 tablet in tub when tub is half full and continue filling.

ADVERSE REACTIONS
None reported.

INTERACTIONS
None reported.

CONTRAINDICATIONS
Contraindicated in patients who are allergic to oatmeal.

OVERDOSE & TREATMENT
No information available.

NURSING CONSIDERATIONS
• Colloidal oatmeal is finely ground raw oatmeal and isn't toxic if ingested.

• Combination products sometimes contain ingredients such as lanolin, to which patients might be hypersensitive. Labels should be read carefully.
• Bath bars are nonsoap, nondetergent products containing mineral oil.
• Patients hypersensitive to oatmeal may experience skin irritation.

PATIENT TEACHING
• Advise patient that colloidal oatmeal should be fully dissolved in tepid water and shouldn't be rinsed from skin; pat dry.
• Caution patient to read carefully ingredients on combination products to avoid inadvertent exposure to agents to which they are hypersensitive.
• Advise patient that oils or lotions can be applied to moist skin after bathing or showering, to limit loss of skin moisture and reduce irritation from clothing.
• Tell patient to seek medical advice if symptoms worsen or don't improve within 1 week.

---

dextranomer
Debrisan

Pregnancy Risk Category NR

HOW SUPPLIED
Beads: 4 g, 25 g, 60 g, 120 g
Dressing pad: 3 g
Paste: 10 g

ACTION
Cleanses wound surfaces by capillary action, drawing wound exudate, bacteria, and contaminants into the beads, thereby enhancing formation of granulation tissue and promoting wound healing.

Route	Onset	Peak	Duration
Topical	Unknown	Unknown	Unknown

INDICATIONS & DOSAGES
Cleaning exudative wounds—
Adults and children: apply to affected area q.d., b.i.d., or more often if drainage is heavy. Apply at least ¼-inch thickness and cover with sterile gauze.

ADVERSE REACTIONS
Skin: transient pain at site, bleeding, erythema, contact dermatitis.

INTERACTIONS
None reported.

CONTRAINDICATIONS
Contraindicated in patients with dry wounds, deep fistulas, sinus tracts, or any area where complete removal of drug isn't certain.

OVERDOSE & TREATMENT
No information available.

NURSING CONSIDERATIONS
• Dextranomer isn't an enzyme and can't be used for dry wounds.
• Wound must be cleansed before applying, leaving area moist. Bandage is applied to hold beads in place; requires room for expansion (1 g of beads absorbs 4 ml of exudate).
• When product is saturated and grayish yellow, irrigate wound and remove beads or paste. Beads must be removed thoroughly, especially before any surgical treatment; vigorous irrigation or soaking may be necessary.

PATIENT TEACHING
• Teach patient how to perform sterile dressing changes.
• Advise patient to avoid getting drug in eyes and to wash hands well after application.
• If dressing becomes dry, tell patient not to remove it without wetting to loosen bandage and beads.
• Caution patient to stop treatment when area is free from exudate.
• Caution patient not to use in areas where complete removal of drug isn't certain; for example, in fistulas or sinus tracts.

dibucaine
Dibucaine, Nupercainal

Pregnancy Risk Category B

HOW SUPPLIED
Cream: 0.5%
Ointment: 1%

ACTION
Inhibits conduction of nerve impulses and decreases cell membrane permeability to ions, anesthetizing local nerve endings.

Route	Onset	Peak	Duration
Topical	Unknown	Unknown	Unknown

INDICATIONS & DOSAGES
Pain and itching from abrasions, sunburn, minor burns, insect bites, and other minor skin conditions—
Adults and children: apply to affected areas, p.r.n. Maximum daily dose of 1% ointment is 30 g for adults and 7.5 g for children.

Pain, itching, and burning caused by hemorrhoids—
Adults: instill 1% ointment into rectum using a rectal applicator each morning and evening and after each bowel movement, p.r.n. Apply additional ointment topically to anal tissues. Maximum daily dose is 30 g.

ADVERSE REACTIONS
Skin: irritation, inflammation, contact dermatitis, cutaneous lesions, urticaria.
Other: *hypersensitivity reactions* (edema, burning, stinging, tenderness).

INTERACTIONS
Drug-drug
Class I antiarrhythmics (procainamide, quinidine): potential toxic effect. Don't use together.

CONTRAINDICATIONS
Contraindicated in patients who are hypersensitive to drug, sulfites, or other amide-type local anesthetics. Also contraindicated for use on large skin areas, on broken skin or mucous membranes, and in eyes.

OVERDOSE & TREATMENT
Ingestion causes systemic toxicity, with hypotension and bradycardia. CNS effects include nervousness, vomiting, seizures, and respiratory distress.

Support airway and treat with vasopressors and anticonvulsants, if necessary.

NURSING CONSIDERATIONS
•Drug is for topical use only, for short periods, and should be stopped immediately if hypersensitivity reaction occurs.
•Drug shouldn't be used by breast-feeding patients.

•In children and elderly patients, dosage should be adjusted according to patient's age, size, and physical condition.

PATIENT TEACHING
•Caution patient that if symptoms persist or worsen after 1 week of treatment, he should contact a doctor for evaluation.
•Explain how to use drug correctly.
•Emphasize need to wash hands thoroughly after use.
•Caution patient to apply drug sparingly to minimize untoward effects.
•Tell patient to keep drug out of reach of children.

diphenhydramine hydrochloride, topical
Anti-itch, Benadryl*, Dermamycin, Diphenhist

Pregnancy Risk Category B

HOW SUPPLIED
Cream: 1%, 2%
Gel: 1%, 2%
Solution: 1%, 2%
Stick: 2%

ACTION
Competes with histamine for H_1-receptor sites on effector cells. Prevents but doesn't reverse histamine-mediated responses, particularly in smooth

---

*Liquid contains alcohol.   **May contain tartrazine.   †Canada   ‡Australia   §U.K.

muscle of the bronchial tree, GI tract, uterus, and blood vessels. Structurally related to local anesthetics, diphenhydramine provides local anesthesia by preventing initiation and transmission of nerve impulses.

Route	Onset	Peak	Duration
Topical	Unknown	Unknown	Unknown

INDICATIONS & DOSAGES
Temporary relief from itching caused by minor skin disorder, sunburn, insect bites, reactions to poison ivy, sumac, or oak—
Adults and children older than age 2: apply to affected area t.i.d. or q.i.d. (or as directed by doctor).

ADVERSE REACTIONS
Skin: local irritation, sensitization (prolonged use).

INTERACTIONS
None reported.

CONTRAINDICATIONS
Contraindicated in patients who are hypersensitive to diphenhydramine or any of its active ingredients. Also contraindicated for use on blistered, raw, or oozing skin and for application near eyes or other mucous membranes (mouth, nose).

OVERDOSE & TREATMENT
Systemic toxicity may develop in children after repeated application of topical diphenhydramine to relieve itching from poison ivy, sumac, or oak. Toxic signs and symptoms in children include CNS stimulation, abnormal eye movements, dry mouth, urine retention, confusion, restlessness, irritability, and slurred speech.

If child has developed systemic toxicity, stop use of product and provide supportive care.

NURSING CONSIDERATIONS
• Benadryl Maximum Strength Spray contains 70% alcohol.
• For external use only; not for use on broken, exposed, or oozing areas of the skin or around eyes or other mucous membranes (mouth, nose).
• Drug shouldn't be used for longer than 1 week or for large areas of the body.

PATIENT TEACHING
• Advise patient to avoid taking other OTC products that may contain diphenhydramine or other antihistamines.
• Caution patient that topical preparations of diphenhydramine are flammable and shouldn't be used near open flames or lighted cigarettes.
• Advise patient to discontinue use of product and contact doc-

tor if skin condition persists or doesn't improve within 1 week.

---

gentian violet
Gentian Violet

Pregnancy Risk Category C

HOW SUPPLIED
Solution: 1%*, 2%*

ACTION
Antifungal and antibacterial with unknown mechanism of action; effective against some gram-positive organisms including *Staphylococcus* species and some pathogenic yeast such as *Candida* species. It's less active against gram-negative bacteria and is ineffective against bacterial spores.

Route	Onset	Peak	Duration
Topical	Unknown	Unknown	Unknown

INDICATIONS & DOSAGES
Topical disinfectant for treatment of Candidiasis albicans *infection—*
Adults and children: apply to affected area with cotton b.i.d. or t.i.d. for 3 days.

ADVERSE REACTIONS
EENT: irritation, ulceration of mucous membranes.
Skin: staining, necrosis.

INTERACTIONS
None known.

CONTRAINDICATIONS
Contraindicated in patients who are hypersensitive to drug or its components; also contraindicated for use on ulcerative lesions.

OVERDOSE & TREATMENT
No information available.

NURSING CONSIDERATIONS
• Gentian violet stains skin and clothing.
• *Alert:* Esophagitis, laryngitis, and tracheitis may occur after swallowing solution used to treat oral candidiasis.
• When used for oral candidiasis, apply to individual lesions to prevent excessive swallowing of drug; place infants face down after application to prevent ingestion.
• Patient should stop use if irritation or sensitization occurs.
• Patient shouldn't use on ulcerative lesions on face because this may cause tattooing.
• Topical product shouldn't be used internally and shouldn't be allowed to contact eyes.
• Patient shouldn't use occlusive dressings.

PATIENT TEACHING
• Advise patient to read carefully and follow all package instructions.

- Tell patient to discontinue use if irritation occurs.
- Advise patient to avoid use of occlusive dressings.
- Caution patient not to allow product to come in contact with eyes.
- Warn patient to avoid swallowing excessive amounts of drug; serious adverse effects may occur.
- Tell parent to place infant face down after applying to oral lesions to prevent excessive ingestion.
- Advise patient that product will stain skin and clothing.
- Advise patient to avoid sexual intercourse during treatment for vaginal disorder.
- Encourage proper hygiene and skin care to prevent spread of infection or reinfection.

---

hydroactive dressings and granules, flexible
DuoDerm, DuoDerm CGF, DuoDerm Extra Thin, Kaltostat, Kaltostat Fortex, IntraSite, Shur-Clens, Sorbsan

Pregnancy Risk Category NR

HOW SUPPLIED
Dressings (inches): 4×4, 6×8, 8×8, 8×12 (sterile); 4×4, 8×8 (adhesive border)

Gel: 2% graft T starch copolymer
Gel dressing (inches): 2.5×2.5, 4×4, 4×5, 6×6, 6×7, 8×8
Granules: 5 g/tube
Pads (inches): 2×2, 3×3, 4×4, 4×8
Paste
Solution: 20% poloxamer 188
Wound-packing fibers

ACTION
Hydroactive substance interacts with tissue exudate to form a gel at the wound surface; permits removal of dressing from wound or ulcer with little or no trauma to newly formed tissue.

Route	Onset	Peak	Duration
Topical	Unknown	Unknown	Unknown

INDICATIONS & DOSAGES
Dermal ulcers, pressure ulcers, superficial wounds minor abrasions, donor sites, second-degree burns, protective dressings, postoperative wounds—
Adults: clean and prepare wound site before application; follow product-specific instructions.

ADVERSE REACTIONS
None reported.

INTERACTIONS
None reported.

Reactions may be *common*, uncommon, *life-threatening*, or COMMON AND LIFE-THREATENING.

CONTRAINDICATIONS
Contraindicated in patients who are hypersensitive to drug or its components. Also contraindicated in those with dermal ulcers involving muscle, tendon, or bone; ulcers resulting from infection, such as tuberculosis, syphilis, or deep fungal infection; active vasculitis, such as polyarteritis nodosa, systemic lupus erythematosus, or cryoglobulinemia; third-degree burns; or clinically infected wounds.

OVERDOSE & TREATMENT
No information available.

NURSING CONSIDERATIONS
• Dressings are designed to be in place for 1 to 7 days.
• Wound odor should dissipate with cleansing.
• With any occlusive dressing, size and depth of wound will increase as dead tissue and exudate are removed.
• If wound appears infected (inflammation, persistent odor despite cleansing, pus), don't use dressing, but contact the doctor.

PATIENT TEACHING
• Advise patient to read carefully and follow package instructions.
• Inform patient that wound odor should dissipate with cleansing.
• Warn patient that size and depth of wound will increase as cleansing progresses.
• Caution patient to contact a doctor if symptoms worsen or signs and symptoms of infection develop.

---

hydrocortisone
Acticort 100, Ala-Cort, Ala-Scalp, Bactine Hydrocortisone, Caldecort, Carmol, Cetacort, Cortaid, Cortizone, Delacort, Dermacort, Dermolate, Dermtex HC, Efcortelan§, Hydrocortisyl, KeriCort, Procort, Scalpicin, Squibb-HC‡, Tegrin-HC, T/Scalp

hydrocortisone acetate
Anusol HC-1, Caldecort Maximum Strength, Cortaid, Cortamed†, Corticaine, Corticreme†, Gynecort, Hydrocortisone Acetate, Lanacort

Pregnancy Risk Category C

HOW SUPPLIED
hydrocortisone
Cream: 0.5%, 1%
Gel: 1%
Liquid: 1%*
Lotion: 1%
Ointment: 0.5%, 1%
Spray: 1%*
Stick roll-on: 1%

---

*Liquid contains alcohol.   **May contain tartrazine.   †Canada   ‡Australia   §U.K.

hydrocortisone acetate
Cream: 0.5%, 1%
Ointment: 0.5%, 1%

ACTION
Unknown; diffuses across cell membranes to form complexes with specific cytoplasmic receptors; anti-inflammatory, antipruritic, vasoconstrictive, and antiproliferative activity.

Route	Onset	Peak	Duration
Topical	Unknown	Unknown	Unknown

INDICATIONS & DOSAGES
Temporary relief from itching caused by minor skin irritation, inflammation, or rash—
Adults and children ages 2 and older: clean area; apply cream, gel, lotion, ointment, or topical solution sparingly to area q.d. to q.i.d.

ADVERSE REACTIONS
GU: glycosuria.
Metabolic: hyperglycemia.
Skin: burning, pruritus, irritation, dryness, erythema, folliculitis, hypertrichosis, hypopigmentation, acneiform eruptions, allergic contact dermatitis, maceration, secondary infection, atrophy, striae, miliaria with occlusive dressings.
Other: hypothalamic-pituitary-adrenal axis suppression, Cushing's syndrome.

INTERACTIONS
None significant.

CONTRAINDICATIONS
Contraindicated in patients who are hypersensitive to drug or its components.

OVERDOSE & TREATMENT
No information available.

NURSING CONSIDERATIONS
- Don't use as monotherapy in primary bacterial infections (impetigo, cellulitis), fungal infections, or viral infections.
- Don't use to treat rosacea, perioral dermatitis, or acne.
- Don't use near eyes.
- Systemic absorption is likely with use of occlusive dressings, prolonged treatment, or extensive body surface treatment.
- Children may absorb larger amounts of drug and be more prone to systemic toxicity.

PATIENT TEACHING
- Advise patient to read carefully and follow package instructions.
- Tell patient to use drug for a maximum of 1 week.
- Instruct patient to stop using the drug and notify a doctor of any lack of improvement or signs of systemic absorption, skin irritation or ulceration, hypersensitivity, or infection.

Reactions may be *common*, uncommon, *life-threatening*, or COMMON AND LIFE-THREATENING.

hydrogen peroxide
Orajel Perioseptic, Peroxyl

Pregnancy Risk Category NR

HOW SUPPLIED
Gel: 1.5%
Solution: 1.5%, 3%

ACTION
Topical antiseptic activity through oxidization; effervescent oxygen production cleanses wounds.

Route	Onset	Peak	Duration
Topical	Unknown	Unknown	Unknown

INDICATIONS & DOSAGES
Cleansing minor gum inflammation resulting from dental procedures, dentures, orthodontic appliances, accidental injury, canker sores, or other irritations of mouth or gums—
Adults and children ages 2 and older: dilute with equal volume of water and rinse oral cavity p.r.n.; or apply gel to affected area, allow to remain for 1 minute, and then rinse and spit out. Use up to q.i.d.

Cleansing minor wounds—
Adults: apply solution to affected area, p.r.n.

ADVERSE REACTIONS
Skin: irritation.

Other: hypertrophy of tongue papillae with prolonged use as mouthwash.

INTERACTIONS
None reported.

CONTRAINDICATIONS
Contraindicated in patients hypersensitive to drug or its components.

OVERDOSE & TREATMENT
Vomiting and diarrhea are common after ingestion; gastric injury occurs rarely after accidental ingestion.

Give patient water or milk to dilute the drug, and contact a doctor immediately.

NURSING CONSIDERATIONS
• Dose and frequency depend on the patient's condition.
• Using drug on intact skin provides no therapeutic value.
• Patient should use concentrated solutions of 20% or more cautiously because they irritate skin and mucous membranes.

PATIENT TEACHING
• Advise patient to follow package instructions and discontinue use immediately if adverse reactions occur.
• Caution patient not to use if he's hypersensitive to any component.

---

*Liquid contains alcohol. **May contain tartrazine. †Canada ‡Australia §U.K.

• Advise patient that product is for external use only; he should avoid contact with eyes.

---

hydroquinone
Alpha Hydrox, Ambi Skin Tone, Eldopaque, Eldoquin, Esoterica, Neostrata AHA Gel for Age Spots and Skin Lightening, Porcelana, Solaquin

Pregnancy Risk Category C

HOW SUPPLIED
Cream: 1.5%, 2%
Gel: 2%

ACTION
Inhibits melanin production by suppressing melanocyte metabolic processes.

Route	Onset	Peak	Duration
Topical	Unknown	Unknown	Unknown

INDICATIONS & DOSAGES
Temporary bleaching of hyperpigmented skin, such as freckles, chloasma, melasma—
Adults and children ages 12 and older: apply b.i.d. to affected area.

ADVERSE REACTIONS
Skin: burning, itching, stinging, transient erythema, dryness.

INTERACTIONS
Drug-lifestyle
Sun exposure: reverses bleaching effect of drug. Tell patient to use sunscreen and avoid unnecessary exposure.

CONTRAINDICATIONS
Contraindicated in patients who are hypersensitive to drug or its components; also contraindicated for use near eyes.

OVERDOSE & TREATMENT
Ingestion has caused dyspnea, anoxia, and respiratory failure. CV effects may include pallor, cyanosis, and CV collapse.

Immediately dilute with 4 to 8 oz (120 to 240 ml) of milk or water (not to exceed 15 ml/kg in a child). Induction of emesis isn't recommended because of the potential for CNS depression and seizures. Maintain airway and support ventilation; provide supportive and symptomatic care. Contact a poison control center or doctor.

NURSING CONSIDERATIONS
• Exposure of skin to UV light can reverse therapeutic effect.
• Perinasal application increases risk of irritation.

PATIENT TEACHING
• Advise patient to protect skin from UV light to avoid aggravation of hyperpigmentation.
• Caution patient to avoid use if pregnancy is planned or suspected.
• Advise patient to read carefully and follow package instructions; explain that product is for external use only.
• Caution patient not to use product near eyes and to avoid using it around nose because it may be irritating.

---

iodine
Iodex, Iodine, Iodine Tincture, Strong Iodine (Lugol's Solution), Strong Iodine Tincture

Pregnancy Risk Category D

HOW SUPPLIED
Ointment: 4.7% iodine with oleic acid, petrolatum
Solution: 2% iodine and 2.4% sodium iodide in purified water; 5% iodine and 10% potassium iodide in water; 2% iodine and 2.4% sodium iodide in 47% alcohol, purified water*; 7% iodine and 5% potassium iodide in 83% alcohol*

ACTION
Antimicrobial. Oxidizes carbohydrates, lipids, proteins, and amino acids, killing the microorganism. Active against bacteria, fungi, yeast, viruses, spores, and protozoa.

Route	Onset	Peak	Duration
Topical	Unknown	Unknown	Unknown

INDICATIONS & DOSAGES
Disinfection of intact skin, decontamination of minor wounds—
Adults and children: apply p.r.n. to affected area.

ADVERSE REACTIONS
Metabolic: iodism.
Skin: irritation, rash, staining.
Other: *hypersensitivity reactions.*

INTERACTIONS
None reported.

CONTRAINDICATIONS
Contraindicated in patients who are hypersensitive to drug or its components.

OVERDOSE & TREATMENT
Oral ingestion may cause severe toxicity, including corrosive gastroenteritis, vomiting, delirium, headache, hypotension, and circulatory collapse.
Irrigating wounds or burns with large amounts of iodine-containing compounds has caused serious or fatal reac-

tions; contact with eyes may cause severe burns.

Ocular and dermal exposures should immediately be irrigated with large amounts of water. Contact a poison control center or doctor.

NURSING CONSIDERATIONS
- Don't cover with occlusive dressing.
- Don't irrigate open wounds with large amounts of iodine solutions.
- Povidone-iodine retains more antiseptic activity in the presence of body secretions, body fluids, or surfactants.
- Sodium thiosulfate may remove iodine stains from skin.

PATIENT TEACHING
- Advise patient that iodine may stain skin or clothing and that sodium thiosulfate may remove stains.
- Advise patient that dose and frequency of use depend on condition and on patient tolerance.
- Instruct patient not to cover affected area with occlusive dressings.
- Caution patient to avoid contact with eyes.

---

isopropyl alcohol
Isopropyl alcohol

Pregnancy Risk Category NR

HOW SUPPLIED
Solution: 70%*

ACTION
Antiseptic and antibacterial; mechanism not defined.

Route	Onset	Peak	Duration
Topical	Unknown	Unknown	Unknown

INDICATIONS & DOSAGES
Skin disinfectant, massage lubricant—
Adults and children: apply to affected area topically, p.r.n.

ADVERSE REACTIONS
CNS: CNS depression.
Skin: irritation, drying.

INTERACTIONS
None reported.

CONTRAINDICATIONS
Contraindicated in patients who are hypersensitive to alcohol; in neonates; and over large body areas in children.

OVERDOSE & TREATMENT
Isopropyl alcohol is rapidly absorbed after ingestion. Respiratory distress, nausea and vomit-

---

ing, hypotension, and dizziness may occur.

Don't induce emesis; lavage may be performed but has limited value. Perform symptomatic and supportive treatment: Monitor vital signs, maintain airway, correct hypoglycemia, and correct hypotension.

To treat ocular contamination, irrigate eye for 15 minutes with tepid water; if symptoms persist 1 hour after irrigation, have patient notify a doctor.

NURSING CONSIDERATIONS
• Patient with skin disorders is at greater risk for drying and irritation of skin.
• Isopropyl alcohol isn't suitable for disinfecting contaminated surfaces.

PATIENT TEACHING
• Caution patient to avoid contact with eyes.
• Advise patient to avoid use if he's hypersensitive to any components.
• Advise parent not to use on neonate and not to apply to large body areas in child.
• Caution patient that product is flammable and to keep away from fire and flame.

ketoconazole
Nizoral A-D

Pregnancy Risk Category C

HOW SUPPLIED
Shampoo: 1%

ACTION
Antifungal. Inhibits purine transport and DNA, RNA, and protein synthesis. Increases cell-wall permeability, making fungus more susceptible to osmotic pressure.

Route	Onset	Peak	Duration
Topical	Unknown	Unknown	Unknown

INDICATIONS & DOSAGES
Control of flaking, scaling, and itching associated with dandruff—
Adults and children ages 12 and older: wet hair, lather, and massage for 1 minute. Rinse and repeat. Patient should use shampoo twice a week for up to 8 weeks, with at least 3 days between each use, and then p.r.n. to control dandruff.

ADVERSE REACTIONS
Skin: irritation, pruritus, stinging, hair loss, abnormal hair texture, scalp pustules, oiliness or dryness of hair or scalp.

INTERACTIONS
Drug-drug
Topical corticosteroids: may increase absorption of corticosteroid. Don't use together.

CONTRAINDICATIONS
Contraindicated in patients hypersensitive to drug or its components.

OVERDOSE & TREATMENT
If ingested, provide supportive treatment. Gastric lavage and induced emesis usually aren't necessary.

NURSING CONSIDERATIONS
• Most patients show improvement soon after treatment begins.
• Safe use in children younger than age 2 hasn't been established. Consider for use in children only when benefits outweigh risks.
• Drug may appear in breast milk. Recommend cautious use or an alternative feeding method.

PATIENT TEACHING
• Advise patient to read carefully and follow package instructions and to stop use if hypersensitivity reaction occurs.
• Advise patient to contact a doctor if condition worsens or doesn't improve in 2 to 4 weeks, or if rash appears.

• Warn patient that shampoo applied to permanent-waved hair removes curl.
• Warn patient to avoid contact of drug with eyes and to avoid use on broken or inflamed skin.

lidocaine hydrochloride, topical
Burn-O-Gel, DermaFlex, ELA-Max, Solarcaine, Xylocaine, Zilactin-L, Zilactin-B

Pregnancy Risk Category B

HOW SUPPLIED
Cream: 0.5%
Gel: 0.5%, 2.5%
Liquid: 2.5%
Ointment: 2.5%
Spray: 0.5%

ACTION
Inhibits nerve conduction and pain perception by changing permeability of nerve cell membrane.

Route	Onset	Peak	Duration
Topical	Unknown	Unknown	Unknown

INDICATIONS & DOSAGES
Topical anesthesia in local skin disorders, including pruritus and pain caused by minor burns, chickenpox, prickly heat, abrasions, sunburn, dermal exposure to toxic plants, insect

bites, and eczema. May be combined with topical antiseptics to help prevent bacterial contamination in minor wounds—
Adults: apply to affected area p.r.n.
Local analgesia for canker sores, fever blisters, and cold sores—
Adults: dosage varies according to location of application and formulation. Follow specific product packaging instructions.

ADVERSE REACTIONS
EENT: stinging with oral use.
Skin: itching, vasodilation.

INTERACTIONS
None reported.

CONTRAINDICATIONS
Contraindicated in patients who are allergic or hypersensitive to local anesthetics (such as lidocaine or benzocaine) and in patients who have methemoglobinemia.

OVERDOSE & TREATMENT
Cardiac arrhythmias, seizures, and coma with respiratory depression may occur in severe oral or topical overdose.

Emesis is contraindicated after oral ingestion. Maintain airway and support ventilation; provide supportive and sympto-matic care. Contact a poison control center or doctor.

NURSING CONSIDERATIONS
• Topical lidocaine is poorly absorbed through intact skin but readily absorbed through mucous membranes; absorption increases through breaks in the skin (such as abrasions or ulcers).
• Don't use in the eyes, over large areas of the body, or on deep wounds, puncture wounds, animal bites, or serious burns.
• Don't use in large quantities, particularly over raw or blistered areas.
• A dressing may be applied over treated area.

PATIENT TEACHING
• Advise patient not to use if allergic to local anesthetics such as lidocaine or benzocaine.
• Advise patient to read carefully and follow package instructions.
• Caution patient that if symptoms persist or worsen after 1 week of treatment, he should contact the doctor for evaluation.
• Warn patient not to use in large quantities, particularly over raw surfaces or blistered areas.
• Advise patient that to minimize the risk of aspiration or of biting tongue or mucosa, he

should wait 1 hour after oral use to eat, drink, or chew gum.

---

miconazole nitrate
Cruex, Desenex, Fungoid Tincture, Lotrimin AF Antifungal Aerosol Powder Spray, Lotrimin AF Antifungal Jock-Itch Aerosol Powder Spray, Lotrimin AF Antifungal Liquid Spray, Lotrimin AF Antifungal Powder, Micatin, Zeasorb-AF

Pregnancy Risk Category C

HOW SUPPLIED
Cream: 2%
Powder: 2%
Spray powder: 2%

ACTION
Fungicidal. Disrupts cell membrane permeability. Alters mitochondrial activity and peroxisomal enzymes.

Route	Onset	Peak	Duration
Topical	Unknown	Unknown	Unknown

INDICATIONS & DOSAGES
Tinea corporis, tinea cruris, tinea pedis; cutaneous candidiasis; common dermatophyte infections—
Adults and children ages 2 and older: apply sparingly b.i.d. for 2 to 4 weeks. Powder can be used liberally over af-

fected area. For spray, hold 4 to 6 inches from skin and spray over affected area b.i.d.

ADVERSE REACTIONS
Skin: irritation, burning, maceration, allergic contact dermatitis.

INTERACTIONS
None significant.

CONTRAINDICATIONS
Contraindicated in patients who are hypersensitive to drug or its components.

OVERDOSE & TREATMENT
No information available.

NURSING CONSIDERATIONS
• Area should be cleaned before application of product.
• Don't use occlusive dressings.

PATIENT TEACHING
• Warn patient to discontinue drug if sensitivity or chemical irritation occurs.
• Advise patient to read carefully and follow product instruction, not to exceed recommended maximum duration, and to immediately discontinue use if adverse symptoms occur.
• Instruct patient to notify a doctor if symptoms persist or worsen at end of therapy.

- Instruct patient to apply sparingly in skin-fold areas and rub in well to prevent maceration.
- Tell patient with tinea pedis to apply product between toes, wear well-fitting, ventilated shoes, and change socks daily.
- Advise patient to avoid inhaling spray or spraying in eyes.
- Tell patient to use for 2 weeks for tinea cruris and tinea corporis, and for 4 weeks for tinea pedis.

---

minoxidil, topical
Minoxidil for Men, Rogaine, Rogaine Extra Strength

Pregnancy Risk Category C

HOW SUPPLIED
Solution: 2%*, 5%*

ACTION
Stimulates hair growth, possibly by dilating arterial microcapillaries around hair follicles.

Route	Onset	Peak	Duration
Topical	Unknown	Unknown	Unknown

INDICATIONS & DOSAGES
Androgenetic alopecia—
Adults: apply 1 ml solution to affected area b.i.d.

ADVERSE REACTIONS
Skin: irritant dermatitis, allergic contact dermatitis, eczema, hypertrichosis, local erythema, pruritus, dry skin or scalp, flaking, alopecia, exacerbation of hair loss, facial hair growth (women).

INTERACTIONS
Drug-drug
Petroleum jelly, topical corticosteroids, topical retinoids, other drugs that may enhance skin absorption: increases risk of systemic effects of minoxidil. Patient shouldn't apply minoxidil if using other drugs.

CONTRAINDICATIONS
Contraindicated in patients who are hypersensitive to drug or its components. Also, use of the 5% solution is contraindicated in women.

OVERDOSE & TREATMENT
No information available.

NURSING CONSIDERATIONS
- Absorption of drug through irritated skin increases risk of adverse systemic effects.
- Treatment works best in patients with balding area smaller than 4 inches (10 cm) that developed within past 10 years.
- About 40% of patients will experience moderate to dense hair growth.
- Patient shouldn't use if scalp is inflamed, red, infected, irritated, or painful.

• Topical minoxidil shouldn't be used by breast-feeding women.
• Safety and effectiveness haven't been established for patients younger than age 18.

PATIENT TEACHING
• Advise patient to read carefully and follow package instructions.
• Inform patient that using more than 1 application daily won't result in increased hair growth but may increase adverse reactions.
• Caution patient not to double the dose if one is missed.
• Advise patient that therapy will be prolonged and will continue for at least 2 to 4 months before clinical effects appear and that drug must be used daily for optimal results. If hair doesn't grow back in 8 months in women or 12 months in men (4 months if using 5% solution), patient should consult a doctor.
• Inform patient that discontinuing drug may result in loss of new hair growth; new hair growth is usually fine and may be colorless but will resemble existing hair after continued treatment.

---

neomycin sulfate
Myciguent, Neomycin

Pregnancy Risk Category C

HOW SUPPLIED
Cream: 3.5 mg/g
Ointment: 3.5 mg/g

ACTION
Aminoglycoside that inhibits protein synthesis in gram-negative organisms and some species of *Staphylococcus*.

Route	Onset	Peak	Duration
Topical	Unknown	Unknown	Unknown

INDICATIONS & DOSAGES
Prevention of infection at site of minor skin breaks (cuts, burns, wounds, scrapes)—
Adults and children: clean area, apply thin film q.d. to t.i.d. for up to 1 week.

ADVERSE REACTIONS
EENT: ototoxicity.
GU: *nephrotoxicity.*
Skin: contact dermatitis, burning, erythema, rash, urticaria.

INTERACTIONS
None significant.

CONTRAINDICATIONS
Contraindicated in patients who are hypersensitive to drug or its components.

OVERDOSE & TREATMENT
No information available.

NURSING CONSIDERATIONS
• Drug shouldn't be used more than once daily on burns covering more than 20% of body surface.
• Prolonged use may result in overgrowth of nonsusceptible organisms.
• In products containing corticosteroids, use of occlusive dressings increases corticosteroid absorption and likelihood of systemic effects.
• Systemic absorption is enhanced on denuded or abraded areas.
• Substantial absorption may occur in infants with abraded diaper rash.

PATIENT TEACHING
• Tell patient to discontinue drug and seek medical advice if no improvement occurs or if condition worsens.
• Caution patient with kidney or hearing problems about potential for ototoxicity or nephrotoxicity with use of neomycin.
• Tell patient to notify a doctor if any adverse reactions, especially systemic reactions, occur.
• Instruct patient not to use drug for longer than 1 week, unless otherwise directed.
• Tell patient not to use drug for deep wounds, puncture wounds, animal bites, or serious burns without medical advice.

---

permethrin
Nix

Pregnancy Risk Category B

HOW SUPPLIED
Spray (furniture and bedding): 0.25%
Topical liquid (cream rinse): 1%

ACTION
Disrupts sodium channel current of nerve cell membrane of parasite causing delayed repolarization and resulting in paralysis. Effective against lice, ticks, mites, and fleas.

Route	Onset	Peak	Duration
Topical	10-15 min	Unknown	10 days

INDICATIONS & DOSAGES
Single-application treatment of infestation with head lice and lice eggs (nits)—
Adults and children ages 2 and older: use after hair has been washed with shampoo, rinsed with water, and towel-dried. Apply 30 to 60 ml of liquid to saturate the hair and scalp. Allow drug to remain on hair for 10 minutes before rinsing off with water. If live lice are observed more than 1 week

after treatment, repeat same procedure.

ADVERSE REACTIONS
Skin: pruritus, edema, erythema, rash.

INTERACTIONS
None significant.

CONTRAINDICATIONS
Contraindicated in patients who are hypersensitive to pyrethrins, chrysanthemums, or components of drug.

OVERDOSE & TREATMENT
With accidental ingestion, perform gastric lavage and use general supportive measures.

NURSING CONSIDERATIONS
• A single treatment is usually sufficient. Combing of nits doesn't increase effectiveness of treatment; fine-tooth comb is for cosmetic use, as desired.
• If lice remain 1 week or longer after initial application, repeat the treatment for lice.
• Posttreatment infestation occurs in less than 1% of patients and isn't the result of patient noncompliance.
• Safety and efficacy for use in children younger than age 2 haven't been established.

PATIENT TEACHING
• Caution patient to read carefully and follow package instructions.
• Explain that treatment may temporarily worsen symptoms of head lice infestation, such as pruritus, erythema, and edema.
• Advise patient or parent to wash bed linens daily (machine washing with hot water and machine drying for at least 20 minutes on hot cycle). Hairbrush, comb, and hats can be washed daily in hot water until infestation is eliminated. Nonwashable items should be sealed in plastic bag for 2 weeks or sprayed with product designed to eliminate lice and their nits.
• Warn patient not to use drug on eyelashes or eyebrows.
• Tell parent to inform school or daycare center and to check other family members for infestation.

---

povidone-iodine
ACU-dyne, Aerodine, Betadine, Betagen, Biodine Topical, Etodine, Iodex, Iodex-P, Minidyne, Operand, Polydine, Povidine

Pregnancy Risk Category C

HOW SUPPLIED
Aerosol: 0.5%, 5%
Cleanser: 7.5%

Cream: 5%
Ointment: 1%, 4.7%, 10%
Shampoo: 7.5%
Solution: 1%, 10%

ACTION
The bactericidal activity of iodine, but less potent; a broad-spectrum antimicrobial agent that liberates free iodine.

Route	Onset	Peak	Duration
Topical	Unknown	Unknown	Unknown

INDICATIONS & DOSAGES
Antiseptic—
Adults: apply thin film to affected area p.r.n. Treated areas may be bandaged. For cleanser, apply enough to work up a lather; allow lather to remain for 3 minutes; then rinse. Repeat b.i.d. to t.i.d.

Relief from scaling and itching caused by dandruff—
Adults: apply shampoo to wet hair and scalp; use warm water to lather. Rinse and repeat. Massage gently and leave on for 5 minutes. Rinse with warm water. Repeat twice weekly until improvement is noted, and then once a week.

ADVERSE REACTIONS
Skin: rash, irritation.

INTERACTIONS
None reported.

CONTRAINDICATIONS
Contraindicated in patients who are hypersensitive to iodine.

OVERDOSE & TREATMENT
No information available.

NURSING CONSIDERATIONS
• Patient allergic or hypersensitive to iodine shouldn't use this product.
• Product concentrations vary widely; specific product information should be carefully reviewed before use.
• It's not known if drug appears in breast milk. Urge patient to stop breast-feeding temporarily or stop drug use.

PATIENT TEACHING
• Caution patient to avoid product contact with eyes and not to apply over large areas of the body.
• Advise patient to read carefully and follow product instruction and to stop use and consult a doctor if the symptoms persist or worsen or if infection occurs.
• Tell patient not to use for deep or puncture wounds without medical advice.

---

*Liquid contains alcohol.   **May contain tartrazine.   †Canada   ‡Australia   §U.K.

pramoxine hydrochloride
Itch-X, PrameGel, Prax,
Tronothone HCl

Pregnancy Risk Category C

HOW SUPPLIED
Cream: 1%
Gel: 1%
Lotion: 1%
Spray: 1%

ACTION
Local anesthetic that inhibits
conduction of nerve impulses
from sensory nerves.

Route	Onset	Peak	Duration
Topical	3-5 min	Unknown	Unknown

INDICATIONS & DOSAGES
*Temporary relief from pain and
itching in local skin disorder—*
Adults: clean affected area and
apply thin layer to skin t.i.d. to
q.i.d.

ADVERSE REACTIONS
Skin: irritation, contact dermatitis.

INTERACTIONS
None reported.

CONTRAINDICATIONS
Contraindicated in patients who
are hypersensitive to drug or its
components; also contraindicated when local infection occurs at site.

OVERDOSE & TREATMENT
No information available.

NURSING CONSIDERATIONS
● Some combination products
may contain ingredients that
can cause hypersensitivity reactions.
● The lowest possible dosage for
symptom relief will reduce the
risk of systemic absorption and
related adverse effects.
● Precautions should be taken to
prevent children from transferring medication to their mouths
after application.

PATIENT TEACHING
● Advise patient not to use on
large areas of the body, especially if skin is broken or
abraded.
● Caution patient not to get
pramoxine in eyes, mouth, or
nose.
● Advise patient to read carefully and follow product information.

pyrethrins
A-200, Barc, Blue, End Lice,
Pronto, Pyrinyl, R & C, RID,
Tisit, Triple X

Pregnancy Risk Category C

HOW SUPPLIED
Shampoo: pyrethrins 0.2% and piperonyl butoxide 2%; pyrethrins 0.3% and piperonyl butoxide 3%; pyrethrins 0.33% and piperonyl butoxide 4%
Topical gel: pyrethrins 0.3% and piperonyl butoxide 3%
Topical solution: pyrethrins 0.18% and piperonyl butoxide 2%; pyrethrins 0.2%, piperonyl butoxide 2%, and deodorized kerosene 0.8%; pyrethrins 0.3% and piperonyl butoxide 3%; pyrethrins 0.3% and piperonyl butoxide 2%

ACTION
Contact poison that disrupts parasitic nervous system, causing paralysis and death of parasites.

Route	Onset	Peak	Duration
Topical	Unknown	Unknown	Unknown

INDICATIONS & DOSAGES
Infestations of lice (head, body, and pubic) and their eggs—
Adults and children: apply to hair, scalp, or other infested areas until entirely wet. Leave on for 10 minutes but no longer. Wash thoroughly with warm water and soap or shampoo. Dead lice and eggs can be removed with fine-tooth comb. Treatment repeated if needed in 7 to 10 days to kill newly hatched lice; not to exceed two applications within 24 hours.

ADVERSE REACTIONS
Skin: irritation, pruritus, erythema, edema.

INTERACTIONS
None significant.

CONTRAINDICATIONS
Contraindicated in patients who are hypersensitive to drug, ragweed, or chrysanthemums.

OVERDOSE & TREATMENT
Ingestion of 5 to 50 mg of pyrethrins produces no toxicity. Ingestion of piperonyl butoxide may cause nausea, vomiting, diarrhea, CNS depression, and hemorrhagic enteritis.

After ingestion of pyrethrins and piperonyl butoxide, treat with immediate gastric lavage and saline cathartics, followed by supportive and symptomatic care.

NURSING CONSIDERATIONS
• To treat eyebrows or eyelashes, patient should apply an occlusive ophthalmic ointment to the eyelid margins twice daily for 10 days.
• Tell patient to avoid contact with face, eyes, mucous membranes, and urethral meatus.

- If accidental contact with eyes occurs, patient should flush thoroughly with water.
- Drug shouldn't be used on inflamed, raw, or weeping skin.
- Family members should be checked daily for at least 2 weeks for infestation.
- Drug isn't effective against scabies.
- Use cautiously in infants and small children.

PATIENT TEACHING
- Instruct patient not to apply to open areas, acutely inflamed skin, eyebrows or eyelashes, or face, eyes, mucous membranes, or urethral meatus. If accidental contact with eyes occurs, advise patient to flush with water and seek medical advice.
- Tell patient to stop using drug, wash it off skin, and seek medical advice immediately if skin irritation develops. All preparations contain petroleum distillates.
- Instruct patient to change and sterilize all clothing and bed linens after drug is washed off body. Washable items should be disinfected by machine washing in hot water and drying on hot cycle for at least 20 minutes. Other items can be dry cleaned, sealed in plastic bags for 2 weeks, or treated with products made for this purpose.

- Urge patient to warn other family members and sexual contacts about infestation. Sexual contacts should be treated simultaneously.

---

pyrithione zinc
American Crew, Denorex Advanced Formula, DHS Zinc, Head & Shoulders, Head & Shoulders Dry Scalp, Pantene Pro-V Shampoo True Confidence Antidandruff, Pert Plus Dandruff Control, Sebulon, Zincon, ZNP Bar

Pregnancy Risk Category NR

HOW SUPPLIED
Shampoo: 1%, 2%
Soap: 2%

ACTION
Cytostatic agent that reduces cell turnover rate, skin scaling, and sloughing. Strongly binds to hair and external skin layers.

Route	Onset	Peak	Duration
Topical	Unknown	Unknown	Unknown

INDICATIONS & DOSAGES
Control of seborrheic dermatitis (scalp and body), control of dry scalp—
Adults: apply to wet hair and scalp, lather, and rinse. May be repeated twice weekly.

Nursing Nonprescription Drug Handbook
Photoguide to tablets and capsules

This photoguide provides full-color photographs of some of the most common OTC tablets and capsules in the United States. Shown in actual size, the drugs are organized alphabetically by trade name for quick reference.

ADVIL

Advil 200-mg Tablets, Caplets, Gel Caplets, Liqui-Gels

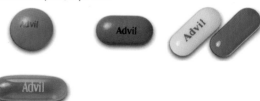

Advil Cold & Sinus Caplets, Tablets

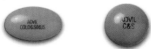

Advil Migraine 200-mg Liquid Filled Capsules

Children's Advil 50-mg Chewable Tablets: fruit and grape

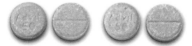

Junior Strength Advil 100-mg Coated Tablets, Chewable Tablets: fruit and grape

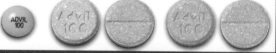

ALEVE

Aleve 220-mg Tablets, Caplets, Gelcaps

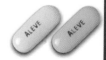

ALKA-SELTZER

Alka-Seltzer Gas Relief Maximum Strength Liquid Softgels

Alka-Seltzer Original, Lemon-Lime, Cherry Effervescent Tablets

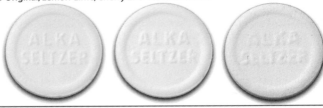

Alka-Seltzer Plus Cold & Cough Liqui-Gels

Alka-Seltzer Plus Cold & Flu Non-drowsy Liqui-Gels

Alka-Seltzer Plus Cold & Sinus Non-drowsy Liqui-Gels

Alka-Seltzer Plus Cold Liqui-Gels

Alka-Seltzer Plus Night-Time Cold Liqui-Gels

ANACIN

Aspirin-free Anacin Extra Strength 500-mg Tablets

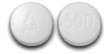

AXID

Axid AR 75-mg Tablets

BAYER

Aspirin Regimen Bayer Adult Low Strength 81-mg Enteric Coated Tablets

Aspirin Regimen Bayer Adult Low Strength 81-mg with Calcium Caplets

Aspirin Regimen Bayer Children's 81-mg Chewable Tablets: cherry and orange

Aspirin Regimen Bayer Regular Strength 325-mg Enteric Coated Caplets

Extra Strength Bayer Aspirin 500-mg Caplets, Gelcaps

Extra Strength Bayer Aspirin Arthritis Pain Regimen 500-mg Caplets

Extra Strength Bayer Plus 500-mg Caplets

Extra Strength Bayer PM Aspirin Plus Sleep Aid Caplets

Genuine Bayer Aspirin 325-mg Tablets, Caplets, Gelcaps

BENADRYL

Benadryl Allergy Kapseals

Benadryl Allergy Ultratab Tablets

Benadryl Allergy/Cold Tablets

Benadryl Allergy/Congestion Tablets

Benadryl Allergy & Sinus Fastmelt Dissolving Tablets: cherry

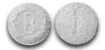

Benadryl Allergy/Sinus Headache Caplets, Gelcaps

 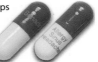

Benadryl Dye-Free Allergy Liqui-gels Softgels

CALTRATE 600

Caltrate 600 Tablets

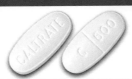

Caltrate 600 + D Tablets

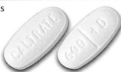

Caltrate 600 Plus Chewable Tablets: assorted fruit flavors

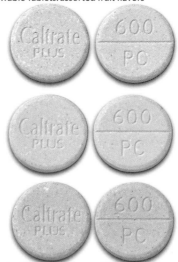

CENTRUM

Centrum Silver Tablets

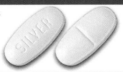

Centrum Tablets

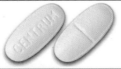

CHLOR-TRIMETON

Chlor-Trimeton Allergy 4-Hour Tablets

Chlor-Trimeton Allergy 8-Hour Tablets

Chlor-Trimeton Allergy 12-Hour Tablets

Chlor-Trimeton Allergy-D 4-Hour Tablets

Chlor-Trimeton Allergy-D 12-Hour Tablets

CONTAC

Contac 12-Hour Cold Non-Drowsy Caplets

Contac Day & Night Allergy/Sinus Caplets

Contac Day & Night Cold/Flu Caplets

Contac Severe Cold & Flu Maximum Strength Caplets

Contac Severe Cold & Flu Non-drowsy Formula Caplets

CORRECTOL

Correctol Tablets, Caplets, Softgels

ECOTRIN

Ecotrin Adult Low Strength 81-mg Tablets

Ecotrin Maximum Strength Arthritis Relief 500-mg Tablets

Ecotrin Regular Strength 325-mg Tablets

EXCEDRIN

Extra Strength Excedrin Tablets, Caplets, Geltabs

Aspirin Free Excedrin Extra Strength Caplets, Geltabs

Aspirin Free Excedrin PM Tablets, Caplets, Geltabs

Excedrin Migraine Tablets, Caplets, Geltabs

EX-LAX

Ex-lax Chocolated Regular Strength Pieces

Ex-lax Gentle Strength Laxative Plus Stool Softener Caplets

Ex-lax Maximum Strength Laxative Pills

Ex-lax Regular Strength Laxative Pills

GAS-X

Gas-X Extra Strength 125-mg Chewable Tablets: cherry and peppermint

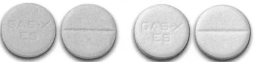

Gas-X Regular Strength 80-mg Chewable Tablets: cherry and peppermint

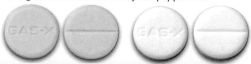

IMODIUM

Imodium A-D Caplets

Imodium Advanced Chewable Tablets: mint

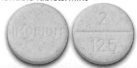

LACTAID

Lactaid Extra Strength Caplets

Lactaid Original Strength Caplets

Lactaid Ultra Caplets, Chewable Tablets: vanilla

MAALOX

Maalox Anti-Gas Extra Strength Tablets: peppermint

Maalox Quick Dissolve Maximum Strength Chewable Tablets: assorted flavors

Maalox Quick Dissolve Regular Strength Chewable Tablets: assorted flavors

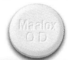 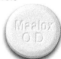

MOTRIN

Children's Motrin 50-mg Chewable Tablets: orange

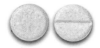

Junior Strength Motrin 100-mg Caplets, Chewable Tablets: orange

Motrin Cold and Flu Caplets

Motrin IB 200-mg Tablets, Caplets, Gelcaps

Motrin Migraine 200-mg Caplets

Motrin Sinus/Headache Non-drowsy formula Caplets

MYLANTA

Mylanta Gas Maximum Strength Chewable Tablets: mint

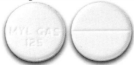

Mylanta Gelcaps

Mylanta Ultra Tabs Tablets: cherry and mint

NICORETTE

Nicorette 2-mg Gum: original, mint, orange

Nicorette 4-mg Gum: original, mint, orange

OS-CAL

Os-cal 500 Tablets

Os-cal 500+D Tablets

PEPCID AC

Pepcid AC Tablets, Chewable Tablets, Gelcaps

PEPTO-BISMOL

Pepto-Bismol Caplets, Chewable Tablets

 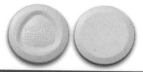

PHILLIPS

Phillips' Liqui-Gels

PRIMATENE

Primatene Tablets

ROBITUSSIN

Robitussin Cold/Cold & Congestion Non-drowsy Formula Caplets and Softgels

Robitussin Cold Multi-Symptom Cold & Flu Non-drowsy Formula Caplets and Softgels

Robitussin Cold Severe Congestion Non-drowsy Formula Softgels

Robitussin Cold Sinus & Congestion Caplets

ROLAIDS

Rolaids Antacid Tablets: peppermint, spearmint, cherry

Rolaids Extra Strength Tablets: fruit

SUDAFED

Children's Sudafed Nasal Decongestant Chewables: orange

Sudafed 12-hour Caplets 120 mg

Sudafed 24-hour Tablets 240 mg

Sudafed Maximum Strength Cold & Allergy Tablets

Sudafed Maximum Strength Nasal Decongestant 30-mg Tablets

Sudafed Maximum Strength Non-Drying Sinus Liquid Caps

Sudafed Maximum Strength Severe Cold Formula Caplets, Tablets

Sudafed Multi-Symptom Cold & Cough Liquid Caps

Sudafed Multi-Symptom Cold & Sinus Liquid Caps

Sudafed Sinus Headache Caplets

TAGAMET

Tagamet HB 200 Tablets

TAVIST

Tavist Allergy Tablets

Tavist Sinus Non-drowsy Caplets

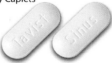

THERAFLU

TheraFlu Maximum Strength Non-drowsy Flu, Cold & Cough Caplets

THERAGRAN-M

Theragran-M Advanced Caplets

TRIAMINIC

Triaminic Softchews Cold & Allergy: orange

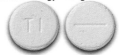

Triaminic Softchews Cold & Cough: cherry

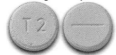

Triaminic Softchews Cough & Sore Throat: grape

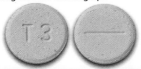

TUMS

Tums Regular Strength Peppermint Tablets

TYLENOL

Children's Tylenol Allergy-D Chewable Tablets: bubble gum

Children's Tylenol Cold Chewable Tablets: grape

Children's Tylenol Cold Plus Cough Chewable Tablets: cherry

Children's Tylenol Sinus Chewable Tablets: fruit burst

Junior Strength Tylenol 160-mg Chewable Tablets: fruit and grape

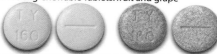

Tylenol Allergy Sinus Maximum Strength Multi-Symptom Gelcaps

Tylenol Arthritis Extended Relief 650-mg Caplets

Tylenol Cold Multi-Symptom Complete Formula Caplets

Tylenol Extra Strength 500-mg Caplets, Gelcaps, Geltabs, Tablets

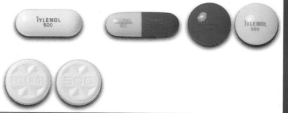

Tylenol Flu Maximum Strength NightTime Gelcaps

Tylenol PM Extra Strength Caplets, Gelcaps, Geltabs

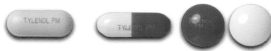

Tylenol Regular Strength 325-mg Tablets

Tylenol Sinus Non-drowsy Maximum Strength Caplets, Gelcaps, Geltabs

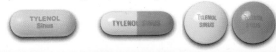

VICKS

Vicks DayQuil LiquiCaps

Vicks NyQuil LiquiCaps

ZANTAC 75

Zantac 75 tablets

ADVERSE REACTIONS
Skin: irritation.

INTERACTIONS
None reported.

CONTRAINDICATIONS
Contraindicated in patients who are hypersensitive to drug or its components.

OVERDOSE & TREATMENT
No information available.

NURSING CONSIDERATIONS
• May temporarily discolor bleached, tinted, gray, or permed hair.

PATIENT TEACHING
• Advise patient to read carefully and follow product information.
• Caution patient to avoid contact with eyes, eyelids, and mucous membranes; rinse thoroughly if exposure occurs.
• Advise patient prolonged rinsing will reduce risk of discoloration of bleached, tinted, gray, or permed hair.
• Tell patient to seek medical advice if improvement doesn't occur after regular use of product.
• Notify patient that scalp may tingle during use of some products.

salicylic acid
Aveeno Acne Treatment, Biore Acne Products, Clean & Clear Products, Clearasil Products, Clear Away, Compound W, DuoFilm, DuoPlant, Fostex, Freezone, Fung-O, Gordofilm, Keralyt, Maximum Strength Wart Remover, Mediplast, Mosco, Noxzema Anti-Acne Products, Occlusal HP, Off-Ezy Corn & Callus Remover Kit, Off-Ezy Wart Remover, Oxy Clean Acne Products, Panscol, Psor-a-set, Sal-Acid, Salactic Film, Sal-Plant, Stri-Dex Acne Products, Trans-Ver-Sal AdultPatch, Trans-Ver-Sal PediaPatch, Trans-Ver-Sal PlantarPatch, Wart-Off

Pregnancy Risk Category C

HOW SUPPLIED
Cake: 2%, 3%
Cream: 2%, 17%
Gel: 2%, 5%
Lotion: 2%, 3%
Ointment: 3%
Plaster: 15%, 40%
Pledgets: 0.5%, 2%
Shampoo: 2%, 3%, 4%
Soap: 0.5%
Solution: 0.5%, 1.8%, 2%, 3%, 13.6%, 16.7%, 17%

---

*Liquid contains alcohol.   **May contain tartrazine.   †Canada   ‡Australia   §U.K.

ACTION
Salicylic acid has a potent kera-tolytic action and a slight anti-septic action when applied to the skin. In low concentrations, the drug has keratoplastic activ-ity (correction of abnormal ker-atinization), and in concentra-tions of 1% or more, the drug has keratolytic activity (causing skin to peel). By dissolving an intercellular cement substance, the drug causes desquamation of the horny layer of skin, but doesn't affect the structure of the viable epidermis. The ker-atolytic action causes the corni-fied epithelium to swell, soften, macerate, and then desquamate.

Route	Onset	Peak	Duration
Topical	1 hr	5 hr	Unknown

INDICATIONS & DOSAGES
Removal of excessive keratin in hyperkeratotic skin disorders, including common warts and plantar warts, calluses, corns—
Adults: for warts, apply 5% to 17% product to wart q.d. or b.i.d. For corns and calluses, apply 12% to 17.6% product, 1 drop at a time, allowing com-plete drying between drops, un-til each corn or callus is cov-ered. Or, apply 12% to 40% plaster, pad, or disk to corn or callus, leave in place for 48 hours, and then remove. Maxi-mum 5 applications in 14 days.

Acne—
Adults: apply 0.5% to 2% product to affected area q.d. to t.i.d. Or, wash with soap or cleanser b.i.d.

Seborrheic dermatitis, psoria-sis, dandruff—
Adults: apply 1.8% to 3% product in a thin layer to the af-fected area q.d. to b.i.d. Or, use shampoo twice weekly.

ADVERSE REACTIONS
Skin: irritation.

INTERACTIONS
Drug-drug
Abrasive medicated soaps, acne preparations, isotretinoin, preparations that contain alco-hol: may increase dryness or ir-ritation of the skin. Tell patient to monitor closely and stop us-ing together if reaction occurs.

CONTRAINDICATIONS
Contraindicated in patients who are hypersensitive to salicylic acid. Also contraindicated in children younger than age 2 and in patients with diabetes or im-paired circulation. Not for use on moles, birthmarks, warts with hair growing from them, genital or facial warts, warts on mucous membranes, irritated skin, or skin that is infected or reddened.

Reactions may be *common*, uncommon, *life-threatening*, or COMMON AND LIFE-THREATENING.

OVERDOSE & TREATMENT
No information available.

NURSING CONSIDERATIONS
• Repeated applications may cause irritation to the skin.
• Contact with clothing, fabrics, plastics, wood, metal, or other materials may cause damage and should be avoided.
• Drug shouldn't be used along with other topical acne drugs, unless otherwise directed by a doctor.
• Drug isn't recommended for use in children younger than age 2.

PATIENT TEACHING
• Advise patient to read carefully and follow package instructions.
• Caution patient to avoid contact with eyes, face, genitals, mucous membranes, and normal skin surrounding warts.
• Inform patient that medication may cause reddening or scaling of skin when used on open skin lesions.
• Advise patient that contact with clothing, fabrics, plastics, wood, metal, or other materials may damage them; urge patient to avoid such contact.
• Advise patient treating warts, corns, or calluses to avoid contact with adjacent tissue. Petrolatum may be applied around lesion to prevent contact with healthy skin.
• Tell patient to soak warts for 5 minutes, corns or calluses for 15 to 30 minutes in warm water before treatment, then remove loose tissue with wash cloth, soft brush or emery board, and dry the area thoroughly before applying product. Don't rub hard enough to cause bleeding.
• Advise patient to seek medical advice for warts that aren't improved within 12 weeks, or corns or calluses that aren't improved in 14 days.
• Tell patient using plaster, pad, or disk to treat corns or calluses to soak foot in warm water for 15 to 30 minutes after removing product.

---

selenium sulfide
Head & Shoulders Intensive Treatment Dandruff Shampoo, Selsun Blue, Selsun Gold for Women

Pregnancy Risk Category C

HOW SUPPLIED
Shampoo: 1%

ACTION
Cytostatic effect on cells of epidermis and follicular epithelium, resulting in reduced corneocyte production and scaling.

Route	Onset	Peak	Duration
Topical	Unknown	Unknown	Unknown

INDICATIONS & DOSAGES
Dandruff, seborrheic dermatitis of the scalp—
Adults: massage vigorously as a shampoo into wet scalp, rinse thoroughly, and repeat application. Use up to twice weekly and less frequently after symptoms are controlled.

ADVERSE REACTIONS
Skin: irritation, contact dermatitis, hair discoloration, hair loss, scalp dryness, scalp oiliness.

INTERACTIONS
None reported.

CONTRAINDICATIONS
Contraindicated in patients who are hypersensitive to drug or its components.

OVERDOSE & TREATMENT
None reported; low toxicity if ingested.
   No treatment needed.

NURSING CONSIDERATIONS
• For external use only; patient should avoid contact with eyes.
• If using before or after bleaching, tinting, or permanent waving, patient should rinse hair for at least 5 minutes in cool running water after use.

PATIENT TEACHING
• Advise patient to read carefully and follow package instructions.
• Caution patient not to apply more frequently than required to maintain control.
• Advise patient to wash hands after treatment.
• Caution patient to avoid contact with eyes and not to use on acutely inflamed skin.
• Advise patient to discontinue use if irritation occurs.
• Advise patient using medication after bleaching, tinting, or permanent waving to rinse hair for at least 5 minutes in cool running water after use.
• Advise patient that product may damage jewelry; remove before using.

sodium hypochlorite
Dakin's ½ Strength, Dakin's Full Strength

Pregnancy Risk Category NR

HOW SUPPLIED
Solution: 0.25%, 0.5%

ACTION
Germicidal, deodorizing, and bleaching agent, effective against vegetative bacteria and viruses, somewhat effective against spores and fungi.

Route	Onset	Peak	Duration
Topical	Unknown	Unknown	Unknown

INDICATIONS & DOSAGES
Local skin antiseptic—
Adults: apply thin film to clean, affected area.

ADVERSE REACTIONS
Skin: local irritation.

INTERACTIONS
None reported.

CONTRAINDICATIONS
Contraindicated in patients who are hypersensitive to drug or its components.

OVERDOSE & TREATMENT
No information available.

NURSING CONSIDERATIONS
• Dakin's solution is prepared from liquid household bleach diluted 10:1 before use.
• Solutions are relatively unstable and should be prepared fresh daily.
• Isotonic solutions used for baths in burn patients may be prepared with another tenfold dilution.

PATIENT TEACHING
• Caution patient that chemical burns may occur, that he should avoid contact with eyes, and that he should discontinue use immediately if adverse signs or symptoms develop.
• Advise patient that individual products should be reviewed for their use and dosage guidelines, and that dose and frequency of use depend on the condition, area to be treated, and tolerance.

sulfur
Acne Lotion 10, Fostril, Liquimat, SAStid Soap, Sulfoam Medicated Antidandruff, Sulfo-Lo, Sulfur Soap, Sulmasque, Sulpho-Lac, Sulpho-Lac Acne Medication, ZAPZYT Cleansing Bar

Pregnancy Risk Category C

HOW SUPPLIED
Cake: 3%, 5%, 10%
Cream: 5%
Lotion: 2%, 4%, 10%
Mask: 6.4%
Shampoo: 2%
Soap: 3%, 5%

ACTION
Keratolytic with peeling and drying actions. Although it may help to resolve comedones, it may also promote the development of new ones by increasing horny cell adhesion.

Route	Onset	Peak	Duration
Topical	2 hr	8 hr	24 hr

INDICATIONS & DOSAGES
Treatment of acne vulgaris—
Adults and children ages 12 and older: apply 1% to 8% cream, lotion, or soap q.d. to t.i.d.

Seborrheic dermatitis—
Adults: massage 2% to 5% lotion or shampoo into scalp, rinse, and repeat. Use twice weekly.

ADVERSE REACTIONS
Skin: local irritation, dry skin, dermatitis.

INTERACTIONS
None reported.

CONTRAINDICATIONS
Contraindicated in patients who are hypersensitive to drug or its components.

OVERDOSE & TREATMENT
No information available.

NURSING CONSIDERATIONS
• Topical sulfur-containing preparations shouldn't be used near the eyes; if contact occurs, patient should rinse thoroughly with water.
• Allergic reactions occur rarely.
• Repeated applications may cause irritation to the skin.
• Sulfur ointment stains clothing, bedding, and metal, including jewelry.
• Topical preparations containing sulfur shouldn't be used in children younger than age 2 except under the direction and supervision of a doctor.

PATIENT TEACHING
• Advise patient to read carefully and follow product instruction.
• Tell patient using drug for acne to begin with one treatment daily, to prevent excessive drying, and then to increase as needed and tolerated.
• Caution patient to keep away from eyes and to flush immediately with water if contact occurs.
• Inform patient that product may cause irritation of the skin; if this occurs, patient should discontinue use and notify a doctor.
• Inform patient that product may stain clothing, bedding, and metal, including jewelry.

---

terbinafine hydrochloride
Lamisil AT

Pregnancy Risk Category B

HOW SUPPLIED
Cream: 1%
Solution: 1%
Spray: 1%

ACTION
Fungicidal that selectively inhibits an early step in synthesis of sterols used by fungi for cell-wall synthesis.

Route	Onset	Peak	Duration
Topical	Unknown	Unknown	Unknown

INDICATIONS & DOSAGES
Treatment of itching, burning, cracking, and scaling from tinea pedis between the toes—
Adults and children older than age 12: apply b.i.d. (morning and evening) for 1 week.

Treatment of itching, burning, cracking, and scaling from tinea pedis on the bottom or sides of the feet—
Adults and children older than age 12: apply b.i.d. (morning and evening) for 2 weeks.

Treatment of itching, burning, cracking, and scaling from tinea corporis and tinea cruris—
Adults, and children older than age 12: apply q.d. for 1 week.

ADVERSE REACTIONS
Skin: rash, blistering, oozing, burning, or itching.

INTERACTIONS
None significant.

CONTRAINDICATIONS
Contraindicated in patients who are hypersensitive to drug or its components.

OVERDOSE & TREATMENT
Overdose with a topical terbinafine is unlikely because of the limited systemic absorption. Oral terbinafine overdose causes nausea, vomiting, abdominal pain, dizziness, rash, urinary frequency, and headache.

Treatment is supportive.

NURSING CONSIDERATIONS
• Drug is for external use and shouldn't be used in the mouth or eyes.
• Topical terbinafine shouldn't be used to treat fungal infections of the nails or scalp or to treat vaginal yeast infections.
• Therapy shouldn't exceed 4 weeks.
• Drug appears in breast milk. A decision to discontinue either breast-feeding or drug must be made, taking into account the importance of drug to the mother. Women who are breast-feeding shouldn't apply terbinafine cream to the breast.
• Safety and efficacy in children younger than age 12 haven't been established.

PATIENT TEACHING
• Urge patient to use drug for the full treatment period, even if symptoms may have improved.
• Instruct patient to wash the infected skin with soap and water and dry completely before applying medication.
• Tell patient to wash his hands after applying medication.
• Caution patient to stop drug and call doctor if irritation, redness, itching, burning, blistering, swelling, oozing, or sensitivity develops.
• Tell patient to notify doctor if no improvement occurs in 4 weeks for tinea pedis or 2 weeks for tinea cruris or tinea corporis.
• Tell patient treating tinea pedis to apply drug between toes, wear well-fitting ventilated shoes, and change socks daily.
• Instruct patient not to wear occlusive dressings, unless directed by a doctor.

---

tetracaine hydrochloride
Pontocaine, Supracaine†,
Viractin

Pregnancy Risk Category C

HOW SUPPLIED
Cream: 1%, 2%
Gel: 2%
Ointment: 1%

ACTION
A local anesthetic that changes the nerve's permeability to sodium ions to slow the transmission of nerve impulses along sensory nerves; this causes an inability to propagate an action potential.

Route	Onset	Peak	Duration
Topical	3-10 min	3-8 min	30-60 min

INDICATIONS & DOSAGES
Minor skin disorders such as burns, sunburns, insect bites or stings, contact dermatitis, minor wounds (cuts and scratches)—
Adults and children ages 2 and older: apply to the affected area t.i.d. to q.i.d.

Cold sores and fever blisters (Viractin)—
Adults and children ages 2 and older: apply to affected area not more than t.i.d. to q.i.d.

ADVERSE REACTIONS
Skin: contact dermatitis, rash, urticaria, edema, burning, stinging, tenderness.

INTERACTIONS
Drug-drug
Class I antiarrhythmics: may cause toxic effects. Advise patient not to use together.

Reactions may be *common*, uncommon, *life-threatening*, or COMMON AND LIFE-THREATENING.

CONTRAINDICATIONS
Contraindicated in patients hypersensitive to drug or to para-aminobenzoic acid (PABA) or its derivatives.

OVERDOSE & TREATMENT
No information available.

NURSING CONSIDERATIONS
• Drug should be used cautiously by patients receiving class I antiarrhythmics.
• Adverse reactions are dose-related.

PATIENT TEACHING
• Advise patient to read carefully and follow package instructions.
• Caution patient that product isn't intended for prolonged use.
• Advise patient to use lowest dose possible to obtain symptom relief.

---

tetracycline hydrochloride
Achromycin

chlortetracycline hydrochloride
Aureomycin

Pregnancy Risk Category B

HOW SUPPLIED
Ointment: 3%

ACTION
The exact mechanism of action is unknown; tetracyclines are broad-spectrum bacteriostatic agents that inhibit protein synthesis by blocking the binding of aminoacyl tRNA to the mRNA ribosome complex.

Route	Onset	Peak	Duration
Topical	Unknown	Unknown	Unknown

INDICATIONS & DOSAGES
Minor bacterial skin infections by streptococci, staphylococci, and other susceptible organisms—
Adults: apply thin film to the affected area b.i.d. to t.i.d., morning and evening.

Prophylaxis of minor bacterial skin infections and treatment of dermal ulcer—
Adults: apply thin film to the affected area b.i.d. to t.i.d., morning and evening.

ADVERSE REACTIONS
Skin: burning or stinging sensation upon application, yellowing of the skin.

INTERACTIONS
None reported.

CONTRAINDICATIONS
Contraindicated in patients who are hypersensitive to drug or its components.

---

*Liquid contains alcohol.   **May contain tartrazine.   †Canada   ‡Australia   §U.K.

OVERDOSE & TREATMENT
No information available.

NURSING CONSIDERATIONS
• Yellowing of the skin with application can be eliminated by washing.
• Product is for topical use only; patient should avoid using around the eyes, nose, and mouth.
• Normal use of cosmetics is permissible.
• The treated areas may be covered with gauze, if needed.

PATIENT TEACHING
• Advise patient that product is for topical use only, avoid using around the eyes, nose, and mouth.
• Advise patient to wash, rinse, and dry the area before putting on the medicine and to use only enough ointment to cover the affected area and surrounding skin.
• Inform patient that transient burning and stinging may occur.
• Tell patient not to use for longer than 1 week and to contact doctor if symptoms persist or worsen.
• Advise patient not to use for deep or puncture wounds, animal bites, or serious burns, unless directed by doctor.

thimerosal
Aeroaid, Mersol

Pregnancy Risk Category NR

HOW SUPPLIED
Solution: 1:1000
Spray: 1:1000
Tincture: 1:1000*

ACTION
Organomercurial antiseptic that has sustained bacteriostatic and fungistatic activity against some common pathogens.

Route	Onset	Peak	Duration
Topical	Unknown	Unknown	Unknown

INDICATIONS & DOSAGES
Antisepsis for minor cuts, scratches, wounds, abrasions—
Adults: apply to area q.d. to t.i.d.

ADVERSE REACTIONS
Skin: erythema, papular and vesicular eruptions over application area.
Other: *hypersensitivity reactions.*

INTERACTIONS
Drug-drug
Heavy metal salts, iodine, potassium permanganate: incompatible with these drugs. Discourage use together or immediately after application.

CONTRAINDICATIONS
Contraindicated in patients who are hypersensitive to drug or its components.

OVERDOSE & TREATMENT
No information available.

If patient ingests tincture, provide supportive treatment because of 50% alcohol content.

NURSING CONSIDERATIONS
• Frequent or prolonged use may cause serious mercury poisoning.
• Drug is incompatible with iodine, heavy metal salts, and potassium permanganate.
• Frequent or prolonged use or application to large areas may cause serious mercury poisoning.
• Therapy should be discontinued if redness, swelling, pain, infection, rash, or irritation persists or increases.
• Product shouldn't be allowed to contact eyes.

PATIENT TEACHING
• Advise patient to read carefully and follow product information.
• Caution patient to avoid contact with eyes.
• Advise patient that if redness, swelling, pain, infection, rash, or irritation persists or increases, he should discontinue drug and consult a doctor.
• Caution patient not to use in combination with or immediately after the application of strong acids, salts of heavy metals, potassium permanganate, and iodine.

tolnaftate
Absorbine Jr., Aftate for Athlete's Foot, Aftate for Jock Itch, Dr. Scholl's Athlete's Foot, Genaspor, Odor-Eaters Spray, Quinsana Plus, Tinactin, Ting

Pregnancy Risk Category B

HOW SUPPLIED
Cream: 1%
Powder: 1%
Pump spray liquid: 1%* (36% alcohol)
Solution: 1%
Spray powder: 1%* (14% alcohol)

ACTION
Unknown; distorts the hyphae and stunts mycelial growth in susceptible fungi.

Route	Onset	Peak	Duration
Topical	Unknown	Unknown	Unknown

INDICATIONS & DOSAGES

Superficial fungal infections of the skin; infections caused by common pathogenic fungi; tinea pedis, tinea cruris, tinea corporis—

Adults and children ages 12 or older: apply small amount of cream or 2 to 3 drops of solution to cover area; same amount of cream or solution to cover toes and interdigital webs of one foot; or gel, powder, or spray to cover affected area. Apply drug and massage gently into skin b.i.d. for 2 to 6 weeks.

ADVERSE REACTIONS

Skin: irritation.

INTERACTIONS

None significant.

CONTRAINDICATIONS

Contraindicated in patients who are hypersensitive to drug or its components.

OVERDOSE & TREATMENT

No information available.

NURSING CONSIDERATIONS

• Don't use to treat fungal infections of hair or nails; tolnaftate is ineffective against these fungi.
• Drug is odorless and greaseless; it won't stain or discolor skin, hair, nails, or clothing.
• Powder or aerosol may be used inside socks and shoes of persons susceptible to tinea infections.
• Ointments, creams, and liquid are primarily used for treatment; powder and aerosol are adjuncts unless infection is very mild.
• Additional courses of drug may be necessary to treat infections.

PATIENT TEACHING

• Teach patient to clean area and dry thoroughly before applying drug.
• Tell patient to use drug for full treatment period prescribed, even if condition has improved. Treatment should continue for at least 2 weeks after symptoms have resolved.
• Advise patient to use only small quantity of cream or lotion; treated area shouldn't be wet with solution.
• Advise patient to seek medical advice if no improvement occurs after 10 days or if condition worsens.
• Advise patient to wear shoes and cotton socks that fit well and to change footwear daily.
• Tell patient to keep drug away from eyes.

Reactions may be *common*, uncommon, *life-threatening*, or COMMON AND LIFE-THREATENING.

triclosan, irgasan
Basis All Clear Bar, Cetaphil, Clean & Clear Cleanser, Clean & Smooth, Clearasil Daily Face Wash, Dial Antibacterial, Jergen's Antibacterial, Lever 2000, no more germies, San Francisco Soap, Septi-Soft, Septisol, Softsoap Antibacterial, Stridex Face Wash, Suave Antibacterial

Pregnancy Risk Category NR

HOW SUPPLIED
Liquid: 0.3%, 0.6%
Soap: 0.25%
Solution: 0.25%, 1%

ACTION
A *bis*-phenol disinfectant, triclosan is bacteriostatic and has activity against a wide range of both gram-positive and gram-negative bacteria.

Route	Onset	Peak	Duration
Topical	Unknown	Unknown	Unknown

INDICATIONS & DOSAGES
Skin cleanser—
Adults: use as daily soap.

Health care personnel hand-wash and skin germ-killer (Septisol)—
Adults: dispense a small amount (5 ml) on hands; rub thoroughly for 30 seconds, rinse well, dry.

ADVERSE REACTIONS
None reported.

INTERACTIONS
None known.

CONTRAINDICATIONS
Contraindicated on burned or denuded skin and on mucous membranes.

OVERDOSE & TREATMENT
No information available.

NURSING CONSIDERATIONS
• Septisol and Septisoft shouldn't be used routinely or over large portions of body.

PATIENT TEACHING
• Caution patient not to use Septisol or Septisoft routinely for prophylaxis and not to use on burned or denuded skin.
• Advise patient to read carefully and follow product information.
• Advise patient that dose and frequency are dependent on area of treatment, tolerance, and dose form.

---

*Liquid contains alcohol.   **May contain tartrazine.   †Canada   ‡Australia   §U.K.

undecylenic acid and derivatives
FungiCure, Fungi-Nail

Pregnancy Risk Category NR

HOW SUPPLIED
Solution: 10%, 25%

ACTION
Antifungal and antibacterial; action unspecified.

Route	Onset	Peak	Duration
Topical	Unknown	Unknown	Unknown

INDICATIONS & DOSAGES
Ringworm or athlete's foot affecting fingers or toes—
Adults and children ages 2 and older: apply b.i.d., p.r.n., or as directed, after cleaning and drying the affected area. Four weeks of treatment is usually necessary for athlete's foot or ringworm.

ADVERSE REACTIONS
None reported.

INTERACTIONS
Skin: allergic reaction.

CONTRAINDICATIONS
Contraindicated in patients who are hypersensitive to drug or its components.

OVERDOSE & TREATMENT
No information available.

NURSING CONSIDERATIONS
• Product is for external use only.
• Ointments and creams are used as primary therapy; powder is generally used as adjunctive therapy.
• Area should be cleansed and dried before treatment.

PATIENT TEACHING
• Caution patient to avoid contact with eyes or mucous membranes and to avoid inhaling these products.
• Caution patient to carefully monitor symptoms when using drug on blistered, raw, or oozing skin.
• Advise patient that drug must be used for the full treatment duration, even when symptoms have abated.
• Caution patient to discontinue use and contact a doctor if symptoms persist or become worse.
• Tell patient with tinea pedis to wear well-fitting, ventilated shoes and to change socks daily.

urea (carbamide)
Aquacare, Carmol 10,
Carmol 20, Gormel Crème,
Lanaphilic, Nutraplus, Ultra
Mide 25, Ureacin-10,
Ureacin-20

Pregnancy Risk Category NR

HOW SUPPLIED
Cream: 10%, 20%
Lotion: 10%, 25%
Ointment: 10%

ACTION
Topical emollient that promotes
hydration and removes excess
keratin in dry and hyperkeratotic skin by helping to remove
scales and crusts. It may also
decrease itching.

Route	Onset	Peak	Duration
Topical	Unknown	Unknown	Unknown

INDICATIONS & DOSAGES
Moisturizing of dry skin—
Adults: apply thin film to affected area q.d. to t.i.d.; rub in
completely.

ADVERSE REACTIONS
Skin: transient stinging, burning, local irritation.

INTERACTIONS
None reported.

CONTRAINDICATIONS
No information available.

OVERDOSE & TREATMENT
None reported.

NURSING CONSIDERATIONS
• Product is for external use and
shouldn't be used near the eyes.
• Some preparations contain
sulfites that can cause allergic-
type reactions including anaphylaxis or asthmatic attacks in
certain susceptible people.
• Transient stinging, burning, or
local irritation may occur, especially if applied to the face or to
broken or inflamed skin.

PATIENT TEACHING
• Inform patient that therapeutic
effect may be enhanced by applying the urea preparation to
the skin while it is still moist.
• Caution patient that product is
for external use only and to
avoid contact with eyes.
• Advise patient to discontinue
use if irritation or rash occurs
and to contact a doctor immediately if shortness of breath or
breathing difficulty occurs.
• Caution patient to keep drug
out of reach of children.

---

*Liquid contains alcohol.   **May contain tartrazine.   †Canada   ‡Australia   §U.K.

vitamins A, D, and E, topical
A & D, Lazer Creme, Lobana Derm-Aide

Pregnancy Risk Category NR

HOW SUPPLIED
Cream
Lotion
Ointment

ACTION
Emollient that provides relief from minor skin irritations.

Route	Onset	Peak	Duration
Topical	Unknown	Unknown	Unknown

INDICATIONS & DOSAGES
Minor burns (including sun and wind), abrasions, chapped or chafed skin, and other minor noninfected irritations of the skin, including diaper rash, urine scald, lasered skin, and irritations associated with ileostomy and colostomy drainage—
Adults and children: apply thin film to cover the affected area q.d. to b.i.d. Repeat p.r.n.

ADVERSE REACTIONS
Skin: stinging, burning, itching, irritation.

INTERACTIONS
None reported.

CONTRAINDICATIONS
Contraindicated in patients who are hypersensitive to drug or its components. Not for use near eyes or on deep wounds, infections, or lacerations.

OVERDOSE & TREATMENT
No information available.

NURSING CONSIDERATIONS
• Patient shouldn't use around eyes or on deep wounds, puncture wounds, infections, or lacerations.

PATIENT TEACHING
• Tell patient to clean area before using and not to apply if signs of infection develop.
• Caution patient to keep out of eyes.
• Caution patient that if symptoms persist or worsen after 1 week of treatment, he should contact a doctor for evaluation.
• Inform patient that these products are for external use only.

witch hazel (hamamelis water)
A•E•R, Good Sense, Witch Hazel

Pregnancy Risk Category NR

HOW SUPPLIED
Gel: 50%*
Liquid: 86%

Pads: 50%

ACTION
Astringent that constricts tissue, stopping the flow of secretions.

Route	Onset	Peak	Duration
Topical	Unknown	Unknown	Unknown

INDICATIONS & DOSAGES
Relief from itching caused by minor skin irritation—
Adults: apply locally q.d. to six times daily p.r.n.

ADVERSE REACTIONS
None reported.

INTERACTIONS
None reported.

CONTRAINDICATIONS
Contraindicated in patients who are hypersensitive to drug or its components.

OVERDOSE & TREATMENT
No information available.

NURSING CONSIDERATIONS
• Drug is prepared from twigs of *Hamamelis virginiana,* which is considered nontoxic and has been used to soothe skin.
• Symptoms that persist should be evaluated by a doctor.

PATIENT TEACHING
• Advise patient to read carefully and follow package instructions.
• Advise patient that drug is for external use only.
• Caution patient that if symptoms persist or worsen, he should contact the doctor for evaluation.

zinc oxide
Balmex, Boudreaux's Butt Paste, Caldesene Baby, Caldesene Protecting, California Baby, Desitin, Earth Friendly Baby, Johnson's Diaper Rash, Little Forest

Pregnancy Risk Category B

HOW SUPPLIED
Cream: 2%, 4%
Ointment: 11.3%, 12%, 16%, 40%
Powders: 4%

ACTION
Mild astringent.

Route	Onset	Peak	Duration
Topical	Immediate	Unknown	Unknown

INDICATIONS & DOSAGES
Treatment for irritated skin (eczema, prickly heat, varicose

veins, around colostomies and ileostomies, diaper rash)—
Adults, children, infants: apply thin film to generous layer on affected area. Repeat p.r.n.

Prevention of sunburn—
Adults, children, infants: apply generous layer to nose, ears, and other areas of skin p.r.n. 30 minutes before sun exposure. Reapply after swimming, sweating, or other activities that may result in the washing away or removal of the sunscreen.

ADVERSE REACTIONS
Skin: rash, pruritus, skin discoloration.

INTERACTIONS
None reported.

CONTRAINDICATIONS
Contraindicated in patients who are hypersensitive to drug.

OVERDOSE & TREATMENT
No information available .

NURSING CONSIDERATIONS
● Drug is considered nontoxic.
● Persistent symptoms should be evaluated by a doctor.
● Combination products containing this drug may also contain other ingredients that can increase the risk of adverse reactions.

PATIENT TEACHING
● Advise patient to read product ingredient list and to read and follow package instructions.
● Caution patient that if symptoms persist or worsen, he should contact the doctor for evaluation.
● Advise patient to clean area thoroughly before applying drug.

Reactions may be *common*, uncommon, *life-threatening*, or COMMON AND LIFE-THREATENING.

Combination products

Brand name and active ingredients	Indications and dosages	Nursing considerations
Aveeno Anti-Itch • calamine 3% • camphor 4.7% • pramoxine 1%	*Relieves itching caused by poison ivy, oak, or sumac, insect bites, allergic itches, or chickenpox* **Adults and children ages 2 and older:** apply to affected area up to q.i.d.	• Patient should avoid getting in eyes. • If symptoms don't improve or if they recur within 1 week, patient should notify doctor.
Aveeno Daily Moisturizing Lotion • colloidal oatmeal 1% • dimethicone 1.25%	*Relieves scaling, chapping, and itching caused by dry skin* **Adults and children:** apply to hands and body p.r.n.	• Product is for external use only.
Bactine Antiseptic Liquid, Bactine Antiseptic-Analgesic Spray • benzalkonium chloride 0.13% • lidocaine hydrochloride 2.5%	*Prevents infection and provides temporary relief from minor cuts, scrapes, and burns* **Adults and children ages 2 and older:** apply small amount to affected area q.d. to q.i.d.	• Patient should clean area before use. • Patient may cover with bandage or sterile gauze after allowing product to dry. • Patient should avoid getting in eyes. • Patient shouldn't use over large areas of body. • If symptoms worsen, persist for longer than 1 week, or recur, patient should notify doctor. • Patient should notify doctor about deep or puncture wounds, animal bites, or serious burns.

(continued)

Combination products *(continued)*

Brand name and active ingredients	Indications and dosages	Nursing considerations
Band-Aid Fast Relief Calamine Spray • benzocaine 5.25% • calamine 14.5% • camphor 0.77%	*Relieves itching and pain caused by skin irritation, rash, poison ivy, oak, or sumac, and insect bites* **Adults and children ages 2 and older:** apply to affected area up to q.i.d.	• Patient should avoid getting in eyes. • Patient should notify doctor if symptoms don't improve or if they persist for longer than 1 week.
Band-Aid Hurt Free Wash • benzalkonium chloride 0.13% • lidocaine hydrochloride 2.5%	*Cleans minor cuts, scrapes, and wounds; relieves pain, and prevents infections* **Adults and children ages 2 and older:** flush affected area up to q.i.d.	• Patient may cover with bandage or sterile gauze after allowing product to dry. • Patient should avoid getting in eyes. • Patient shouldn't use over large areas of body. • If symptoms worsen, persist for longer than 1 week, or recur, patient should notify doctor. • Patient should notify doctor about deep or puncture wounds, animal bites, or serious burns.
Benadryl Extra Strength Itch Relief Spray, Itch Stopping Cream, Itch Stopping Gel, Itch Relief Stick • diphenhydramine 2% • zinc acetate 0.1%	*Relieves itching and pain caused by insect bites, minor skin irritation, and rash caused by poison ivy, oak, or sumac; dries weeping caused by poison ivy, oak, or sumac*	• Patient shouldn't use on chickenpox, measles, or large areas of skin. • Patient should avoid getting in eyes. • If symptoms worsen, are unimproved after 1 week, or if they recur, patient should notify doctor. • Patient shouldn't use drug with other products containing diphenhydramine.

Combination products *(continued)*

Brand name and active ingredients	Indications and dosages	Nursing considerations
Benadryl Extra Strength Itch Relief Spray, Itch Stopping Cream, Itch Stopping Gel, Itch Relief Stick *(continued)*	**Adults and children ages 12 and older:** apply to affected area up to q.i.d.	• Itch-relief stick may be used in children age 6 and older.
Betadine Antibiotic Moisturizing Ointment • bacitracin zinc 500 IU • polymyxin B sulfate 10,000 IU **Polysporin First Aid Antibiotic Ointment** • bacitracin zinc 500 IU • polymyxin B sulfate 10,000 IU **Neosporin First Aid Antibiotic Ointment** • bacitracin 400 U • neomycin 3.5 mg • polymyxin B 5,000 U	*Prevents infections of minor cuts, scrapes, and burns* **Adults and children:** apply amount equal to the surface area of the tip of the finger to affected area q.d. to q.i.d.	• Patient should clean area before use. • Patient may cover with bandage or sterile gauze. • Patient should avoid getting in eyes. • Patient shouldn't use over large areas of body. • If symptoms persist or worsen or if rash or allergic reaction occurs, patient should notify doctor. • Patient shouldn't use for longer than 1 week.
Caladryl • calamine 8% • pramoxine hydrochloride 1%	*Relieves itching and pain caused by poison ivy, oak, or sumac, insect bites, and minor skin irritations* **Adults and children ages 2 and older:** apply to affected area t.i.d. to q.i.d.	• Patient should clean and dry affected area before use. • Patient should avoid getting in eyes. • If symptoms aren't improved or recur within 1 week, patient should notify doctor. *(continued)*

Combination products *(continued)*

Brand name and active ingredients	Indications and dosages	Nursing considerations
Domeboro Powder and Tablets, Bluboro Powder, Boropak Powder, Pedi-Boro Soak Paks • aluminum sulfate • calcium acetate **MG217 Medicated** • coal tar 2% • colloidal sulfur 1.1% • salicylic acid 1.5% **P&S Plus** • coal tar solution 8% • salicylic acid 2%	*Relieves inflammatory conditions of the skin* **Adults and children:** 1 packet or tablet in a pint of water produces a modified 1:40 Burow's solution. Apply every 15 to 30 minutes, 4 to 6 times daily.	• Product is for external use only. • Patient should avoid getting in eyes. • Patient shouldn't use plastic or other impervious material to prevent evaporation. • If symptoms persist for longer than 1 week, patient should discontinue use and notify doctor.
Esoterica Skin Discoloration Fade Cream, SPF 10 • benzophenon-3 2.5% • hydroquinone 2% • octyl dimethyl PABA 3.3%	*To fade freckles and age spots* **Adults and children ages 12 and older:** apply thin layer to affected areas b.i.d.	• Patient shouldn't apply to inflamed or broken skin. • Patient should use for at least 6 weeks. • Patient should discontinue use after discoloration is gone. If discoloration reappears, patient should restart. • Patient shouldn't use with products containing resorcinol, phenol, or salicylic acid, unless directed by doctor. • Patient should limit sun exposure during and after treatment. • Patient should avoid using near eyes. • Drug may temporarily irritate or darken skin. If symptoms continue, patient should contact doctor.

Combination products (continued)

Brand name and active ingredients	Indications and dosages	Nursing considerations
Foille Medicated First Aid Ointment • benzocaine 5% • chloroxylenol 0.1%	*Prevents infection and relieves pain caused by sunburn* **Adults and children ages 2 and older:** apply at first sign of heat and redness. *Prevents infection and relieves pain caused by minor burns* **Adults and children ages 2 and older:** apply liberally over burn area. *Prevents infection and relieves pain caused by minor cuts and scrapes* **Adults and children ages 2 and older:** apply to affected area up to q.i.d.	• For burns, patient should immediately place burned area in cool water for several minutes before applying drug. • Patient should notify doctor about severe burns or puncture wounds, recurring symptoms, or symptoms persisting for longer than 1 week.
Fougara Triple Antibiotic Ointment • bacitracin 400 U • neomycin sulfate 3.5 mg • polymyxin B sulfate 5,000 U	*Prevents infections of minor cuts, scrapes, and burns* **Adults and children:** apply amount equal to the surface	• Patient should clean area before use. • Patient may cover with bandage or sterile gauze. • Patient should avoid getting in eyes. • Patient shouldn't use over large areas of body. *(continued)*

Combination products *(continued)*

Brand name and active ingredients	Indications and dosages	Nursing considerations
Fougara Triple Antibiotic Ointment *(continued)*	area of the tip of the finger to affected area q.d. to q.i.d.	• If symptoms persist or worsen or if rash or allergic reaction occurs, patient should notify doctor. • Patient shouldn't use for longer than 1 week. • Patient should notify doctor about deep or puncture wounds, animal bites, or serious burns.
Gold Bond Anti-Itch Cream • menthol 1% • pramoxine 1%	*Relieves itching caused by dry skin* **Adults and children ages 2 and older:** apply to affected area up to q.i.d.	• Patient should avoid getting in eyes. • If symptoms worsen, persist for longer than 1 week, or recur, patient should notify doctor.
Lanacane Maximum Strength Anti-Itch Cream • benzocaine 20% • benzethonium chloride 0.1%	*Prevents infection and relieves pain and itching of sunburn, insect bites, poison ivy, and other irritations* **Adults and children ages 2 and older:** apply to affected area q.d. to q.i.d.	• Patient should clean area before use. • Patient should avoid getting in eyes. • Patient should notify doctor about severe burns or puncture wounds, recurring symptoms, or symptoms persisting for longer than 1 week.
Neosporin Plus Pain Relief Maximum Strength First Aid Antibiotic Ointment • bacitracin 500 U • neomycin 3.5 mg	*Prevents infection and relieves pain or discomfort of cuts, scrapes, and burns*	• Patient should clean area before use. • Patient may cover with bandage or sterile gauze. • Patient should avoid getting in eyes. • Patient shouldn't use over large areas of body.

Combination products *(continued)*

Brand name and active ingredients	Indications and dosages	Nursing considerations
Neosporin Plus Pain Relief Maximum Strength First Aid Antibiotic Ointment *(continued)* • polymyxin B 10,000 U • pramoxine hydrochloride 10 mg	**Adults and children ages 2 and older:** apply amount equal to the surface area of the tip of the finger to affected area q.d. to q.i.d.	• If symptoms persist or worsen or if rash or allergic reaction occurs, patient should notify doctor. • Patient shouldn't use for longer than 1 week.
Neutrogena TGel • neutar 2% • solubilized coal tar extract 0.5%	*Controls symptoms of dandruff, psoriasis, and seborrheic dermatitis* **Adults:** massage liberal amount into scalp. Leave on for several minutes, rinse, and repeat. Use twice weekly.	• Patient should avoid getting in eyes. • Patient should notify doctor if symptoms are unimproved or if they worsen with regular use. • Patient should avoid sun exposure for 24 hours after use. • Patient shouldn't use for prolonged periods with prescriptions or UV therapy for psoriasis, or over large areas of the body without medical advice. • Drug may discolor gray, blond, bleached, or tinted hair.
Polysporin Powder • bacitracin 500 U • polymyxin B 10,000 U	*Prevents infections of minor cuts, scrapes, and burns* **Adults and children:** apply a light dusting of powder to affected area q.d. to q.i.d.	• Patient should clean area before use. • Patient may cover with bandage or sterile gauze. • Patient should avoid getting in eyes. • Patient shouldn't use over large areas of body. • If symptoms persist or worsen or if rash or allergic reaction occurs, patient should notify doctor. • Patient shouldn't use for longer than 1 week.

(continued)

Combination products *(continued)*

Brand name and active ingredients	Indications and dosages	Nursing considerations
Sebulex Shampoo • salicylic acid 2% • sulfur 2%	*Relieves symptoms caused by dandruff* **Adults:** massage into wet scalp. Leave on for 5 minutes, rinse, and repeat. Use daily or every other day.	• Patient should avoid getting in eyes. • Patient should notify doctor if irritation occurs. • Use of product once or twice weekly may maintain symptom relief.

8

Respiratory system

The primary function of the respiratory system is to exchange gases between the atmosphere and the blood. With inhalation, air enters the lungs and oxygen moves into adjacent blood vessels. At the same time, carbon dioxide (CO_2) moves out of the blood and into the lungs for exhalation. Besides providing gas exchange, the respiratory system also permits speech and helps to regulate acid-base balance.

Anatomy

Respiratory function is accomplished not only by the lungs and airways but also by the bones of the thorax, the respiratory muscles, and the central nervous system (CNS). The structures of the respiratory system are divided into upper and lower segments.

Upper respiratory system

Upper respiratory structures include the nose, mouth, pharynx, epiglottis, and larynx. These structures warm, filter, and humidify inhaled air. They also provide an important defense mechanism for the respiratory system. The nose contains tiny hairs and a mucus layer that trap dust, dirt, and large airborne particles that might otherwise be inhaled into the lungs, causing irritation or infection.

The epiglottis closes over the larynx during swallowing to prevent food or fluids from entering the lower airways. The bony outer portion of the larynx protects the softer vocal folds, which allow speech.

Lower respiratory system

The lower respiratory system includes the conducting airways and the gas exchange units of the lungs. Conducting airways include the trachea, the right and left main-stem bronchi, the lobar bronchi, the segmental and subsegmental bronchial tubes, and the terminal bronchioles. The main functions of these airways are to conduct air from the upper airways to the gas exchange units and to protect the delicate gas exchange units from inhaled irritants. The epithelial lining of the conducting airways is covered with a thin layer of mucus that traps small particles inhaled into the lungs.

Microscopic hairlike structures called cilia grow from the epithelium and, through a continuous waving action, propel the mucus layer upward toward larger airways, where the mucus can be coughed or cleared from the lungs.

The gas exchange units consist of the respiratory bronchioles, alveolar ducts, alveoli, and pulmonary capillaries. The walls of these structures are so thin and their surface area is so immense that individual oxygen molecules cross from the air into the blood and CO_2 molecules from the blood to the air in a quarter of a second. The heart transports oxygenated blood to the body tissues for use in cellular metabolism.

Thorax, respiratory muscles, and brainstem

Thoracic bones include the ribs, sternum, clavicles, vertebrae, and scapulae. Respiratory muscles include the diaphragm, intercostal muscles, and accessory muscles in the neck and abdomen. The medulla in the brainstem stimulates respiration and controls the basic rhythm of respiration. The central controller in the medulla sends signals via the phrenic and intercostal nerves to the diaphragm and intercostal muscles, causing the muscles to contract. When they contract, the thorax enlarges, which enlarges the lungs as well. Air flows into the lungs because of the negative pressure created by this enlargement.

Then, an intrinsic mechanism causes the signal from the medulla to stop. The pneumotaxic center in the pons also signals the inspiratory area of the medulla oblongata to stop the inspiratory stimulus and limit the inhalation time. A third signal controlling inhalation is the apneustic area in the pons. Stretch receptors in the lungs sense when the lungs become inflated. Impulses are then sent to the inspiratory and apneustic areas, and inhalation is inhibited. This reflex is called the Hering-Breuer inflation reflex.

During expiration, which is passive, the muscles relax and the natural recoil of the lungs causes them to return to their resting size.

Chemosensitive areas in the medulla monitor the pH of cerebrospinal fluid and signal the central controller to increase or decrease the rate and depth of ventilation to maintain the appropriate pH. Chemoreceptors in the carotid and aortic sinuses are sensitive to changes in CO_2 and oxygen levels in the blood. The partial pressure of carbon dioxide (Pa_{CO_2}) in arterial blood is about 40 mm Hg. If the Pa_{CO_2} level rises, the chemosensitive area and the chemoreceptors are stimulated, which in turn stimulates the inspiratory area and increases the respiration rate. Hyperventilation allows the body to expel the excess CO_2 until the level returns to normal. If the arterial Pa_{CO_2} falls below 40 mm Hg, the chemosensitive area and chemoreceptors aren't stimulated, and the inspiratory area maintains a slower rate until the Pa_{CO_2} level returns to normal.

Each lung is encased in a membrane called the visceral pleura. The inside of the thoracic cavity is lined with a membrane called the parietal pleura. A thin layer of pleural fluid between these two pleural layers allows the membranes to slide over each other during breathing but not to separate. Because the natural tendency of the lungs is to recoil to a smaller size and the natural tendency of the thorax is to expand, negative pressure exists between the pleurae in a potential space called the pleural cavity. The negative pressure causes the walls of the lungs to be pulled outward during inspiration, increasing lung volume.

When the thoracic bones, respiratory muscles, brainstem, and lungs are functioning normally, this process of breathing is effortless and involuntary. But conditions such as upper respiratory tract infection, influenza, allergic rhinitis, sore throat, laryngitis, acute bronchitis, and asthma can lead to many distressing signs and symptoms, including sneezing, runny nose, congested nasal passages, hoarseness, cough, mucus production, dyspnea, and chest pain. These symptoms commonly occur with benign, self-limiting conditions that respond well to home remedies and over-the-counter (OTC) medications, but they can also signify serious acute and chronic conditions that should receive professional medical treatment.

Upper respiratory tract infection

An upper respiratory tract infection, also called the common cold, is usually caused by a virus that attacks the mucous membranes of the upper respiratory structures. The mucous membranes become inflamed and swollen and initially produce a thin, watery discharge that later becomes thick and opaque.

Signs and symptoms
Usual signs and symptoms include a runny nose, congestion, sneezing, sore throat, cough, itchy eyes, fever less than 100° F (37.8° C), headache, and fatigue.

Serious conditions
Signs and symptoms of upper respiratory tract infection usually last 5 to 7 days; if they last longer than that, other conditions may be the problem. For example, the patient may have acute sinusitis caused by a bacterial infection, especially if he has pain or tenderness just above or below the eyes. If aspirin and decongestants don't relieve the pain and pressure in 48 hours, the patient should contact a doctor.

Complications
Patients who use decongestant nasal sprays for longer than 3 days may develop rebound nasal congestion when they try to stop using the spray. Discourage patients with asthma or chronic obstructive pulmonary disease (COPD) from using antihistamines because the drying effect of these drugs may cause bronchial mucus plugging.

Prolonged use of aspirin and ibuprofen may cause gastrointestinal (GI) distress and ulcers. Aspirin increases the clotting time of blood and may increase the risk of bleeding. Overuse of ibuprofen may cause renal failure.

Nursing considerations
• A common cold typically needs no medical attention. Because viruses aren't susceptible to antibiotics, discourage patients from calling their doctors to obtain antibiotics.
• Cold signs and symptoms usually last 5 to 7 days. If they persist longer than that, begin to suspect other causes.
• Patients who have COPD or asthma may have worsening of their chronic disease if they develop a cold.

Patient teaching
• Tell the patient to drink plenty of fluids.
• Tell an adult patient to relieve cold signs and symptoms with aspirin, acetaminophen, or ibuprofen. Children and teenagers should avoid aspirin because of the danger of developing Reye's syndrome.
• Instruct the patient to take decongestants for nasal congestion.
• Urge the patient not to use decongestant nasal sprays for longer than 3 days. Tell the patient to use a saline nasal spray instead.

• Advise the patient to get plenty of rest.
• Tell the patient to cover his nose and mouth when coughing and sneezing to avoid spreading infection.
• Teach the patient to wash his hands after coughing or blowing his nose.

Influenza

Influenza, or the flu, is a viral infection that affects primarily the respiratory system. The virus invades mucous membranes of both the upper and lower respiratory tract, causing inflammation and swelling. The virus also has broad systemic effects that go beyond the respiratory system.

Signs and symptoms

Influenza is characterized by a runny nose, congestion, sore throat, cough, fever over 100° F (37.8° C), headache, and severe aching of muscles and joints.

Serious conditions

For otherwise healthy people, the flu is a serious illness that causes discomfort and loss of work time. For people with underlying chronic conditions, the flu can be life-threatening.

Complications

Pneumonia, respiratory failure, and adult respiratory distress syndrome can be complications of influenza. A cough that produces discolored sputum, persistent fever over 100° F (37.8° C) after 2 to 3 days, or dyspnea should cause concern.

Patients who use decongestant nasal sprays for longer than 3 days may develop rebound nasal congestion when they try to stop using the spray. Discourage patients with asthma or COPD from using antihistamines because the drying effect of these drugs may cause bronchial mucus plugging.

Prolonged use of aspirin and ibuprofen may cause GI distress and ulcers. Aspirin increases the clotting time of blood and may increase the risk of bleeding. Overuse of ibuprofen may cause renal failure.

Nursing considerations

• Prevention is very important because influenza can become life-threatening, especially in certain groups of people. Encourage anyone at high risk for influenza or flu-related complications to get a flu vaccination every autumn. These people include health care workers; patients with chronic respiratory disease, cardiovascular (CV) disease, renal disease, or diabetes; and immunosuppressed patients, such as organ transplant, cancer, and AIDS patients.

• Previously healthy patients shouldn't need medical attention for influenza. Because viruses aren't susceptible to antibiotics, discourage patients from asking a doctor for an antibiotic.

• Influenza signs and symptoms usually last 5 to 7 days. If they persist longer than that, begin to suspect other causes.

• Patients who have chronic respiratory diseases may need hospitalization because of the severity of their symptoms.

Patient teaching

• Tell the patient to drink plenty of fluids.

• Tell an adult patient to relieve influenza signs and symptoms with aspirin, acetaminophen, or ibuprofen. Children and teenagers should avoid aspirin because of the danger of developing Reye's syndrome.

• Instruct the patient to take decongestants for nasal congestion.

• Advise the patient not to use decongestant nasal sprays for longer than 3 days. Tell the patient to use a saline nasal spray instead.

• Advise the patient to get plenty of rest and to stay home from work.

• Tell the patient to cover his nose and mouth when coughing and sneezing to avoid spreading infection.

• Advise the patient to wash his hands after coughing or blowing his nose.

• Instruct the patient to call a doctor if fever, dyspnea, or productive cough persists.

Allergic rhinitis

Various pollens, molds, dusts and other irritants may cause an allergic reaction in the nose, sinuses, and nasopharynx, resulting in inflammation, swelling, and watery discharge of the mucous membranes.

Signs and symptoms

Sneezing, itchy eyes and nose, frequent watery discharge from the nose, and headache are symptoms of allergic rhinitis. These symptoms occur when the person is exposed to the substance causing the allergic reaction, either in a specific situation (such as exposure to dog or cat dander) or a particular season of the year (such as exposure to ragweed in the late summer and fall).

Serious conditions

A patient who has allergic rhinitis may also have asthma. If so, tell the patient to consult a doctor if wheezing or dyspnea occurs. Nasal discharge that becomes thick or discolored may indicate a bacterial sinus infection; tell the patient to notify a doctor so that an antibiotic can be prescribed.

Complications

A patient who uses a decongestant nasal spray for longer than 3 days may develop rebound nasal congestion when he stops using the spray. Discourage a patient with asthma or COPD from using antihistamines because the drying effect of these drugs may cause bronchial mucus plugging.

Prolonged use of aspirin and ibuprofen may cause GI distress and ulcers. Aspirin increases the clotting time of blood and may increase the risk of bleeding. Overuse of ibuprofen may cause renal failure.

Nursing considerations

• Tell the patient to consult a doctor if an OTC medication used to treat allergic rhinitis produces incomplete relief or excessive drowsiness. Medications available only by prescription may be more effective in relieving the symptoms.

Patient teaching

• Instruct the patient to take antihistamines and decongestants for a runny nose and itchy, watering eyes.
• Advise the patient not to use decongestant nasal sprays for longer than 3 days. Tell the patient to use saline nasal spray instead.
• Tell an adult patient to relieve headache with aspirin, acetaminophen, or ibuprofen. Children and teenagers should avoid aspirin because of the danger of developing Reye's syndrome.
• Tell the patient to drink plenty of fluids.
• Advise the patient to try to identify and avoid the causative agent, if possible.

Sore throat

Infection or irritation of the pharynx can cause a painful sore throat. Inflammation and swelling occur in the mucous membranes of the pharynx and possibly in the tonsils. A sore throat often accompanies a cold.

Signs and symptoms

Painful swallowing, a runny nose, congestion, fever less than 100° F (37.8° C), swollen lymph nodes in the neck, and a cough are signs and symptoms that commonly accompany a sore throat.

Serious conditions

Most sore throats are caused by viral infections that respond well to home remedies, but several other causes of sore throat may require different types of treatment. Sore throat caused by streptococcal bacteria ("strep throat") must be treated with antibiotics.

Mononucleosis causes sore throat and fatigue more severe than those caused by the common cold. Because it's caused by a virus, mononucleosis doesn't respond to antibiotics, but most affected patients seek medical attention anyway because of the severity and persistence of their symptoms. Teenagers and young adults are most likely to get mononucleosis.

The sore throat caused by recurrent tonsillitis may require removal of the tonsils to eliminate the pain. Smoking and alcohol consumption may also cause a sore throat. Continued irritation from the smoke or alcohol may lead to throat cancer. Mumps may also cause sore throat, along with swollen glands under the jaw.

Complications

A sore throat caused by a viral infection should clear in several days. If it persists, suspect other causes.

Prolonged use of aspirin and ibuprofen may cause GI distress and ulcers. Aspirin increases the clotting time of blood and may increase the risk of bleeding. Overuse of ibuprofen may cause renal failure.

Nursing considerations

• If the patient is a smoker, counsel him about other health consequences related to smoking.
• If the patient consumes alcohol, counsel him about other health consequences related to alcohol.

Patient teaching

• Advise the patient that gargling with warm saltwater may help to soothe his sore throat.
• Instruct the patient that throat lozenges and anesthetic sprays may also help to relieve pain.
• Tell an adult patient to relieve pain with aspirin, acetaminophen, or ibuprofen. Children and teenagers should avoid aspirin because of the danger of developing Reye's syndrome.
• Advise the patient not to smoke or drink alcohol.

Laryngitis

Laryngitis is loss of voice or hoarseness caused by inflammation of the vocal cords. It usually results from a viral infection, overuse of the voice, or inhaled irritants.

Signs and symptoms

Hoarseness, a change in voice, or an inability to make sound are the usual changes that occur with laryngitis. Sore throat may also occur.

Serious conditions

Persistent hoarseness may be a symptom of benign or malignant vocal cord nodules. Hypothyroidism may also cause hoarseness.

Complications

Hoarseness caused by viral infection or overuse of the voice should disappear within a week. If the hoarseness persists or recurs, suspect other causes.

Prolonged use of aspirin and ibuprofen may cause GI distress and ulcers. Aspirin increases the clotting time of blood and may increase the risk of bleeding. Overuse of ibuprofen may cause renal failure.

Nursing considerations

• Smoking and alcohol increase the risk of vocal cord cancer.

• If a patient has persistent or recurrent hoarseness, encourage him to contact a doctor, especially if he has no other signs or symptoms of viral upper respiratory tract infection.

Patient teaching

• Advise the patient to rest the voice as much as possible.
• Tell the patient to drink plenty of fluids.
• Tell an adult patient to relieve pain with aspirin, acetaminophen, or ibuprofen. Children and teenagers should avoid aspirin because of the danger of developing Reye's syndrome.
• Advise the patient not to smoke or drink alcohol.
• Tell the patient to contact a doctor if the hoarseness lasts longer than 1 week or recurs.

Acute bronchitis

Acute bronchitis may be caused by either a viral or bacterial infection. The organism invades the mucous membranes of the bronchial tubes, causing inflammation, swelling, and increased mucus production.

Signs and symptoms

Acute bronchitis causes cough, which may be dry or may produce mucus and, sometimes, fever. Symptoms of an upper respiratory tract infection may accompany or precede bronchitis.

Serious conditions

Although cough is the primary symptom of acute bronchitis, it also accompanies many other serious conditions. If the person is a smoker, for example, suspect chronic bronchitis. In this situation, the patient probably will report that the cough has been present for many weeks, even months or years, and that it produces sputum.

The chronic or recurrent cough that sometimes occurs in patients with asthma can be confused with acute bronchitis, especially if the patient also has an upper respiratory tract infection. Cough, often occurring with a high fever and shortness of breath, is also a symptom of pneumonia, an infection in the parenchyma of the lungs.

Cough is commonly the primary symptom in lung cancer, tuberculosis, pulmonary fibrosis, and unusual lung infections. Sudden onset of dry, harsh cough may occur if a patient inhales a foreign object. Cough and shortness of breath may accompany congestive heart failure.

Complications

The greatest danger of prolonged use of OTC drugs is that the patient's illness may be caused by something far more serious than acute bronchitis. Cough is a serious symptom that shouldn't be ignored. Whenever a cough can't be attributed to an upper respiratory tract infection or acute bronchitis, or when it persists for several weeks, the patient should consult a doctor.

The drying effects of antihistamines may, with prolonged use, cause mucus plugging in small airways.

Nursing considerations

● The fever caused by acute bronchitis shouldn't last longer than 3 or 4 days, the cough no longer than 7 to 10 days. Tell the patient to consult a doctor if either symptom exceeds these periods.
● If a patient develops wheezing, dyspnea, or hemoptysis (coughing up blood), tell him to contact a doctor.
● Patients with severe coughing episodes may experience chest pain from muscle strain.
● Ask about the nature of the patient's chest pain; usually it will be an aching pain that worsens with coughing or deep breathing. You may be able to

elicit the pain by palpating the chest wall.

• If the patient smokes, urge him to quit because smokers have a much higher risk of developing serious lung problems than nonsmokers.

• Acute bronchitis caused by a bacterial infection must be treated with antibiotics. If sputum is foul-smelling, green, or rust-colored, suspect bacterial infection.

Patient teaching

• Tell the patient to drink plenty of fluids.

• Advise the patient to inhale steam from a hot shower or basin filled with hot water.

• Advise the patient to stop smoking, if appropriate.

• Tell the patient that cough preparations may help to ease his cough.

• Tell an adult patient to relieve fever and pain with aspirin, acetaminophen, or ibuprofen. Children and teenagers should avoid aspirin because of the danger of developing Reye's syndrome.

• Advise the patient to avoid antihistamines if his cough is productive.

• Instruct the patient to call his doctor if he coughs up blood or if phlegm becomes foul-smelling, rust-colored, or green.

Asthma

Asthma is a chronic disorder characterized by inflammation of the airways and bronchospasm. Exposure to an asthma trigger begins an immediate response in which mast cells in the airways release histamine, prostaglandins, and leukotrienes, leading to bronchoconstriction. In a later response, eosinophils and lymphocytes cause inflammation in the airway mucous membranes. Mucus plugging, disruption of the ciliated epithelium, and smooth muscle hypertrophy also occur.

Signs and symptoms

Wheezing, dyspnea, chest tightness, and cough are the characteristic symptoms of asthma. Signs and symptoms typically are intermittent, with asymptomatic periods sandwiched between asthma attacks. Triggers for these attacks include inhaled allergens (dust mites, pollen, molds), exercise, cold air, air pollution, smoke, viral upper respiratory tract infections, and beta blocker therapy.

Serious conditions

Asthma is a serious medical condition that patients shouldn't try to treat on their own. Other conditions with signs and symptoms similar to those of asthma are congestive heart failure, aspiration of a foreign body, vocal dysfunction, and panic disorders.

Complications
Asthma can't be adequately treated with OTC drugs. That's because OTC bronchodilators aren't as effective as prescribed bronchodilators, and they have many adverse cardiac effects. Corticosteroids, which are essential in treating persistent asthma, aren't available without a prescription.

An inadequately treated acute asthma attack can lead to respiratory failure, respiratory arrest, and even death. Asthma that has been inadequately treated for many years may lead to permanent airway damage.

Nursing considerations
• If a patient has asthma symptoms, tell him to contact a doctor immediately; urge him to visit an emergency department if he has acute respiratory distress.
• Discourage use of OTC or herbal remedies in place of professional medical care and prescribed medications.
• Help the patient to identify asthma triggers.

• Pursed-lip breathing may help to control shortness of breath.

Patient teaching
• Teach the patient that wheezing, coughing, chest tightness, and shortness of breath are signs and symptoms of asthma. Urge the patient to see his doctor if he has these symptoms.
• Help the patient to identify the situations that trigger his asthma attacks.
• Teach the patient to remain calm during asthma attacks.
• Instruct the patient to breathe slowly and deeply during an attack and to use pursed-lip breathing to control shortness of breath.

**brompheniramine maleate
chlorpheniramine maleate
clemastine fumarate
dextromethorphan
   hydrobromide
diphenhydramine
   hydrochloride
ephedrine sulfate
epinephrine
guaifenesin
triprolidine hydrochloride**

**brompheniramine
maleate**
Bromphen*, Chlorphed,
Dimetane*, Dimetane
Extentabs

Pregnancy Risk Category C

HOW SUPPLIED
Tablets: 4 mg, 8 mg, 12 mg
Tablets (extended-release):
8 mg, 12 mg
Elixir: 2 mg/5 ml*

ACTION
Competes with histamine for
H_1-receptor sites on effector
cells. Prevents, but doesn't reverse, histamine-mediated responses.

Route	Onset	Peak	Duration
P.O.	15-60 min	2-5 hr	3-24 hr

INDICATIONS & DOSAGES
Rhinitis, allergy symptoms—
**Adults and children ages 12
and older:** 4 mg P.O. q 4 to 6

hours; or 8 or 12 mg extended-
release P.O. q 8 to 12 hours or
12 hours, respectively. Maximum oral dose is 24 mg daily.
Children ages 6 to 11: 2 mg
P.O. q 4 to 6 hours, or 8 or 12
mg extended-release P.O. q 12
hours. Maximum dose is 12 mg
daily. The extended-release
preparation isn't recommended
for home use in children
younger than age 12.
Children younger than age 6:
0.5 mg/kg P.O. daily in divided
doses t.i.d. or q.i.d.

ADVERSE REACTIONS
CNS: dizziness, tremors, irri-
tability, insomnia, syncope,
drowsiness, stimulation.
CV: hypotension, palpitations.
GI: anorexia, nausea, vomiting,
dry mouth and throat.
GU: urinary retention.
Hematologic: *thrombocytope-
nia, agranulocytosis.*
Skin: urticaria, rash.

INTERACTIONS
Drug-drug
CNS depressants: increases sedation. Advise patient to use together cautiously.
MAO inhibitors: increases anticholinergic effects. Advise patient to avoid using together.

Drug-lifestyle
Alcohol use: increases CNS depression. Advise patient to avoid using together.

CONTRAINDICATIONS
Contraindicated in patients who are hypersensitive to drug's ingredients and in patients with acute asthma, severe hypertension, coronary artery disease, angle-closure glaucoma, urinary retention, symptomatic prostatic hyperplasia, pyloroduodenal obstruction, or peptic ulcer. Also contraindicated within 2 weeks of MAO inhibitor therapy.

OVERDOSE & TREATMENT
Signs and symptoms of overdose may include those of CNS depression (sedation, reduced mental alertness, apnea, and CV collapse) or those of CNS stimulation (insomnia, hallucinations, tremors, or seizures). Anticholinergic symptoms, such as dry mouth, flushed skin, fixed and dilated pupils, and GI symptoms, are common, especially in children.

Treat overdose by inducing emesis with ipecac syrup (in conscious patients), followed by activated charcoal to reduce further drug absorption. Use gastric lavage if patient is unconscious or if ipecac fails. Treat hypotension with vasopressors, and control seizures

with diazepam or phenytoin I.V. Don't give stimulants.

NURSING CONSIDERATIONS
• Use cautiously in elderly patients and in those with increased intraocular pressure, diabetes, ischemic heart disease, hyperthyroidism, hypertension, bronchial asthma, and prostatic hyperplasia.
• Monitor blood count during long-term therapy, as ordered; observe for signs of blood dyscrasias.
• Drug can prevent, reduce, or mask positive diagnostic skin test response. Advise patient to discontinue drug 4 days before test.
• Children younger than age 6 should use only as directed by doctor.

PATIENT TEACHING
• Instruct patient to reduce GI distress by taking drug with food or milk.
• Warn patient to avoid alcohol and activities that require alertness until drug's CNS effects are known.
• Advise patient to notify a doctor if unusual bleeding or bruising occurs.
• Tell patient that coffee or tea may reduce drowsiness but that he should use cautiously if palpitations develop. This drug

---

Reactions may be *common*, uncommon, *life-threatening*, or COMMON AND LIFE-THREATENING.

causes less drowsiness than some other antihistamines.

• Inform patient that sugarless gum, sugarless sour hard candy, or ice chips may relieve dry mouth.

• Tell patient to notify a doctor if tolerance develops because a different antihistamine may need to be prescribed.

chlorpheniramine maleate
Aller-Chlor*, Chlo-Amine, Chlorate, Chlor-Niramine, Chlor-100, Chlor-Trimeton*, Chlor-Trimeton 12 Hour Relief, Chlor-Tripolon†, Gen-Allerate, Novo-Pheniram†, Pfeiffer's Allergy, Piriton§, Teldrin

Pregnancy Risk Category B

HOW SUPPLIED
Tablets: 4 mg, 8 mg, 12 mg
Tablets (chewable): 2 mg
Tablets (timed-release): 8 mg, 12 mg
Capsules (timed-release): 6 mg, 8 mg, 12 mg
Syrup: 2 mg/5 ml*

ACTION
Competes with histamine for H_1-receptor sites on effector cells. It prevents, but doesn't reverse, histamine-mediated responses.

Route	Onset	Peak	Duration
P.O.	15-60 min	2-6 hr	24 hr

INDICATIONS & DOSAGES
Rhinitis, allergy symptoms—
Adults and children ages 12 and older: 4 mg P.O. q 4 to 6 hours, not to exceed 24 mg/day; or 8 or 12 mg timed-release P.O. q 12 hours in the morning and evening, not to exceed 24 mg daily.
Children ages 6 to 11: 2 mg P.O. q 4 to 6 hours, not to exceed 12 mg daily. Or, may give 8 mg timed-release P.O. h.s., as directed by a doctor.
Children ages 2 to 5: 1 mg P.O. q 4 to 6 hours, not to exceed 6 mg daily.

ADVERSE REACTIONS
CNS: stimulation, sedation, drowsiness, excitability (in children).
CV: hypotension, palpitations, weak pulse.
GI: epigastric distress, dry mouth.
GU: urinary retention.
Respiratory: thick bronchial secretions.
Skin: rash, urticaria.

INTERACTIONS
Drug-drug
CNS depressants: increases sedation. Advise patient to use together cautiously.

MAO inhibitors: increases anticholinergic effects. Advise patient to avoid using together.

Drug-lifestyle
Alcohol use: increases CNS depression. Advise patient to avoid using together.

CONTRAINDICATIONS
Contraindicated in patients having acute asthmatic attacks; in patients with angle-closure glaucoma, symptomatic prostatic hyperplasia, pyloroduodenal obstruction, or bladder neck obstruction; and in patients taking MAO inhibitors. Antihistamines aren't recommended for breast-feeding women because small amounts of drug appear in breast milk.

OVERDOSE & TREATMENT
Signs and symptoms of overdose may include either CNS depression (sedation, reduced mental alertness, apnea, and CV collapse) or CNS stimulation (insomnia, hallucinations, tremors, and seizures). Atropine-like symptoms, such as dry mouth, flushed skin, fixed and dilated pupils, and GI symptoms are common, especially in children.

Treat overdose by inducing emesis with ipecac syrup (in conscious patient), followed by activated charcoal to reduce further drug absorption. Use gastric lavage if patient is unconscious or if ipecac fails. Treat hypotension with vasopressors, and control seizures with diazepam or phenytoin. Don't give stimulants. Administering ammonium chloride or vitamin C to acidify urine will promote drug excretion.

NURSING CONSIDERATIONS
• Use cautiously in elderly patients and those with increased intraocular pressure, hyperthyroidism, CV or renal disease, hypertension, bronchial asthma, urine retention, prostatic hyperplasia, and stenosing peptic ulcerations.
• Ask patient about use of other prescription or OTC drugs.
• Monitor patient for adverse reactions or worsening condition.
• Antihistamines can prevent, reduce, or mask positive diagnostic skin test response. Advise patient to discontinue drug 4 days before test.
• Drug shouldn't be used in children younger than age 6 unless directed by doctor.

PATIENT TEACHING
• Warn patient to avoid alcohol and driving or other activities that require alertness until drug's CNS effects are known.
• Tell patient that coffee or tea may reduce drowsiness.

Reactions may be *common*, uncommon, *life-threatening*, or COMMON AND LIFE-THREATENING.

- Inform patient that sugarless gum, sugarless sour hard candy, or ice chips may relieve dry mouth.
- Instruct patient to notify doctor if tolerance develops because a different antihistamine may need to be prescribed.
- Tell parent that drug shouldn't be used in children younger than age 6 unless directed by doctor; extended-release preparations shouldn't be used in children younger than age 12, unless directed.

---

clemastine fumarate
Antihist-1, Tavist, Tavist-1

Pregnancy Risk Category B

HOW SUPPLIED
Tablets: 1.34 mg, 2.68 mg
Syrup: 0.67 mg/5 ml*

ACTION
Competes with histamine for H_1-receptor sites on effector cells. It prevents, but doesn't reverse, histamine-mediated responses.

Route	Onset	Peak	Duration
P.O.	15-60 min	5-7 hr	12 hr

INDICATIONS & DOSAGES
Rhinitis, allergy symptoms—
Adults and children ages 12 and older: 1.34 mg P.O. q 12 hours, or 2.68 mg P.O q.d. to t.i.d., p.r.n. Don't exceed daily dose of 8.04 mg.
Children ages 6 to 11: 0.67 to 1.34 mg P.O. b.i.d. Don't exceed daily dose of 4.02 mg.

ADVERSE REACTIONS
CNS: sedation, drowsiness, *seizures,* nervousness, tremor, confusion, restlessness, vertigo, headache, sleepiness, dizziness, fatigue.
CV: hypotension, palpitations, tachycardia.
GI: epigastric distress, anorexia, diarrhea, nausea, vomiting, constipation, dry mouth.
GU: urine retention, urinary frequency.
Hematologic: hemolytic anemia, *thrombocytopenia, agranulocytosis.*
Respiratory: thick bronchial secretions.
Skin: rash, urticaria, photosensitivity, diaphoresis.
Other: *anaphylactic shock.*

INTERACTIONS
Drug-drug
CNS depressants: increases sedation. Advise patient to use together cautiously.
MAO inhibitors: increases anticholinergic effects. Advise patient to avoid using together.

Drug-lifestyle
Alcohol use: increases CNS depression. Advise patient to avoid using together.
Sun exposure: photosensitivity reactions may occur. Tell patient to use sunblock and avoid prolonged sun exposure.

CONTRAINDICATIONS
Contraindicated in patients who are hypersensitive to this drug or to other antihistamines of similar chemical structure and in patients with acute asthma, angle-closure glaucoma, stenosing peptic ulcer, symptomatic prostatic hyperplasia, bladder neck obstruction, or pyloroduodenal obstruction. Also contraindicated in neonates, premature infants, and breast-feeding women. Avoid use in those taking MAO inhibitors.

OVERDOSE & TREATMENT
Signs and symptoms of overdose may include either CNS depression (sedation, reduced mental alertness, apnea, and CV collapse) or CNS stimulation (insomnia, hallucinations, tremors, or seizures). Anticholinergic symptoms, such as dry mouth, flushed skin, fixed and dilated pupils and GI symptoms are common, especially in children.

Treat overdose by inducing emesis with ipecac syrup (in conscious patient), followed by activated charcoal to reduce further drug absorption. Use gastric lavage if patient is unconscious or if ipecac fails. Treat hypotension with vasopressors, and control seizures with diazepam or phenytoin. Don't give stimulants.

NURSING CONSIDERATIONS
● Use cautiously in elderly patients and in those with increased intraocular pressure, hyperthyroidism, CV disease, hypertension, bronchial asthma, and prostatic hyperplasia.
● Children younger than age 12 should use only as directed by a doctor.
● Monitor blood counts during long-term therapy, as ordered; observe for signs of blood dyscrasias.
● Antihistamines can prevent, reduce, or mask positive diagnostic skin test response. Advise patient to discontinue drug 4 days before test.

PATIENT TEACHING
● Warn patient to avoid alcohol and driving or other activities that require alertness until drug's CNS effects are known.
● Tell patient that coffee or tea may reduce drowsiness but that he should use cautiously if palpitations develop.

Reactions may be *common*, uncommon, *life-threatening*, or COMMON AND LIFE-THREATENING.

- Inform patient that sugarless gum, sugarless sour hard candy, or ice chips may relieve dry mouth.
- Warn patient of possible photosensitivity reactions. Advise use of a sunblock.
- Tell patient to notify health care provider if tolerance develops because a different antihistamine may need to be prescribed.

dextromethorphan hydrobromide

Balminil D.M., Benylin DM, Broncho-Grippol-DM†, Buckley's DM, Children's Hold, Delsym, DM Syrup, Hold, Koffex DM†, Mediquell, Neo-DM†, Ornex-DM 15, Ornex-DM 30, Pertussin Cough Suppressant, Pertussin CS, Pertussin ES, Robidex†, Robitussin Pediatric, Sedatuss†, St. Joseph Cough Suppressant for Children, Sucrets Cough Control Formula, Trocal, Vicks Formula 44-d Pediatric Formula

Pregnancy Risk Category C

HOW SUPPLIED
Liquid (extended-release):
30 mg/5 ml
Lozenges: 5 mg, 7.5 mg

Solution: 3.5 mg/5 ml, 5 mg/ 5 ml*, 7.5 mg/5 ml, 10 mg/ 5 ml*, 15 mg/5 ml*, 15 mg/ 15 ml*

ACTION
Antitussive that suppresses the cough reflex by direct action on the cough center in the medulla.

Route	Onset	Peak	Duration
P.O.	< 0.5 hr	Unknown	3-6 hr

INDICATIONS & DOSAGES
Nonproductive cough—
Adults and children ages 12 and older: 10 to 20 mg P.O. q 4 hours, or 30 mg q 6 to 8 hours. Or, 60 mg extended-release liquid b.i.d. Maximum dose is 120 mg daily.
Children ages 6 to 11: 5 to 10 mg P.O. q 4 hours, or 15 mg q 6 to 8 hours. Or, 30 mg extended-release liquid b.i.d. Maximum dose is 60 mg daily.
Children ages 2 to 5: 2.5 to 5 mg P.O. q 4 hours, or 7.5 mg q 6 to 8 hours. Or, 15 mg extended-release liquid b.i.d. Maximum dose is 30 mg daily.
Children younger than age 2: dosages must be individualized.

ADVERSE REACTIONS
CNS: drowsiness, dizziness.
GI: nausea, vomiting, stomach pain.

INTERACTIONS
Drug-drug
MAO inhibitors: increases risk of hypotension, coma, hyperpyrexia, and death. Advise patient to avoid using together.
Selegiline: increases risk of confusion, coma, hyperpyrexia. Advise patient to avoid using together.

Drug-herb
Parsley: may promote or produce serotonin syndrome. Advise patient to avoid using together.

CONTRAINDICATIONS
Contraindicated in patients currently taking MAO inhibitors or within 2 weeks of discontinuing MAO inhibitors.

OVERDOSE & TREATMENT
Signs and symptoms of overdose may include nausea, vomiting, drowsiness, dizziness, blurred vision, nystagmus, shallow respirations, urine retention, toxic psychosis, stupor, and coma.

Treatment of overdose involves administering activated charcoal to reduce drug absorption and I.V. naloxone to support respiration. Other symptoms are treated supportively.

NURSING CONSIDERATIONS
● Urge cautious use in atopic children, sedated or debilitated patients, and patients confined to the supine position. Also urge caution if patient is sensitive to aspirin or tartrazine dyes.
● Dextromethorphan shouldn't be used when cough is a valuable diagnostic sign or is beneficial (as after thoracic surgery).
● Dextromethorphan 15 to 30 mg is equivalent to 8 to 15 mg codeine as an antitussive.
● Drug produces no analgesia or addiction and little or no CNS depression.
● Use drug with chest percussion and vibration.
● Monitor cough type and frequency.

PATIENT TEACHING
● Instruct patient to take exactly as prescribed.
● Tell patient to report adverse reactions.
● Tell patient not to use drug for cough caused by emphysema, asthma, or smoking.
● *Alert:* Make sure patient understands that persistent cough may indicate a serious condition and that he should contact a doctor if cough lasts longer than 1 week, recurs frequently, or is accompanied by high fever, rash, or severe headache.

Reactions may be *common*, uncommon, *life-threatening*, or COMMON AND LIFE-THREATENING.

diphenhydramine hydrochloride

Allerdryl†, AllerMax Caplets, Allermed, Banophen, Banophen Caplets, Beldin, Belix, Benadryl, Benadryl 25, Benadryl Kapseals, Benylin Cough, Bydramine Cough, Diphenadryl, Diphen Cough, Diphenhist, Diphenhist Captabs, Dormarex 2, Genahist, Gen-D-phen, Hydramine, Hydramine Cough, Hydramyn, Nidryl, Nordryl, Nordryl Cough, Tusstat, Uni-Bent Cough

Pregnancy Risk Category B

HOW SUPPLIED
Tablets: 25 mg, 50 mg
Capsules: 25 mg, 50 mg
Elixir: 12.5 mg/5 ml (14% alcohol)*
Syrup: 12.5 mg/5 ml*

ACTION
Competes with histamine for H_1-receptor sites on effector cells. Prevents, but doesn't reverse, histamine-mediated responses, particularly histamine's effects on the smooth muscle of the bronchial tubes, GI tract, uterus, and blood vessels. Structurally related to local anesthetics, diphenhydramine provides local anesthesia by preventing initiation and transmission of nerve impulses. Also suppresses cough reflex by a direct effect in the medulla of the brain.

Route	Onset	Peak	Duration
P.O.	15 min	1-4 hr	6-8 hr

INDICATIONS & DOSAGES
Rhinitis, allergy symptoms, motion sickness—
Adults and children ages 12 and older: 25 to 50 mg P.O. q 4 to 6 hours, not to exceed 300 mg daily.
Children ages 6 to 11: 12.5 to 25 mg P.O. q 4 to 6 hours. Maximum dose is 150 mg daily.

Rhinitis, allergy symptoms—
Children ages 2 to 5: 6.25 mg q 4 to 6 hours. Maximum dose is 37.5 mg daily, as directed by a doctor.

Nonproductive cough—
Adults and children ages 12 and older: 25 mg P.O. q 4 hours. Maximum dose is 150 mg daily.
Children ages 6 to 11: 12.5 mg P.O. q 4 hours. Maximum dose is 75 mg daily.
Children ages 2 to 5: 6.25 mg P.O. q 4 hours. Maximum dose is 37.5 mg daily, as directed by a doctor.

ADVERSE REACTIONS

CNS: drowsiness, confusion, insomnia, headache, vertigo, sedation, sleepiness, dizziness, incoordination, fatigue, restlessness, tremor, nervousness, *seizures.*

CV: palpitations, hypotension, tachycardia.

EENT: diplopia, blurred vision, nasal congestion, tinnitus.

GI: nausea, vomiting, diarrhea, dry mouth, constipation, epigastric distress, anorexia.

GU: dysuria, urine retention, urinary frequency.

Hematologic: hemolytic anemia, *thrombocytopenia, agranulocytosis.*

Respiratory: thickening of bronchial secretions.

Skin: urticaria, photosensitivity, rash.

Other: *anaphylactic shock.*

INTERACTIONS

Drug-drug

CNS depressants: increases sedation. Advise patient to use together cautiously.

MAO inhibitors: increases anticholinergic effects. Advise patient to avoid using together.

Metoprolol: inhibits metabolism and enhances effects of beta blocker. Advise patient to avoid using together.

Drug-lifestyle

Alcohol use: increases CNS depression. Advise patient to avoid using together.

Sun exposure: photosensitivity reactions may occur. Tell patient to use sunblock and avoid prolonged sun exposure.

CONTRAINDICATIONS

Contraindicated in patients who are hypersensitive to drug and in those with angle-closure glaucoma, stenosing peptic ulcer, symptomatic prostatic hyperplasia, bladder neck obstruction, or pyloroduodenal obstruction; also contraindicated during acute asthmatic attacks and in newborns, premature neonates, and breast-feeding women. Patients taking MAO inhibitors shouldn't take this drug.

OVERDOSE & TREATMENT

Drowsiness is the usual symptom of overdose. Seizures, coma, and respiratory depression may occur with a profound overdose. Anticholinergic symptoms, such as dry mouth, flushed skin, fixed and dilated pupils, and GI symptoms, are common, especially in children.

Treat overdose by inducing emesis with ipecac syrup (in conscious patient), followed by activated charcoal to reduce further drug absorption. Use gastric lavage if patient is un-

---

Reactions may be *common*, uncommon, *life-threatening*, or COMMON AND LIFE-THREATENING.

conscious or if ipecac fails. Treat hypotension with vasopressors, and control seizures with diazepam or phenytoin. Don't give stimulants.

NURSING CONSIDERATIONS
• Urge extreme caution in patients with prostatic hyperplasia, asthma, or COPD, increased intraocular pressure, hyperthyroidism, CV disease, and hypertension.
• Children younger than age 6 should use only as directed by a doctor.
• Younger children may be stimulated rather than sedated by diphenhydramine.
• Antihistamines can prevent, reduce, or mask positive diagnostic skin test response. Advise patient to discontinue drug 4 days before test.
• *Alert:* Don't confuse diphenhydramine with dimenhydrinate, or Benadryl with Bentyl, Benylin, or benazepril.

PATIENT TEACHING
• Instruct patient to take drug 30 minutes before travel to prevent motion sickness.
• Tell patient to take diphenhydramine with food or milk to reduce GI distress.
• Warn patient to avoid alcohol and driving or other hazardous activities that require alertness until drug's CNS effects are known.
• Tell patient that coffee or tea may reduce drowsiness but that he should use cautiously if palpitations develop.
• Inform patient that sugarless gum, sugarless sour hard candy, or ice chips may relieve dry mouth.
• Tell patient to notify doctor if tolerance develops because a different antihistamine may need to be prescribed.
• Diphenhydramine is contained in many OTC sleep and cold products. Advise patient to consult doctor before using these products.
• Warn patient of possible photosensitivity reactions. Advise use of a sunblock.

---

ephedrine sulfate

Pregnancy Risk Category C

HOW SUPPLIED
Capsules: 25 mg

ACTION
Stimulates alpha and beta receptors and is a direct- and indirect-acting sympathomimetic. Relaxes bronchial smooth muscle by $beta_2$-receptor stimulation.

Route	Onset	Peak	Duration
P.O.	15-60 min	Unknown	3-5 hr

INDICATIONS & DOSAGES
Bronchodilation—
Adults and children ages 12 and older: 12.5 to 25 mg P.O. q 4 hours, not to exceed 150 mg in 24 hours.
Children ages 6 to 11: 6.25 to 12.5 mg P.O. q 4 hours, not to exceed 75 mg in 24 hours.
Children ages 2 to 5: 2 to 3 mg/kg or 100 mg/m^2 P.O. daily in four to six divided doses.

ADVERSE REACTIONS
CNS: insomnia, nervousness, dizziness, headache, muscle weakness, euphoria, confusion, delirium, tremor, *cerebral hemorrhage.*
CV: palpitations, tachycardia, hypertension, precordial pain, *arrhythmias.*
EENT: dry nose and throat.
GI: nausea, vomiting, anorexia.
GU: urine retention, painful urination from visceral sphincter spasm.
Skin: diaphoresis.

INTERACTIONS
Drug-drug
Acetazolamide: increases serum ephedrine levels. Monitor patient for toxicity.
Alpha blockers: unopposed beta-adrenergic effects, resulting in hypotension. Advise patient to avoid using together.
Antihypertensives: decreases effects. Tell patient to monitor blood pressure.
Beta blockers: unopposed alpha-adrenergic effects, resulting in hypertension. Tell patient to monitor blood pressure.
Cardiac glycosides, general anesthetics (halogenated hydrocarbons): increases risk of ventricular arrhythmias. Monitor electrocardiogram (ECG) closely.
Ergot alkaloids: decreases vasoconstrictor activity. Monitor patient closely.
Guanadrel, guanethidine: decreases pressor effects of ephedrine. Monitor patient closely.
Levodopa: enhances risk of ventricular arrhythmias. Monitor ECG closely.
MAO inhibitors, tricyclic antidepressants: when given with sympathomimetics, may cause hypertensive crisis. Tell patient to monitor blood pressure closely.
Methyldopa, reserpine: may inhibit ephedrine effects. Monitor patient carefully.

CONTRAINDICATIONS
Contraindicated in patients who are hypersensitive to ephedrine and other sympathomimetics and in those with porphyria, severe coronary artery disease,

arrhythmias, angle-closure glaucoma, psychoneurosis, angina pectoris, substantial organic heart disease, or CV disease; also contraindicated in those receiving MAO inhibitors or general anesthesia with cyclopropane or halothane.

OVERDOSE & TREATMENT

Signs and symptoms of overdose include exaggeration of common adverse reactions, especially arrhythmias, extreme tremor or seizures, nausea and vomiting, fever, and CNS and respiratory depression.

Treatment requires supportive and symptomatic measures. If patient is conscious, induce emesis with ipecac and follow with activated charcoal. If patient is depressed or hyperactive, perform gastric lavage. Maintain airway and blood pressure. Don't administer vasopressors. Monitor vital signs closely.

A beta blocker (such as propranolol) may be used to treat arrhythmias. A cardioselective beta blocker is recommended in asthmatic patients. Phentolamine may be used for hypertension, paraldehyde or diazepam for seizures, and dexamethasone for pyrexia.

NURSING CONSIDERATIONS

• Urge extreme caution in elderly patients and in those with hypertension, hyperthyroidism, nervous or excitable states, diabetes, or prostatic hyperplasia.
• Ephedrine should be used in children younger than age 12 only under the direction of a doctor.
• *Alert:* Hypoxia, hypercapnia, and acidosis, which may reduce effectiveness or increase adverse reactions, must be identified and corrected before or during ephedrine therapy.
• To prevent insomnia, tell patient to avoid taking within 2 hours of bedtime.
• Ephedrine may be misused for its stimulant properties; its distribution is regulated by law.
• People with eating disorders may misuse drug for its anorexiant effects.
• *Alert:* Don't confuse ephedrine with epinephrine.

PATIENT TEACHING

• Tell patient taking oral form of drug at home to take last dose of day at least 2 hours before bedtime.
• Warn patient not to take OTC drugs or herbs that contain ephedrine (such as ma huang) without informing doctor.
• Warn patient about the adverse effects caused by misuse and abuse of ephedrine.

---

*Liquid contains alcohol.   **May contain tartrazine.   †Canada   ‡Australia   §U.K.

epinephrine (adrenaline)
Bronkaid Mist, Bronkaid Mistometer†, Primatene Mist

epinephrine bitartrate
AsthmaHaler Mist, Bronitin Mist, Bronkaid Mist, Primatene Mist Suspension

epinephrine hydrochloride
AsthmaNefrin, MicroNefrin, Nephron

Pregnancy Risk Category C

HOW SUPPLIED
Aerosol inhaler: 160 mcg, 200 mcg, 220 mcg, 250 mcg/metered spray
Nebulizer inhaler: 1% (1:100)†, 1.25%†, 2.25%†

ACTION
Stimulates alpha and beta receptors in the sympathetic nervous system. Relaxes bronchial smooth muscle by beta$_2$-receptor stimulation.

Route	Onset	Peak	Duration
Inhalation	1-5 min	Unknown	1-3 hr

INDICATIONS & DOSAGES
Acute asthma attacks—
Adults and children ages 4 and older: 160 to 250 mcg (metered aerosol), which is equivalent to 1 inhalation, repeated once if needed after at least 1 minute; subsequent doses shouldn't be administered for at least 3 hours. Or, 1% (1:100) solution of epinephrine or 2.25% solution of racepinephrine administered with a hand-bulb nebulizer as 1 to 3 deep inhalations, repeated q 3 hours, p.r.n.

ADVERSE REACTIONS
CNS: nervousness, tremor, vertigo, pain, headache, disorientation, agitation, drowsiness, fear, pallor, dizziness, weakness, *cerebral hemorrhage, CVA.*
CV: palpitations, widened pulse pressure, hypertension, tachycardia, *ventricular fibrillation, shock,* anginal pain, ECG changes (including a decreased T-wave amplitude).
GI: nausea, vomiting.
GU: increased BUN level.
Metabolic: increased serum glucose and serum lactic acid levels.
Respiratory: dyspnea.
Skin: urticaria.

INTERACTIONS
Drug-drug
Alpha blockers: hypotension caused by unopposed beta-adrenergic effects. Advise patient to avoid using together.
Antihistamines, thyroid hormones, tricyclic antidepressants: when given with sympathomimetics, may cause severe

---

Reactions may be *common*, uncommon, *life-threatening*, or COMMON AND LIFE-THREATENING.

adverse cardiac effects. Tell patient to avoid using together.
Beta blockers, such as propranolol: may cause vasoconstriction and reflex bradycardia. Monitor patient carefully.
Cardiac glycosides, general anesthetics (halogenated hydrocarbons): increases risk of ventricular arrhythmias. Monitor ECG closely.
Doxapram, mazindol, methylphenidate: enhances CNS stimulation or pressor effects. Monitor patient closely.
Ergot alkaloids: decreases vasoconstrictor activity. Monitor patient closely.
Guanadrel, guanethidine: enhances pressor effects of epinephrine. Monitor patient closely.
Levodopa: enhances risk of arrhythmias. Monitor ECG closely.
MAO inhibitors: increases risk of hypertensive crisis. Tell patient to monitor blood pressure closely.

CONTRAINDICATIONS
Contraindicated in patients with angle-closure glaucoma, shock (other than anaphylactic shock), organic brain damage, cardiac dilation, arrhythmias, coronary insufficiency, or cerebral arteriosclerosis. Also contraindicated in patients receiving general anesthesia with halogenated hydrocarbons or cyclopropane and

in patients in labor (may delay second stage).
Some commercial products contain sulfites and are contraindicated in patients with sulfite allergies except when epinephrine is being used for treatment of serious allergic reactions or other emergency situations.

OVERDOSE & TREATMENT
Signs and symptoms of overdose may include a sharp increase in systolic and diastolic blood pressure, a rise in venous pressure, severe anxiety, an irregular heartbeat, severe nausea or vomiting, unusual paleness and cold skin, pulmonary edema, renal failure, and metabolic acidosis.
Treatment includes symptomatic and supportive measures, because epinephrine is rapidly inactivated in the body. Monitor vital signs closely. Trimethaphan or phentolamine may be needed for hypotension; beta blockers (such as propranolol) for arrhythmias.

NURSING CONSIDERATIONS
• Urge extreme caution in patients with long-standing bronchial asthma and emphysema who have developed degenerative heart disease. Also urge caution in elderly patients and in those with hyperthyroidism, CV disease, hypertension, psychoneurosis, and diabetes.

- Drug increases rigidity and tremor in patients with Parkinson's disease.
- Tell patient to notify doctor if adverse reactions develop; dosage adjustment or drug discontinuance may be warranted.
- Epinephrine is rapidly destroyed by oxidizing agents, such as iodine, chromates, nitrites, oxygen, and salts of easily reducible metals (such as iron).
- Epinephrine therapy interferes with tests for urinary catecholamines.
- *Alert:* Don't confuse epinephrine with ephedrine.

PATIENT TEACHING
- Teach patient to perform oral inhalation correctly. Give the following instructions for using a metered-dose inhaler:
– Shake the canister.
– Clear your nasal passages and throat.
– Breathe out, expelling as much air from your lungs as possible.
– Place the mouthpiece well into your mouth and inhale deeply as you release a dose from inhaler.
– Hold your breath for several seconds, remove mouthpiece, and exhale slowly. Or, the inhaler may be held about 1 inch (two finger-widths) from the patient's open mouth; the patient inhales while a dose is released.
- If more than 1 inhalation is ordered, advise patient to wait at least 2 minutes before repeating procedure.
- Tell patient that use with a metered-dose inhaler may improve drug delivery to the lungs.
- If patient is also using a corticosteroid inhaler, instruct him to use the bronchodilator first and then wait about 5 minutes before using the corticosteroid. This allows the bronchodilator to open the air passages for maximum effectiveness.
- Instruct patient to wash inhaler with warm, soapy water at least once weekly and to remove the canister before washing.
- Advise patient to seek medical assistance immediately if he receives no relief within 20 minutes or if condition worsens.

guaifenesin (glyceryl guaiacolate)
Anti-Tuss* Balminil Expectorant†, Breonesin, Gee-Gee, GG-Cen*, Glyate*, Glycotuss, Glytuss, Guiatuss*, Hytuss, Hytuss-2X, Naldecon Senior EX, Resyl†, Robitussin*, Scot-Tussin Expectorant, Uni-tussin*

Pregnancy Risk Category C

HOW SUPPLIED
Tablets: 100 mg, 200 mg
Capsules: 200 mg
Solution: 100 mg/5 ml*,
200 mg/5 ml

ACTION
Increases production of respiratory tract fluids to help liquefy and reduce the viscosity of tenacious secretions.

Route	Onset	Peak	Duration
P.O.	Unknown	Unknown	Unknown

INDICATIONS & DOSAGES
Expectorant—
Adults and children ages 12 and older: 200 to 400 mg P.O. q 4 hours. Maximum dose is 2,400 mg daily.
Children ages 6 to 11: 100 to 200 mg P.O. q 4 hours. Maximum dose is 1,200 mg daily.
Children ages 2 to 5: 50 to 100 mg P.O. q 4 hours. Maximum dose is 600 mg daily.

ADVERSE REACTIONS
CNS: dizziness, headache.
GI: vomiting, nausea.
Skin: rash.

INTERACTIONS
None reported.

CONTRAINDICATIONS
Contraindicated in patients who are hypersensitive to drug.

OVERDOSE & TREATMENT
None reported.

NURSING CONSIDERATIONS
• Drug is used to liquefy thick, tenacious sputum. There is evidence that guaifenesin is effective as an expectorant but no evidence to support its role as an antitussive.
• Monitor cough type and frequency.
• Drug may cause color interference with tests for 5-hydroxyindoleacetic acid and vanillylmandelic acid.
• *Alert:* Don't confuse guaifenesin with guanfacine.

PATIENT TEACHING
• *Alert:* Make sure patient understands that persistent cough may indicate a serious condition and that he should contact a doctor if cough lasts longer than 1 week, recurs frequently, or is accompanied by high fever, rash, or severe headache.
• Inform patient that drug shouldn't be used for chronic or persistent cough, such as that caused by smoking, asthma, chronic bronchitis, or emphysema.
• Advise patient to take each dose with 8 ounces of water; increasing fluid intake may prove beneficial.
• Encourage deep-breathing exercises.

---

*Liquid contains alcohol.   **May contain tartrazine.   †Canada   ‡Australia   §U.K.

triprolidine hydrochloride
Actidil

Pregnancy Risk Category C

HOW SUPPLIED
Tablets: 2.5 mg
Syrup: 1.25 mg/5 ml*

ACTION
Competes with histamine for H_1-receptor sites on effector cells and prevents, but doesn't reverse, histamine-mediated responses.

Route	Onset	Peak	Duration
P.O.	15-60 min	2-3 hr	4-8 hr

INDICATIONS & DOSAGES
Colds and seasonal allergy symptoms, chronic urticaria—
Adults and children ages 12 and older: 2.5 mg P.O. q 4 to 6 hours. Maximum daily dose is 10 mg.
Children ages 6 to 11: 1.25 mg P.O. q 4 to 6 hours. Maximum daily dose is 5 mg.
Children ages 4 to 5: 0.938 mg P.O. q 4 to 6 hours. Maximum daily dose is 3.744 mg.
Children ages 2 to 3: 0.625 mg P.O. q 4 to 6 hours. Maximum daily dose is 2.5 mg.
Children ages 4 months to 2 years: 0.313 mg P.O. q 4 to 6 hours. Maximum daily dose is 1.252 mg.

ADVERSE REACTIONS
CNS: drowsiness, dizziness, confusion, restlessness, insomnia, headache, sedation, sleepiness, incoordination, fatigue, anxiety, nervousness, tremor, *seizures,* stimulation.
CV: hypotension, palpitations, tachycardia.
EENT: dry nose and throat.
GI: anorexia, diarrhea, constipation, nausea, vomiting, dry mouth, epigastric distress.
GU: urinary frequency, urine retention.
Hematologic: hemolytic anemia, *thrombocytopenia, agranulocytosis.*
Respiratory: thickening of bronchial secretions.
Skin: urticaria, rash, photosensitivity, diaphoresis.
Other: *anaphylactic shock,* chills.

INTERACTIONS
Drug-drug
CNS depressants: increases sedation. Advise patient to use together cautiously.
MAO inhibitors: increases anticholinergic effects. Advise patient to avoid using together.

Drug-lifestyle
Alcohol use: increases CNS depression. Advise patient to avoid using together.
Sun exposure: may cause photosensitivity reactions. Tell pa-

Reactions may be *common,* uncommon, *life-threatening,* or COMMON AND LIFE-THREATENING.

tient to use sunblock and avoid prolonged sun exposure.

CONTRAINDICATIONS

Contraindicated in patients who are hypersensitive to drug and in those with acute asthma, angle-closure glaucoma, stenosing peptic ulcer, symptomatic prostatic hyperplasia, bladder neck obstruction, or pyloroduodenal obstruction; also contraindicated in neonates, premature infants, and breast-feeding women. Contraindicated in patients taking MAO inhibitors.

OVERDOSE & TREATMENT

Signs and symptoms of overdose may include CNS depression (sedation, reduced mental alertness, apnea, and CV collapse) or CNS stimulation (insomnia, hallucinations, tremors, or seizures). Anticholinergic effects, such as dry mouth, flushed skin, fixed and dilated pupils, and GI symptoms are common, especially in children.

Treat overdose by inducing emesis with ipecac syrup (in conscious patient), followed by activated charcoal to reduce further drug absorption. Use gastric lavage if patient is unconscious or if ipecac fails. Treat hypotension with vasopressors, and control seizures with diazepam or phenytoin. Don't give stimulants.

NURSING CONSIDERATIONS

• Urge extreme caution in patient with increased intraocular pressure, hyperthyroidism, CV disease, hypertension, bronchial asthma, and prostatic hyperplasia.
• Children younger than age 6 should use only as directed by a doctor.
• Antihistamines can prevent, reduce, or mask positive diagnostic skin test response. Advise patient to discontinue drug 4 days before test.

PATIENT TEACHING

• Tell patient to take with food or milk to reduce GI distress.
• Warn patient to avoid alcohol and tasks that require alertness until CNS effects are known.
• Tell the patient that coffee or tea may reduce drowsiness.
• Inform the patient that sugarless gum, sugarless sour hard candy, or ice chips may relieve dry mouth.
• Warn the patient of possible photosensitivity reactions. Advise use of a sunblock.

Combination products

Brand name and active ingredients	Indications and dosages	Nursing considerations
Actifed Cold & Sinus • acetaminophen 500 mg • chlorpheniramine 2 mg • pseudoephedrine 30 mg	*Relief from congestion caused by cold or sinusitis; sinus congestion and pressure; minor aches and pains, headache, fever caused by cold; runny nose, sneezing, itching of nose and throat, itchy, watery eyes caused by hay fever* **Adults and children ages 12 and older:** 2 caplets P.O. q 6 hr. Maximum 8 caplets q 24 hr.	• Tell patient not to take drug within 2 weeks of an MAO inhibitor. • Advise patient to notify doctor if he becomes nervous, dizzy, or sleepless; if symptoms persist after 3 days; or if he has a fever. • Tell patient not to take drug for longer than 10 days. • Warn patient not to take drug if he has heart disease, hypertension, thyroid disease, diabetes, emphysema, chronic bronchitis, glaucoma, or difficulty urinating caused by an enlarged prostate, unless directed by a doctor. • Drug may cause excitability in children. • Warn patient to use caution while driving or operating heavy machinery because drug may cause drowsiness. • Tell patient to avoid alcohol while taking drug. If patient consumes more than three alcoholic beverages daily, tell him to consult a doctor before taking drug. • Urge patient not to take drug with sedatives or tranquilizers unless directed by a doctor.
Allerest • chlorpheniramine 2 mg • pseudoephedrine 30 mg	*Relief from runny nose, sneezing, itchy nose and throat; itchy, watery eyes caused by hay fever or allergies;*	• Tell patient not to take drug within 2 weeks of an MAO inhibitor. • Urge patient to notify doctor if symptoms persist after 7 days or if he has a fever.

Combination products *(continued)*

Brand name and active ingredients	Indications and dosages	Nursing considerations
Allerest *(continued)*	*nasal and sinus congestion* **Adults and children ages 12 and older:** 2 tablets P.O. q 4 to 6 hr. Maximum 8 tablets q 24 hr. **Children ages 6 to 11:** 1 tablet P.O. q 4 to 6 hr. Maximum 4 tablets q 24 hr.	• Tell patient not to take drug if he has heart disease, hypertension, thyroid disease, diabetes, emphysema, chronic bronchitis, glau-coma, or difficulty urinating caused by an enlarged prostate, unless directed by a doctor. • Drug may cause excitability in children. • Tell patient that drug may cause drowsiness and that he should use caution when driving or operating heavy machinery. • Tell patient to avoid alcohol while taking drug. • Warn patient not to take drug with sedatives or tranquilizers unless directed by a doctor.
Benadryl Allergy Congestion • diphenhydramine 25 mg • pseudoephedrine 60 mg	*Relief from runny nose, sneezing, itchy nose and throat, itchy, watery eyes caused by allergies; runny nose, sneezing, congestion caused by cold* **Adults and children ages 12 and older:** 1 tablet P.O. q 4 to 6 hr p.r.n. Maximum 4 tablets q 24 hr.	• Tell patient not to take drug within 2 weeks of an MAO inhibitor. • Tell patient not to exceed recommended dosage. • Advise patient not to take drug if he has emphysema, bronchitis, heart disease, hypertension, thyroid disease, diabetes, breathing problems, chronic cough, cough caused by smoking, or difficulty urinating caused by enlarged prostate, unless directed by a doctor. • Tell patient to notify doctor if he becomes nervous, dizzy, or sleepless.

(continued)

Combination products *(continued)*

Brand name and active ingredients	Indications and dosages	Nursing considerations
Benadryl Allergy Congestion *(continued)*		• Inform patient that drug may cause drowsiness and that he shouldn't take it when driving or drinking alcoholic beverages. • Urge patient not to take drug with sedatives or tranquilizers unless directed by a doctor. • Tell patient that drug may cause excitability in children.
Benadryl Allergy/Sinus Headache • acetaminophen 500 mg • diphenhydramine 12.5 mg • pseudoephedrine 30 mg **Benadryl Severe Allergy/Sinus Headache** • acetaminophen 500 mg • diphenhydramine 25 mg • pseudoephedrine 30 mg	*Relief from headache, rhinorrhea, aches and pains, itchy nose and throat, itchy watery eyes caused by allergies; congestion caused by cold* **Adults and children ages 12 and older:** 2 caplets P.O. q 6 hr p.r.n. Maximum 8 caplets q 24 hr.	• Tell patient not to take drug within 2 weeks of an MAO inhibitor. • Advise patient not to exceed recommended dosage. • Urge patient not to take drug if he has emphysema, bronchitis, heart disease, hypertension, thyroid disease, diabetes, breathing problems, chronic cough, cough caused by smoking, or difficulty urinating caused by enlarged prostate, unless directed by a doctor. • Tell patient not to take drug for longer than 10 days. • Advise patient to notify doctor if symptoms aren't improved, new symptoms occur, or symptoms are accompanied by fever after 3 days. • Inform patient that drug may cause drowsiness and that he shouldn't take it when driving or drinking alcoholic beverages. • Urge patient not to take drug with sedatives or tran-

Combination products *(continued)*

Brand name and active ingredients	Indications and dosages	Nursing considerations
Benadryl Allergy/Sinus Headache *(continued)*		quilizers unless directed by a doctor. • Advise patient that drug may cause excitability in children.
Benylin Expectorant Formula • dextromethorphan 5 mg/5 ml • guaifenesin 100 mg/5 ml	*Relief from cough caused by cold; loosening of phlegm and thinning of bronchial secretions* **Adults and children ages 12 and older:** 4 tsp P.O. q 4 hr. Maximum 6 doses q 24 hr. **Children ages 6 to 11:** 2 tsp P.O. q 4 hr. Maximum 6 doses q 24 hr. **Children ages 2 to 5:** 1 tsp P.O. q 4 hr. Maximum 6 doses q 24 hr.	• Tell patient not to take drug within 2 weeks of an MAO inhibitor. • Urge patient to notify doctor if cough lasts longer than 7 days or is accompanied by fever, rash, or headache. • Advise patient not to take drug for cough caused by asthma, smoking, bronchitis or emphysema, or for cough accompanied by excessive phlegm, unless directed by a doctor.
Bronkaid • ephedrine sulfate 25 mg • guaifenesin 400 mg	*Relief from shortness of breath, chest tightness, wheezing, cough caused by asthma; loosening of phlegm and thinning of bronchial secretions* **Adults and children ages 12 and older:** 1 caplet P.O. q 4 hr p.r.n. Maximum 6 caplets q 24 hr.	• Tell patient not to take drug unless a diagnosis of asthma has been made by a doctor. • Warn patient not to take drug if he has been hospitalized for asthma or is taking prescription drugs for asthma, unless directed by a doctor. • Warn patient not to take drug if he has heart disease, hypertension, thyroid disease, diabetes, or difficulty urinating caused by enlarged prostate, unless directed by a doctor.

(continued)

Combination products *(continued)*

Brand name and active ingredients	Indications and dosages	Nursing considerations
Bronkaid *(continued)*		• Tell patient to notify doctor if symptoms are the same or worse after 1 hour. • Inform patient that drug may cause nervousness, tremor, sleeplessness, nausea, and loss of appetite. • Tell patient not to take drug within 2 weeks of an MAO inhibitor. • Urge patient to notify doctor if cough lasts longer than 7 days or is accompanied by fever, rash, or headache. • Advise patient not to take drug for cough caused by asthma, smoking, bronchitis, or emphysema, or for cough accompanied by excessive phlegm, unless directed by a doctor.
Children's Tylenol Allergy-D • acetaminophen 80 mg • diphenhydramine hydrochloride 6.25 mg • pseudoephedrine hydrochloride 7.5 mg	*To reduce fever and relieve hay fever and upper respiratory allergy symptoms including stuffy nose, sneezing, sore throat, nasal congestion, itchy watery eyes, runny nose, and itchy throat* **Children who weigh 48 to 95 lb and are over age 6:** 4 tablets P.O. q 4 to 6 hours. Maximum 4 doses q 24 hr.	• Tell parent not to give drug to child for longer than 5 days for pain or 3 days for fever, unless directed by the doctor. • Urge parent to notify doctor if child's fever or pain persists or worsens or if redness or swelling occurs. • If sore throat lasts longer than 2 days, is severe, and is accompanied by fever, headache, nausea, vomiting, or rash, have patient consult doctor immediately. • Tell parent not to give drug to child who has glaucoma, respiratory problems (such as chronic bronchitis), heart

Combination products *(continued)*

Brand name and active ingredients	Indications and dosages	Nursing considerations
Children's Tylenol Allergy-D *(continued)*		disease, hypertension, thyroid disease, or diabetes without consulting doctor. • Advise parent that drug may cause excessive drowsiness. Caution against giving it to a child who takes a sedative. • Tell parent not to give drug with other medications that contain acetaminophen. • Warn parent not to give drug to child within 2 weeks of an MAO inhibitor. • If patient has phenylketonuria, advise patient or parent that each tablet contains 5 mg of phenylalanine. • Remind parent not to use drug if package shows signs of tampering.
Children's Tylenol Cold • acetaminophen 80 mg • chlorpheniramine maleate 0.5 mg • pseudoephedrine hydrochloride 7.5 mg	*For relief of coughs, nasal congestion, runny nose, sore throat, sneezing, minor aches and pains, headaches, and fever* **Children ages 6 to 11 old who weigh 48 to 95 lb:** 4 tablets P.O. q 4 to 6 hours. Maximum 4 doses q 24 hr.	• Tell parent not to give drug to child for longer than 5 days for pain or longer than 3 days for fever, unless directed by the doctor. • Urge parent to notify doctor if child's fever or pain persists or worsens. • Tell parent to stop giving drug and notify a doctor if drug makes child nervous, dizzy, or unable to fall asleep normally. • Tell parent not to give drug to child who has heart disease, hypertension, thyroid disease, or diabetes, without consulting doctor.

(continued)

Combination products *(continued)*

Brand name and active ingredients	Indications and dosages	Nursing considerations
Children's Tylenol Cold *(continued)*		• Advise parent not to give drug with other products that contain acetaminophen. • Warn parent not to give drug to child within 2 weeks an MAO inhibitor. • If patient has phenylketonuria, inform patient or parent that each tablet contains 5 mg of phenylalanine. • Remind parent not to use drug if package shows signs of tampering.
Children's Tylenol Sinus • acetaminophen 80 mg • pseudoephedrine hydrochloride 7.5 mg	*To reduce fever or temporarily relieve minor aches, pains, headaches, sinus congestion, stuffy nose, and sinus pressure* **Children ages 6 to 11:** 4 tablets P.O. q 4 to 6 hours, p.r.n. Maximum 4 doses q 24 hr. **Children ages 2 to 5:** 2 tablets P.O. q 4 to 6 hours, p.r.n. Maximum 4 doses q 24 hr.	• Tell parent not to give drug for longer than 5 days for pain or 3 days for fever, unless directed by a doctor. • Urge parent to contact doctor if child's fever or pain persists or worsens. • Advise parent to stop giving drug and notify doctor if the medication makes child nervous, dizzy, or sleepless. • Tell parent not to give drug to child who has heart disease, hypertension, thyroid disease, or diabetes without consulting doctor. • Advise patient not to give drug with other products that contain acetaminophen. • Warn parent not to give drug to child within 2 weeks of an MAO inhibitor. • If patient has phenylketonuria, inform patient or parent that each tablet contains 5 mg of phenylalanine.

Combination products *(continued)*

Brand name and active ingredients	Indications and dosages	Nursing considerations
Children's Tylenol Sinus *(continued)*		• Remind parent not to use drug if package shows signs of tampering.
Contac Day & Night Cold & Flu • acetaminophen 650 mg • dextromethorphan 30 mg (day caplets) • diphenhydramine 50 mg (night caplets) • pseudoephedrine 60 mg	*Relief from headache, aches and pains, fever, congestion, cough caused by cold or flu* **Adults and children ages 12 and older:** 1 day or night caplet q 6 hr. Maximum 4 caplets q 24 hr.	• Tell patient not to take drug within 2 weeks of an MAO inhibitor. • Urge patient to notify doctor if cough recurs, lasts longer than 7 days, or is accompanied by fever, rash, headache, nausea, swelling, or vomiting. • Tell patient not to take drug if he has emphysema, bronchitis, heart disease, hypertension, thyroid disease, diabetes, or difficulty urinating caused by enlarged prostate, unless directed by a doctor. • Tell patient not to exceed recommended dosage. • Tell patient to notify a doctor if he becomes nervous, dizzy, or sleepless. • Urge patient not to take drug for cough caused by asthma, smoking, bronchitis, or emphysema, or for cough accompanied by excessive phlegm, unless directed by a doctor. • Tell patient that night caplets may cause drowsiness and that he shouldn't take them when driving or drinking alcoholic beverages. • Tell patient not to take drug with sedatives or tranquilizers unless directed by a doctor.

(continued)

Combination products *(continued)*

Brand name and active ingredients	Indications and dosages	Nursing considerations
Contac Maximum Strength Severe Cold and Flu • acetaminophen 500 mg • chlorpheniramine 2 mg • dextromethorphan 15 mg • pseudoephedrine 30 mg	*Relief from congestion, runny nose, sneezing, itchy watery eyes, cough caused by cold; fever, sore throat, headache, aches and pains caused by cold or flu* **Adults and children ages 12 and older:** 2 caplets P.O. q 6 hr p.r.n. Maximum 8 caplets q 24 hr.	• Tell patient not to take drug within 2 weeks of an MAO inhibitor. • Caution patient not to exceed recommended dosage. • Urge patient to notify a doctor if he becomes nervous, dizzy, or sleepless. • Warn patient not to take drug for longer than 10 days. • Advise patient to notify doctor if symptoms last longer than 3 days; new symptoms occur; sore throat is severe, lasts longer than 2 days, or is accompanied by fever, headache, rash, nausea, or vomiting; or cough lasts longer than 7 days or is accompanied by rash, headache, or fever. • Caution patient not to take drug for cough caused by asthma, bronchitis, or emphysema, or for cough accompanied by excessive phlegm. • Advise patient not to take drug if he has emphysema, bronchitis, heart disease, hypertension, thyroid disease, diabetes, glaucoma, or difficulty urinating caused by enlarged prostate, unless directed by a doctor. • Tell patient that maximum-strength formula may cause drowsiness and that he shouldn't take it when driving or drinking alcoholic beverages.

Combination products *(continued)*

Brand name and active ingredients	Indications and dosages	Nursing considerations
Contac Maximum Strength Severe Cold and Flu *(continued)*		• Tell patient not to take drug with sedatives or tranquilizers unless directed by a doctor.
Contac Non-Drowsy Severe Cold & Flu • acetaminophen 325 mg • dextromethorphan 15 mg • pseudoephedrine 30 mg	*Relief from congestion, cough caused by cold; fever sore throat, headache, aches and pains caused by cold or flu* **Adults and children ages 12 and older:** 2 caplets P.O. q 6 hr p.r.n. Maximum 8 caplets q 24 hr.	• Tell patient not to take drug within 2 weeks of an MAO inhibitor. • Caution patient not to exceed recommended dosage. • Tell patient to notify a doctor if he becomes nervous, dizzy, or sleepless. • Urge patient not to take drug for longer than 10 days. • Advise patient to notify doctor if symptoms last longer than 3 days; if new symptoms occur; if sore throat is severe, lasts longer than 2 days, or is accompanied by fever, headache, rash, nausea, or vomiting; or if cough lasts longer than 7 days or is accompanied by rash, headache, or fever. • Caution patient not to take drug for cough caused by asthma, bronchitis, or emphysema, or for cough accompanied by excessive phlegm. • Advise patient not to take drug if he has emphysema, bronchitis, heart disease, hypertension, thyroid disease, diabetes, glaucoma, or difficulty urinating caused by enlarged prostate, unless directed by a doctor.

(continued)

Combination products *(continued)*

Brand name and active ingredients	Indications and dosages	Nursing considerations
Contac Non-Drowsy Severe Cold & Flu *(continued)*		• Tell patient that maximum-strength formula may cause drowsiness and that he shouldn't take it when driving or drinking alcoholic beverages. • Tell patient not to take drug with sedatives or tranquilizers, unless directed by a doctor.
Contac Severe Cold & Flu • acetaminophen 500 mg • chlorpheniramine 2 mg • dextromethorphan 15 mg • pseudoephedrine 30 mg	*Relief from congestion, runny nose, sneezing, itchy and watery eyes, cough caused by colds; fever, sore throat, headache, aches and pains caused by cold or flu* **Adults and children ages 12 and older:** 2 caplets P.O. q 6 hr. Maximum 8 caplets q 24 hr.	• Tell patient not to take within 2 weeks of an MAO inhibitor. • Advise patient to notify doctor if he becomes nervous, dizzy, or sleepless, if symptoms persist after 3 days, or if he has a fever. • Urge patient not to take drug for longer than 10 days. • Warn patient not to take drug if he has heart disease, hypertension, thyroid disease, diabetes, emphysema, chronic bronchitis, glaucoma, or difficulty urinating caused by an enlarged prostate, unless directed by a doctor. • Warn patient not to take drug for chronic cough. Tell him to notify a doctor if cough lasts longer than 7 days or is accompanied by rash, fever, headache, nausea, or vomiting. • Drug may cause excitability in children. • Tell patient that drug may cause drowsiness and that he shouldn't take it when driving or drinking alcoholic

Combination products *(continued)*

Brand name and active ingredients	Indications and dosages	Nursing considerations
Contac Severe Cold & Flu *(continued)*		beverages. If patient consumes more than three alcoholic beverages daily, tell him to consult a doctor before taking drug. • Tell patient not to take drug with sedatives or tranquilizers, unless directed by a doctor.
Coricidin D • acetaminophen 325 mg • chlorpheniramine 2 mg • pseudoephedrine 30 mg	*Relief from runny nose, sneezing, congestion, aches and pains, headache, sinus congestion and pressure, fever caused by cold and flu* **Adults and children ages 12 and older:** 2 tablets P.O. q 4 to 6 hr. Maximum 8 tablets q 24 hr. **Children ages 6 to 11:** 1 tablet P.O. q 4 hr. Maximum 4 tablets q 24 hr.	• Tell patient not to take drug within 2 weeks of an MAO inhibitor. • Urge patient to notify a doctor if he becomes nervous, dizzy, or sleepless; if symptoms are unimproved in 7 days (5 days for children); if new symptoms or redness or swelling occur; or if symptoms are accompanied by fever for longer than 3 days. • Tell patient not to take drug for longer than 10 days or if he has heart disease, hypertension, thyroid disease, diabetes, emphysema, chronic bronchitis, glaucoma, or difficulty urinating caused by enlarged prostate, unless directed by a doctor. • Drug may cause excitability in children. • Tell patient that drug may cause drowsiness and that he shouldn't take it when driving or drinking alcoholic beverages. If patient consumes more than three alcoholic beverages daily, tell him

(continued)

Combination products *(continued)*

Brand name and active ingredients	Indications and dosages	Nursing considerations
Coricidin D *(continued)*		to consult a doctor before taking drug. • Tell patient not to take drug with sedatives or tranquilizers unless directed by a doctor.
Dimetapp • dextromethorphan 10 mg • guaifenesin 200 mg	*Relief from congestion, cough caused by cold; loosening of phlegm and thinning of secretions; congestion caused by allergies or sinusitis* **Adults and children ages 12 and older:** 2 caplets P.O. q 4 hr p.r.n. Maximum 4 doses q 24 hr. **Children ages 6 to 11:** 1 caplet P.O. q 4 hr p.r.n. Maximum 4 doses q 24 hr.	• Tell patient not to take drug within 2 weeks of an MAO inhibitor. • Urge patient not to take drug if he has heart disease, hypertension, thyroid disease, diabetes, difficulty urinating caused by enlarged prostate, cough that produces excessive phlegm, or a chronic cough related to smoking, asthma, bronchitis, or emphysema. • Tell patient to notify doctor if he becomes nervous, dizzy, or sleepless. • Urge patient to consult a doctor if cough lasts longer than 7 days or is accompanied by fever, rash, or headache.
Dimetapp— Children's Cold & Cough • brompheniramine 1 mg • dextromethorphan 5 mg • pseudoephedrine 15 mg	*Relief from cough caused by cold; congestion caused by cold, allergies, or sinusitis; runny nose, sneezing, itchy watery eyes, itchy nose and throat caused by allergies* **Adults and children ages 12 and older:** 4 tsp P.O. q 4 hr	• Tell patient not to take drug within 2 weeks of an MAO inhibitor. • Tell patient not to take drug if he has heart disease, hypertension, thyroid disease, diabetes, difficulty urinating caused by enlarged prostate, cough that produces excessive phlegm, or a chronic cough related to smoking, asthma, bronchitis, or emphysema.

Combination products *(continued)*

Brand name and active ingredients	Indications and dosages	Nursing considerations
Dimetapp— Children's Cold & Cough *(continued)*	p.r.n. Maximum 4 doses q 24 hr. **Children ages 6 to 11:** 2 tsp P.O. q 4 hr p.r.n. Maximum 4 doses q 24 hr.	• Urge patient to notify doctor if he becomes nervous, dizzy, or sleepless. • Tell patient to consult a doctor if cough lasts longer than 7 days or is accompanied by fever, rash, or headache. • Drug may cause excitability in children. • Tell patient that drug may cause drowsiness and that he shouldn't take it when driving or drinking alcoholic beverages. • Tell patient not to take drug with sedatives or tranquilizers, unless directed by a doctor.
Dimetapp— Children's Daytime Non-Drowsy Flu • acetaminophen 160 mg • dextromethorphan 5 mg • pseudoephedrine 15 mg	*Relief from headache, sore throat, fever, aches and pains caused by cold or flu; congestion caused by cold* **Adults and children ages 12 and older:** 4 tsp P.O. q 4 hr p.r.n. Maximum 4 doses q 24 hr. **Children ages 6 to 11:** 2 tsp P.O. q 4 hr p.r.n. Maximum 4 doses q 24 hr. **Children ages 2 to 5:** 1 tsp P.O. q 4 hr p.r.n. Maximum 4 doses q 24 hr.	• Encourage patient to notify doctor if sore throat persists or is accompanied by fever, headache, nausea, or vomiting. • Tell patient not to take drug within 2 weeks of an MAO inhibitor. • Advise patient not to take drug if he has heart disease, hypertension, thyroid disease, diabetes, difficulty urinating caused by enlarged prostate, cough that produces excessive phlegm, or a chronic cough related to smoking, asthma, bronchitis, or emphysema. • Tell patient to notify doctor if he becomes nervous, dizzy, or sleepless; if he has new or worsening symptoms; if fever

(continued)

Combination products *(continued)*

Brand name and active ingredients	Indications and dosages	Nursing considerations
Dimetapp— Children's Daytime Non- Drowsy Flu *(continued)*		lasts longer than 3 days; if he has redness or swelling; or if cough lasts longer than 7 days or is accompanied by fever, rash, or headache. • Tell patient that nighttime formula may cause drowsiness and that he shouldn't take it when driving or drinking alcoholic beverages. If patient consumes more than three alcoholic beverages daily, tell him to consult doctor before taking drug. • Tell patient not to take drug with sedatives or tranquilizers, unless directed by a doctor. • Nighttime formula may cause excitability in children.
Dimetapp— Children's Night- time Flu • acetaminophen 160 mg • brompheniramine 1 mg • dextromethorphan 5 mg • pseudoephedrine 15 mg	*Relief from headache, sore throat, fever, aches and pains, congestion caused by cold or flu; sneezing, itchy eyes and throat, runny nose caused by allergies* **Adults and children ages 12 and older:** 4 tsp P.O. q 4 hr p.r.n. Maximum 4 doses q 24 hr. **Children ages 6 to 11:** 2 tsp P.O. q 4 hr p.r.n. Maximum 4 doses q 24 hr.	• Urge patient to notify doctor if sore throat persists or is accompanied by fever, headache, nausea, or vomiting. • Tell patient not to take drug within 2 weeks of an MAO inhibitor. • Advise patient not to take drug if he has heart disease, hypertension, thyroid disease, diabetes, difficulty urinating caused by enlarged prostate, cough that produces excessive phlegm, or a chronic cough related to smoking, asthma, bronchitis, or emphysema. • Tell patient to notify doctor if he becomes nervous, dizzy, or sleepless; if he has new or

Combination products *(continued)*

Brand name and active ingredients	Indications and dosages	Nursing considerations
Dimetapp— Children's Night- time Flu *(continued)*		worsening symptoms; if fever lasts longer than 3 days; if he has redness or swelling; or if cough lasts longer than 7 days or is accompanied by fever, rash, or headache. • Tell patient that nighttime formula may cause drowsiness and that he shouldn't take it when driving or drinking alcoholic beverages. If patient consumes more than three alcoholic beverages daily, tell him to consult a doctor before taking drug. • Tell patient not to take drug with sedatives or tranquilizers unless directed by a doctor. • Nighttime formula may cause excitability in children.
Primatene Mist • ephedrine hydrochloride 12.5 mg • guaifenesin 200 mg	*Relief from short- ness of breath, chest tightness, wheezing caused by asthma; loosening of phlegm and thin- ning of bronchial secretions* **Adults and children ages 12 and older:** 2 tablets P.O. q 4 hr p.r.n. Maximum 12 tablets q 24 hr.	• Tell patient not to take drug unless a diagnosis of asthma has been made by a doctor. • Warn patient not to take drug if he has been hospitalized for asthma or is taking prescription drugs for asthma, unless directed by a doctor. • Warn patient not to take drug if he has heart disease, hypertension, thyroid disease, diabetes, or difficulty urinating caused by enlarged prostate, unless directed by a doctor. • Tell patient to notify doctor if symptoms are the same or worse after 1 hour.

(continued)

Combination products *(continued)*

Brand name and active ingredients	Indications and dosages	Nursing considerations
Primatene Mist *(continued)*		• Inform patient that drug may cause nervousness, tremor, sleeplessness, nausea, and loss of appetite. • Tell patient not to take drug within 2 weeks of an MAO inhibitor. • Urge patient to notify doctor if cough lasts longer than 7 days or is accompanied by fever, rash, or headache. • Advise patient not to take drug for cough caused by asthma, smoking, bronchitis, or emphysema, or for cough accompanied by excessive phlegm, unless directed by a doctor.
Rhinosyn Liquid • chlorpheniramine 4 mg/5 ml • pseudoephedrine 60 mg/5 ml	*Relief from congestion, runny nose, sneezing, itchy nose and throat, itchy watery eyes caused by hay fever or allergies; runny nose, sneezing and congestion caused by cold* **Adults and children ages 12 and older:** 2 tsp P.O. q 4 to 6 hr. Maximum 8 tsp q 24 hr. **Children ages 6 to 11:** 1 tsp P.O. q 4 to 6 hr. Maximum 4 tsp q 24 hr.	• Tell patient not to take drug within 2 weeks of an MAO inhibitor. • Advise patient to notify doctor if symptoms persist after 7 days, if he has a fever, or if he's nervous, dizzy, or sleepless. • Tell patient not to take drug if he has heart disease, hypertension, thyroid disease, diabetes, emphysema, chronic bronchitis, or difficulty urinating caused by enlarged prostate, unless directed by a doctor. • Drug may cause excitability in children. • Tell patient that drug may cause drowsiness and that he shouldn't take it when

Combination products *(continued)*

Brand name and active ingredients	Indications and dosages	Nursing considerations
Rhinosyn Liquid *(continued)*		driving or drinking alcoholic beverages. • Tell patient not to take drug with sedatives or tranquilizers, unless directed by a doctor.
Robitussin CF • dextromethorphan 10 mg/5 ml • guaifenesin 100 mg/5 ml • pseudoephedrine 30 mg/5 ml	*Loosens phlegm and thins bronchial secretions; congestion, cough* **Adults and children ages 12 and older:** 2 tsp P.O. q 4 hr p.r.n. Maximum 4 doses q 24 hr. **Children ages 6 to 11:** 1 tsp P.O. q 4 hr p.r.n. Maximum 4 doses q 24 hr. **Children ages 2 to 5:** ½ tsp P.O. q 4 hr p.r.n. Maximum 4 doses q 24 hr.	• Tell patient not to take drug within 2 weeks of an MAO inhibitor. • Urge patient or parent to notify doctor if cough lasts longer than 7 days or is accompanied by fever, rash, or headache. • Advise patient not to take drug if he has emphysema, bronchitis, heart disease, hypertension, thyroid disease, diabetes, or difficulty urinating caused by enlarged prostate, unless directed by a doctor. • Warn patient not to exceed recommended dosage. • Tell patient to notify doctor if he becomes nervous, dizzy, or sleepless.
Robitussin DM • dextromethorphan 10 mg/5 ml • guaifenesin 100 mg/5 ml	*Relief from cough caused by cold, loosening of phlegm and thinning of secretions* **Adults and children ages 12 and older:** 2 tsp P.O. q 4 hr p.r.n. Maximum 6 doses q 24 hr. **Children ages 6 to 11:** 1 tsp P.O. q 4 hr p.r.n. Maximum 6 doses q 24 hr.	• Tell patient not to take drug within 2 weeks of an MAO inhibitor. • Urge patient or parent to notify doctor if cough lasts longer than 7 days or is accompanied by fever, rash, or headache. • Tell patient not to take drug for chronic cough caused by asthma, smoking, or emphysema, or for cough accompanied by excessive phlegm.

(continued)

Combination products *(continued)*

Brand name and active ingredients	Indications and dosages	Nursing considerations
Robitussin DM *(continued)*	**Children ages 2 to 5:** ½ tsp P.O. q 4 hr p.r.n. Maximum 6 doses q 24 hr.	
Robitussin DM Infant Drops • dextromethorphan 5 mg/2.5 ml • guaifenesin 100 mg/2.5 ml	*Relief from cough caused by cold, loosening of phlegm, and thinning of secretions* **Children ages 2 to 6 (24 to 47 lb):** 2.5 ml P.O. q 4 hr p.r.n. Maximum 6 doses q 24 hr.	• Tell parent not to give drug within 2 weeks of an MAO inhibitor. • Urge parent to notify doctor if child's cough lasts longer than 7 days or is accompanied by fever, rash, or headache. • Advise parent not to give drug for chronic cough caused by asthma.
Sudafed Cold and Allergy • chlorpheniramine 4 mg • pseudoephedrine 60 mg	*Relief from runny nose, congestion, sneezing caused by cold; runny nose, sneezing, congestion, itchy nose or throat, itchy and watery eyes, congestion caused by hay fever* **Adults and children ages 12 and older:** 1 tablet P.O. q 4 to 6 hr. Maximum 4 doses q 24 hr. **Children ages 6 to 11:** ½ tablet P.O. q 4 to 6 hr. Maximum 4 doses q 24 hr.	• Tell patient not to take drug within 2 weeks of an MAO inhibitor. • Urge patient to notify doctor if symptoms are unimproved in 7 days, if patient has a fever, or if patient becomes nervous, dizzy, or sleepless. • Advise patient not to take drug if he has heart disease, hypertension, thyroid disease, diabetes, emphysema, chronic bronchitis, glaucoma, or difficulty urinating caused by enlarged prostate, unless directed by a doctor. • Drug may cause excitability in children. • Tell patient that drug may cause drowsiness and that he shouldn't take it when driving or drinking alcoholic beverages.

Combination products *(continued)*

Brand name and active ingredients	Indications and dosages	Nursing considerations
Sudafed Cold and Allergy *(continued)*		• Tell patient not to take drug with sedatives or tranquilizers, unless directed by a doctor.
Tylenol Allergy Sinus **Tylenol Sinus, Maximum Strength** • acetaminophen 500 mg • pseudoephedrine hydrochloride 30 mg	*Temporary relief from sinus pain and headache and nasal and sinus congestion* **Adults and children ages 12 and older:** 2 geltabs P.O. q 4 to 6 hours. Maximum 8 geltabs q 24 hr.	• Tell parent not to give drug to child for longer than 5 days for pain or longer than 3 days for fever, unless directed by the doctor. • Advise patient to notify doctor if fever or pain persists or worsens or if redness or swelling is present. • If sore throat lasts longer than 2 days, is severe, or is accompanied by fever, headache, nausea, vomiting, or rash, tell patient to contact doctor immediately. • Advise parent to consult doctor if child's cough lasts longer than 1 week, tends to recur, or is accompanied by fever, rash, or headache. Tell parent not to give drug if cough is accompanied by excessive mucus. • Tell parent not to give drug to child who has glaucoma, respiratory problems (such as chronic bronchitis), heart disease, hypertension, thyroid disease, or diabetes, without consulting doctor. • Inform parent that drug may cause excessive drowsiness and that it shouldn't be given to a child who takes a sedative.

(continued)

Combination products *(continued)*

Brand name and active ingredients	Indications and dosages	Nursing considerations
Tylenol Allergy Sinus **Tylenol Sinus, Maximum Strength** *(continued)*		• Drug may cause excitability in children. • Tell parent not to give drug with other medications that contain acetaminophen. • Warn parent not to give drug to child within 2 weeks of an MAO inhibitor. • Advise patient with phenylketonuria that each tablet contains 4 mg of phenylalanine. • Caution paptient not to use drug if package shows signs of tampering.
Tylenol Allergy Sinus Maximum Strength (caplets, geltabs, and gelcaplets) • acetaminophen 500 mg • chlorpheniramine maleate 2 mg • pseudoephedrine hydrochloride 30 mg	*Relief from nasal congestion, sinus congestion and pressure, sinus pain, headache, runny nose, sneezing, itching of the nose or throat, itchy and watery eyes caused by hay fever or other upper respiratory tract allergies* **Adults and children ages 12 and older:** 2 caplets, gelcaplets, or geltablets q 4 to 6 hr. Maximum 8 caplets, geltablets, or gelcaplets in 24 hr, or as directed by a doctor.	• If patient consumes three or more alcoholic beverages daily, tell him to consult a doctor before taking acetaminophen or other pain relievers or fever reducers. Tell patient that acetaminophen may cause liver damage. • Tell patient not to take drug for pain for longer than 7 days or for fever for longer than 3 days, unless directed by a doctor. • Urge patient to consult a doctor if pain or fever persists or worsens, if new symptoms occur, or if redness or swelling is present. • Drug may cause excitability, especially in children. • If nervousness, dizziness, or sleeplessness develops, advise patient to discontinue drug and consult a doctor.

Combination products *(continued)*

Brand name and active ingredients	Indications and dosages	Nursing considerations
Tylenol Allergy Sinus Maximum Strength (caplets, geltabs, and gelcaplets) *(continued)*		• Tell patient that drug may cause drowsiness and that he shouldn't take it when driving or drinking alcoholic beverages. • Tell patient not to take drug with sedatives or tranquilizers unless directed by a doctor. • Caution patient not to take drug if has a breathing problem (such as emphysema or chronic bronchitis), heart disease, high blood pressure, thyroid disease, diabetes, glaucoma, or difficulty urinating caused by an enlarged prostate, unless directed by a doctor. • Advise patient not to exceed recommended dosage. • Encourage pregnant or breast-feeding patient to consult a doctor before using this product. • Tell patient not to take drug with other products that contain acetaminophen. • Tell patient not to take drug within 2 weeks of an MAO inhibitor.
Tylenol Allergy Sinus Nighttime Maximum Strength	*Relief from nasal congestion, sinus congestion and pressure, sinus pain, headache, runny nose, sneezing, itching of the nose or throat, and itchy and watery eyes*	• If patient consumes three or more alcoholic beverages daily, tell him to consult a doctor before taking acetaminophen or other pain relievers or fever reducers. Tell patient that acetaminophen may cause liver damage. *(continued)*

Combination products *(continued)*

Brand name and active ingredients	Indications and dosages	Nursing considerations
Tylenol Allergy Sinus Nighttime Maximum Strength *(continued)* • acetaminophen 500 mg • diphenhydramine hydrochloride 25 mg • pseudoephedrine hydrochloride 30 mg	*from hay fever or other upper respiratory tract allergies* **Adults and children ages 12 and older:** 2 caplets h.s. May repeat in 4 to 6 hr. Maximum 8 caplets in 24 hr, or as directed by a doctor.	• Tell patient not to take drug for pain that lasts longer than 7 days or for fever that lasts longer than 3 days, unless directed by a doctor. If pain or fever persists or worsens, new symptoms occur, or redness or swelling is present, urge patient to consult a doctor because these could be signs of a serious condition. • Tell patient that drug may cause excitability, especially in children. • If patient becomes nervous, dizzy, or sleepless, recommend that he discontinue drug and consult a doctor. • Tell patient that drug may cause drowsiness and that he shouldn't take it when driving or drinking alcoholic beverages. • Tell patient not to take drug with sedatives or tranquilizers unless directed by a doctor. • Advise patient not to take drug if he has a breathing problem (such as emphysema or chronic bronchitis), heart disease, high blood pressure, thyroid disease, diabetes, glaucoma, or difficulty urinating caused by an enlarged prostate, unless directed by a doctor. • Tell patient not to exceed recommended dosage. • Advise pregnant or breast-feeding patient to consult a doctor before taking drug.

Combination products *(continued)*

Brand name and active ingredients	Indications and dosages	Nursing considerations
Tylenol Allergy Sinus Nighttime Maximum Strength *(continued)*		• Caution patient not to take drug with other products that contain acetaminophen. • Tell patient not to take drug within 2 weeks of an MAO inhibitor.
Tylenol Cold Complete Formula • acetaminophen 325 mg • chlorpheniramine maleate 2 mg • dextromethorphan hydrobromide 15 mg • pseudoephedrine hydrochloride 30 mg	*Relief from cold symptoms: minor aches and pains, headaches, sore throat, nasal congestion, runny nose, coughs, sneezing, itchy and watery eyes, and fever* **Adults and children ages 12 and older:** 2 caplets q 6 hr. Maximum 8 caplets q 24 hr, or as directed by a doctor. **Children ages 6 to 11:** 1 caplet q 6 hr. Maximum 4 caplets q 24 hr, or as directed by a doctor.	• If patient consumes three or more alcoholic beverages daily, tell him to consult a doctor before taking acetaminophen or other pain relievers or fever reducers. Tell patient that acetaminophen may cause liver damage. • Tell patient not to take drug for pain that lasts longer than 7 days or for fever that lasts longer than 3 days, unless directed by a doctor. • Advise patient to consult a doctor if pain or fever persists or worsens, new symptoms develop, or redness or swelling is present. • If sore throat is severe, persists for longer than 2 days, or is accompanied or followed by fever, headache, rash, nausea, or vomiting, urge patient to consult a doctor promptly. • If cough persists for longer than 1 week, tends to recur, or is accompanied by fever, rash, or persistent headache, tell patient to consult a doctor. • Caution patient not to take drug for persistent or chron-

(continued)

Combination products (continued)

Brand name and active ingredients	Indications and dosages	Nursing considerations
Tylenol Cold Complete Formula (continued)		ic cough caused by smoking, asthma, or emphysema, or if cough is accompanied by excessive mucus, unless directed by a doctor. • Warn patient not to exceed recommended dosage. • Tell patient to notify doctor if he becomes nervous, dizzy, or sleepless. • Drug may cause excitability, especially in children. • Advise patient not to take drug if he has emphysema, chronic bronchitis, heart disease, high blood pressure, thyroid disease, diabetes, glaucoma, or difficulty urinating caused by an enlarged prostate, unless directed by a doctor. • Tell patient that drug may cause drowsiness and that he shouldn't take it when driving or drinking alcoholic beverages. • Tell patient not to take drug with sedatives or tranquilizers unless directed by a doctor. • Tell pregnant or breast-feeding patient to consult a doctor before taking this drug. • Urge patient not to take drug with other products that contain acetaminophen. • Tell patient not to take drug within 2 weeks of an MAO inhibitor.

Combination products *(continued)*

Brand name and active ingredients	Indications and dosages	Nursing considerations
Tylenol Cold Non-Drowsy (caplets and gelcaplets) • acetaminophen 325 mg • dextromethorphan hydrobromide 15 mg • pseudoephedrine hydrochloride 30 mg	*Relief from cold symptoms: minor aches and pains, headaches, sore throat, nasal congestion, coughs, and fever* **Adults and children ages 12 and older:** 2 caplets q 6 hr. Maximum 8 caplets q 24 hr, or as directed by a doctor. **Children ages 6 to 11:** 1 caplet q 6 hr. Maximum 4 caplets q 24 hr, or as directed by a doctor.	• If patient consumes three or more alcoholic beverages daily, urge him to consult a doctor before taking acetaminophen or other pain relievers or fever reducers. Tell patient that acetaminophen may cause liver damage. • Tell patient not to take drug for pain that lasts longer than 7 days or for fever that lasts longer than 3 days, unless directed by a doctor. If pain or fever persists or worsens, new symptoms occur, or redness or swelling is present, have patient consult a doctor because these could be signs of a serious condition. • If sore throat is severe, persists longer than 2 days, or is accompanied or followed by fever, headache, rash, nausea, or vomiting, tell patient to consult a doctor promptly. • A persistent cough may be a sign of a serious condition. If cough persists for longer than 1 week, tends to recur, or is accompanied by fever, rash, or persistent headache, have patient consult a doctor. • Tell patient not to take drug for persistent or chronic cough caused by smoking, asthma, or emphysema, or if cough is accompanied by excessive phlegm, unless directed by a doctor.

(continued)

Combination products *(continued)*

Brand name and active ingredients	Indications and dosages	Nursing considerations
Tylenol Cold Non-Drowsy (caplets and gelcaplets) *(continued)*		• Advise patient not to exceed recommended dosage. • Tell patient to notify doctor if he becomes nervous, dizzy, or sleepless. • Tell patient not to take drug if he has heart disease, high blood pressure, thyroid disease, diabetes, or difficulty urinating caused by an enlarged prostate, unless directed by a doctor. • Tell pregnant or breast-feeding patient to consult a doctor before using this product. • Patient shouldn't take drug with other products that contain acetaminophen. • Tell patient not to take drug within 2 weeks of an MAO inhibitor.
Tylenol Cold Severe Congestion • acetaminophen 325 mg • dextromethorphan hydrobromide 15 mg • guaifenesin 200 mg • pseudoephedrine hydrochloride 30 mg	*Relief from cold symptoms: minor aches and pains, headaches, sore throat, nasal congestion, coughs, chest congestion, and fever* **Adults and children ages 12 and older:** 2 caplets q 6 to 8 hr. Maximum 8 caplets q 24 hr, or as directed by a doctor. **Children ages 6 to 11:** 1 caplet q 6 to 8 hr. Maximum 4	• If patient consumes three or more alcoholic beverages daily, urge him to consult a doctor before taking acetaminophen or other pain relievers or fever reducers. Tell patient that acetaminophen may cause liver damage. • Tell patient not to take drug for pain that lasts longer than 7 days or for fever that lasts longer than 3 days, unless directed by a doctor. If pain or fever persists or worsens, new symptoms occur, or redness or swelling is present, have patient consult a doctor

Combination products *(continued)*

Brand name and active ingredients	Indications and dosages	Nursing considerations
Tylenol Cold Severe Congestion *(continued)*	caplets q 24 hr, or as directed by a doctor.	because these could be signs of a serious condition. • Advise patient to consult a doctor promptly if sore throat is severe, persists for longer than 2 days, or is accompanied or followed by fever, headache, rash, nausea, or vomiting. • If cough persists for longer than 1 week, tends to recur, or is accompanied by fever, rash, or persistent headache, patient should consult a doctor. Patient shouldn't take this product for persistent or chronic cough caused by smoking, asthma, or emphysema, or if cough is accompanied by excessive phlegm, unless directed by a doctor. • Warn patient not to exceed recommended dosage. • Tell patient to notify doctor if he becomes nervous, dizzy, or sleepless. • Patient shouldn't take this product if he has heart disease, high blood pressure, thyroid disease, diabetes, or difficulty urinating caused by an enlarged prostate, unless directed by a doctor. • Tell pregnant or breast-feeding patient to consult a doctor before using this product. • Urge patient not to take drug with other products that contain acetaminophen.

(continued)

Combination products *(continued)*

Brand name and active ingredients	Indications and dosages	Nursing considerations
Tylenol Cold Severe Congestion *(continued)*		• Tell patient not to take drug within 2 weeks of an MAO inhibitor.
Tylenol Flu Maximum Strength Nighttime Gelcaplets • acetaminophen 500 mg • diphenhydramine hydrochloride 25 mg • pseudoephedrine hydrochloride 30 mg	*Relief from cold and flu symptoms: minor aches and pains, headaches, sore throat, nasal congestion, runny nose, sneezing, and fever* **Adults and children ages 12 and older:** 2 gelcaplets h.s. May repeat q 6 hr. Maximum 8 gelcaplets in 24 hr, or as directed by a doctor.	• If patient consumes three or more alcoholic beverages daily, he should notify doctor before taking acetaminophen or other pain relievers or fever reducers. Tell patient that acetaminophen may cause liver damage. • Instruct patient not to take for pain that lasts longer than 7 days or for fever that lasts longer than 3 days, unless directed by a doctor. • If pain or fever persists or worsens, if new symptoms occur, or if redness or swelling occurs, tell patient to consult a doctor. • If sore throat is severe, persists for longer than 2 days, is accompanied or followed by a fever, headache, rash, nausea or vomiting, tell patient to consult a doctor promptly. • Tell patient not to exceed recommended dosage. • Tell patient to notify doctor if he becomes nervous, dizzy, or sleepless. • Drug may cause excitability, especially in children. • Instruct patient not to take this product, unless directed by a doctor, if he has a breathing problem such as emphysema or chronic bron-

Combination products *(continued)*

Brand name and active ingredients	Indications and dosages	Nursing considerations
Tylenol Flu Maximum Strength Nighttime Gelcaplets *(continued)*		chitis, or if he has glaucoma or difficulty urinating caused by an enlarged prostate. • Patient shouldn't take this product if he has heart disease, high blood pressure, thyroid disease, or diabetes, unless directed by a doctor. • Tell patient that drug may cause drowsiness and that he shouldn't use when driving or take with alcohol, sedatives, or tranquilizers, unless directed by a doctor. • Tell patient to avoid alcoholic beverages while taking this product. If he also takes sedatives or tranquilizers, patient shouldn't take this product without first consulting the doctor. • Advise patient to use caution when driving a motor vehicle or operating machinery. • Pregnant or breast-feeding patient should consult a doctor before using this product. • Tell patient not to use with other products containing acetaminophen. • Tell patient not to take drug together with or within 2 weeks of taking an MAO inhibitor.
Tylenol Flu Maximum Strength Non-Drowsy	*Relief from cold and flu symptoms: minor aches and pains, headaches, sore throat, nasal*	• Tell patient not to take drug for pain that lasts longer than 7 days or fever that lasts longer than 3 days, unless directed by a doctor.

(continued)

Combination products *(continued)*

Brand name and active ingredients	Indications and dosages	Nursing considerations
Tylenol Flu Maximum Strength Non-Drowsy *(continued)* • acetaminophen 500 mg • dextromethorphan hydrobromide 15 mg • pseudoephedrine hydrochloride 30 mg	*congestion, coughs, and fever reduction* **Adults and children ages 12 and older:** 2 gelcaplets q 6 hr. Maximum 8 gelcaplets q 24 hr, or as directed by a doctor.	• If pain or fever persists or worsens, if new symptoms occur, or if redness or swelling is present, tell patient to consult a doctor. • If sore throat is severe, persists for longer than 2 days, is accompanied or followed by a fever, headache, rash, nausea or vomiting, warn patient to consult a doctor promptly. • If cough persists for longer than 1 week, tends to recur, or is accompanied by fever, rash, or persistent headache, advise patient to consult a doctor. • Tell patient not to take drug for persistent or chronic cough (as from smoking, asthma, or emphysema) or for cough accompanied by excessive mucus, unless directed by a doctor. • Tell patient to notify doctor if he becomes nervous, dizzy, or sleepless. • Advise patient not to take drug if he has heart disease, high blood pressure, thyroid disease, diabetes, or difficulty urinating caused by an enlarged prostate, unless directed by a doctor. • If patient is pregnant or breast-feeding, tell her to consult a doctor before using this product.

Combination products *(continued)*

Brand name and active ingredients	Indications and dosages	Nursing considerations
Tylenol Flu Maximum Strength Non-Drowsy *(continued)*		• Tell patient not to take drug with other products that contain acetaminophen. • Tell patient not to take drug within 2 weeks of an MAO inhibitor.
Tylenol Flu Nighttime Liquid (30 ml = 2 tbs) • acetaminophen 1000 mg • dextromethorphan hydrobromide 30 mg • doxylamine succinate 12.5 mg • pseudoephedrine hydrochloride 60 mg	*Relief from body aches, headache, coughing, nasal congestion, sore throat, runny nose sneezing, and fever* **Adults and children ages 12 and older:** 2 tbs. May repeat q 6 hr. Maximum 4 doses q 24 hr, or as directed by a doctor.	• Tell patient not to take acetaminophen for pain that lasts longer than 7 days or for fever that lasts longer than 3 days, unless directed by a doctor. • If patient consumes three or more alcoholic beverages daily, advise him to consult a doctor before taking acetaminophen or other pain relievers or fever reducers. Tell him that acetaminophen may cause liver damage. • Advise patient to consult a doctor if pain or fever persists or worsens, new symptoms occur, or redness or swelling is present. • If sore throat is severe, persists for longer than 2 days, or is accompanied or followed by fever, headache, rash, nausea, or vomiting, patient should consult a doctor promptly. • If cough persists for longer than 1 week, tends to recur, or is accompanied by fever, rash, or persistent headache, patient should consult a doctor.

(continued)

Combination products *(continued)*

Brand name and active ingredients	Indications and dosages	Nursing considerations
Tylenol Flu Nighttime Liquid *(continued)*		• Patient shouldn't take drug for persistent or chronic cough (as from smoking, asthma, or emphysema), or for cough accompanied by excessive phlegm, unless directed by a doctor. • Tell patient not to exceed recommended dosage. • Tell patient to notify doctor if he becomes nervous, dizzy, or sleepless. • Drug may cause excitability, especially in children. • Warn patient not to take drug if he has a breathing problem (such as emphysema or chronic bronchitis), heart disease, high blood pressure, thyroid disease, diabetes, glaucoma, or difficulty urinating caused by an enlarged prostate, unless directed by a doctor. • Tell patient that drug may cause drowsiness and that he shouldn't take it when driving or drinking alcoholic beverages. • Tell patient not to take drug with sedatives or tranquilizers, unless directed by a doctor. • Urge pregnant or breast-feeding patient to consult a doctor before taking drug. • Tell patient not to take drug with other products that contain acetaminophen. • Tell patient not to take drug within 2 weeks of an MAO inhibitor.

Combination products *(continued)*

Brand name and active ingredients	Indications and dosages	Nursing considerations
Tylenol Severe Allergy • acetaminophen 500 mg • diphenhydramine hydrochloride 12.5 mg	*Relief from itchy, watery eyes, runny nose, sneezing, sore or scratchy throat, and itching of the nose or throat caused by hay fever or other upper respiratory tract allergies* **Adults and children ages 12 and older:** 2 caplets q 4 to 6 hr. Maximum 8 caplets q 24 hr, or as directed by a doctor.	• If patient consumes three or more alcoholic beverages daily, urge him to consult a doctor before taking acetaminophen or other pain relievers or fever reducers. Tell patient that acetaminophen may cause liver damage. • Caution patient not to take drug for pain that lasts longer than 7 days or fever that lasts longer than 3 days unless directed by a doctor. If pain or fever persists or worsens, new symptoms occur, or redness or swelling is present, patient should consult a doctor because these could be signs of a serious condition. • If sore throat is severe, persists for longer than 2 days, or is accompanied or followed by fever, headache, rash, nausea or vomiting, have patient consult a doctor promptly. • Drug may cause excitability, especially in children. Tell patient to discontinue drug and consult a doctor if he becomes nervous, dizzy, or sleepless. • Tell patient that drug may cause drowsiness and that he shouldn't take it when driving or drinking alcoholic beverages. • Tell patient not to take drug with sedatives or tranquilizers unless directed by a doctor.

(continued)

Combination products *(continued)*

Brand name and active ingredients	Indications and dosages	Nursing considerations
Tylenol Severe Allergy *(continued)*		• Caution patient not to take drug if he has a breathing problem (such as emphysema or chronic bronchitis), glaucoma, or difficulty urinating caused by an enlarged prostate, unless directed by a doctor. • Advise patient not to exceed recommended dosage. • Urge pregnant or breast-feeding patient to consult a doctor before using this product. • Tell patient not to take drug with other products that contain acetaminophen.
Tylenol Sinus Nighttime • acetaminophen 500 mg • doxylamine succinate 6.25 mg • pseudoephedrine hydrochloride 30 mg	*Relief from nasal congestion, sinus congestion and pressure, sinus pain, headache, runny nose, and itching of the nose or throat* **Adults and children ages 12 and older:** 2 caplets h.s. May repeat q 4 to 6 hr. Maximum 8 caplets q 24 hr, or as directed by a doctor.	• If patient consumes three or more alcoholic beverages daily, urge him to consult a doctor before taking acetaminophen or other pain relievers or fever reducers. Tell patient that acetaminophen may cause liver damage. • Caution patient not to take drug for pain that lasts longer than 7 days or fever that lasts longer than 3 days, unless directed by a doctor. • Tell patient to consult a doctor if pain or fever persists or worsens, new symptoms occur, or redness or swelling is present, because these could be signs of a serious condition. • Drug may cause excitability, especially in children.

Combination products *(continued)*

Brand name and active ingredients	Indications and dosages	Nursing considerations
Tylenol Sinus Nighttime *(continued)*		• Tell patient to notify doctor if he becomes nervous, dizzy, or sleepless. • Caution patient that drug may cause drowsiness and that he shouldn't take it when driving or drinking alcoholic beverages. • Tell patient not to take drug with sedatives or tranquilizers unless directed by a doctor. • Warn patient not to take drug if he has a breathing problem (such as emphysema or chronic bronchitis), glaucoma, heart disease, high blood pressure, thyroid disease, diabetes, or difficulty urinating caused by an enlarged prostate, unless directed by a doctor. • Urge pregnant or breast-feeding patient to consult doctor before taking drug. • Tell patient not to take drug with other products that contain acetaminophen. • Tell patient not to take drug within 2 weeks of an MAO inhibitor.
Tylenol Sinus Non-Drowsy • acetaminophen 500 mg • pseudoephedrine hydrochloride 30 mg	*Relief from sinus pain and headaches and nasal and sinus congestion* **Adults and children ages 12 and older:** 2 gelcaplets, caplets, or geltablets q 4 to 6 hr. Maximum 8	• If patient consumes three or more alcoholic beverages daily, urge him to consult a doctor before taking acetaminophen or other pain relievers or fever reducers. Tell patient that acetaminophen may cause liver damage.

(continued)

Combination products *(continued)*

Brand name and active ingredients	Indications and dosages	Nursing considerations
Tylenol Sinus Non-Drowsy *(continued)*	gelcaplets, caplets, or geltabs q 24 hr, or as directed by a doctor.	• Tell patient not to take drug for pain that lasts longer than 7 days or fever that lasts longer than 3 days, unless directed by a doctor. • Advise patient to consult a doctor if pain or fever persists or worsens, new symptoms occur, or redness or swelling is present, because these could be signs of a serious condition. • Tell patient to notify doctor if he becomes nervous, dizzy, or sleepless. • Caution patient not to take drug if he has heart disease, high blood pressure, thyroid disease, diabetes, or difficulty urinating caused by an enlarged prostate, unless directed by a doctor. • Advise patient not to exceed recommended dosage. • Urge pregnant or breastfeeding patient to consult a doctor before taking drug. • Advise patient not to take drug with other products that contain acetaminophen. • Tell patient not to take drug within 2 weeks of an MAO inhibitor.
Vicks Formula 44D • pseudoephedrine 60 mg/15 ml • dextromethorphan 30 mg/15 ml	*Relief from cough and congestion caused by cold* **Adults and children ages 12 and older:** 3 tsp or 15 ml P.O. q	• Tell patient not to take drug within 2 weeks of an MAO inhibitor. • Urge patient to notify doctor if cough lasts longer than 7 days or is accompanied by fever, rash, or headache.

Combination products *(continued)*

Brand name and active ingredients	Indications and dosages	Nursing considerations
Vicks Formula 44D *(continued)*	6 hr p.r.n. Maximum 4 doses q 24 hr. **Children ages 6 to 11:** 1½ tsp or 7.5 ml P.O. q 6 hr p.r.n. Maximum 4 doses q 24 hr.	• Advise patient not to take drug if he has emphysema, bronchitis, heart disease, hypertension, thyroid disease, diabetes, breathing problems, chronic cough, cough caused by smoking, or difficulty urinating caused by enlarged prostate, unless directed by a doctor.
Vicks Formula 44E • dextromethorphan 20 mg/15 ml • guaifenesin 200 mg/15 ml	*Relief from cough; loosens phlegm* **Adults and children ages 12 and older (more than 95 lb):** 3 tsp or 15 ml P.O. q 4 hr p.r.n. Maximum 6 doses q 24 hr. **Children ages 6 to 11 (48 to 95 lb):** 1½ tsp or 7.5 ml P.O. q 4 hr p.r.n. Maximum 6 doses q 24 hr.	• Tell patient not to take drug within 2 weeks of an MAO inhibitor. • Urge patient to notify doctor if cough lasts longer than 7 days or is accompanied by fever, rash, or headache. • Caution patient not to take drug for chronic cough caused by asthma, smoking, or emphysema, or for cough accompanied by excessive phlegm.

9

Nutrition

Many people believe that over-the-counter (OTC) nutritional supplements—vitamins and minerals—can remedy nutritional deficiencies and act as effectively as prescription drugs. The average consumer may think that nutritional supplements have undergone the same rigorous scientific scrutiny and trial as prescription drugs. In reality, these supplements don't have to be standardized, and some may contain none of the nutrients they claim to have.

Some very practical OTC nutritional remedies are available today, but they shouldn't be consumed without caution. Most supplements can correct a nutritional imbalance, but various interactions may affect their use. For example, some nutrients found in foods may increase the absorption of certain vitamins and minerals; some foods may prevent or slow their absorption. So nutritional supplements shouldn't be used indiscriminately.

Sometimes it's obvious from extensive research that taking a particular nutritional supplement prevents or treats a deficiency—for example, taking calcium for osteoporosis. In other instances, more research is needed before a direct correlation can be made, as in the case of chromium and diabetes. Yet another scenario is when a particular nutrient is proven beneficial, but the exact dosage or strength hasn't been determined. An example of this is when a person takes vitamin C to relieve common cold symptoms.

Although taking a nutritional supplement isn't usually dangerous, more and more people regularly take several supplements, sometimes at toxic levels and without consideration of the dangers involved. They may mistakenly believe that if a little is good, more is better—and many people are searching for a quick fix for perceived or real nutritional deficiencies. Although it's difficult to reach toxic levels of nutrients by eating food, it's very possible to do so by taking nutrients in the concentrated form of available vitamin and mineral supplements.

Taking a supplement may, in fact, be the best method of treatment for some patients. You must be aware, though, that consumption of OTC vitamins and minerals can mask a patient's medical condition, delaying proper diagnosis or complicating a condition with which the patient has already been diagnosed.

When you take a patient's history, if you ask which medications he's taking, he'll typically list prescribed medications but not OTC medications, and especially not OTC nutritional supplements, because he doesn't think they're important enough to mention. Actually, these supplements can significantly affect the way a patient responds to medical treatment, and they may interfere with the metabolism of other foods and drugs he's taking. So it's imperative during your patient interviews to ask specifically about nutritional supplements and to document this information.

This chapter covers some common nutritional deficiencies for which people take OTC drugs. These conditions include anemia, beriberi, copper deficiency, osteoporosis, pellagra, rickets, and osteomalacia.

Anemia

Anemia is a hemoglobin deficiency—a reduction in the number of red blood cells (RBCs)—that may be caused by many different problems. It causes the oxygen-carrying capacity of blood to decline, which leads to hypoxia. Anemia may be related to an array of deficiencies because many different nutrients affect erythropoiesis (RBC formation). These include iron, folic acid, pyridoxine, and vitamins B_{12}, E, and A. Changes in any of these nutrients can disrupt the balance of RBC synthesis.

Signs and symptoms

Anemia is a sign of an underlying condition. It may result from hormonal disorders, chronic inflammation, chronic renal failure, infection, peptic ulcer disease, hemorrhoids, diverticular disease, heavy menstrual bleeding, repeated pregnancies, liver damage, thyroid disorders, rheumatoid arthritis, bone marrow disease, drug use, or surgery. Early signs and symptoms include loss of appetite, constipation, headaches, irritability, and difficulty concentrating. Later signs and symptoms of anemia are fatigue, lack of energy, shortness of breath, weakness, overall pallor, coldness of the limbs, dizziness, pale lips and conjunctiva, soreness of the mouth, pale and brittle nails, depression, and, in severe cases, loss of menstruation.

Serious conditions

The patient who treats himself for the signs and symptoms listed above may find that he's treating the wrong disorder. There are several types of anemia and each affects different nutrients in the body. Three examples are normocytic anemia, pernicious anemia, and iron-deficiency anemia.

Normocytic anemia

Treatment of normocytic anemia is aimed at the specific diagnosis, such as chronic renal failure or aplastic anemia. Severe anemia may require blood transfusions. Transfusions are usually a temporary remedy until other treatments start to affect the underlying cause. Supplemental nutrients wouldn't be helpful in this situation—and could possibly cause harm. Repeated transfusions may cause iron toxicity because the body has no way to eliminate the excess iron. A patient receiving numerous transfusions should be advised to follow a low-iron diet.

Pernicious anemia

The classic form of megaloblastic anemia is pernicious anemia, caused by the inability to produce sufficient intrinsic factor. Although it takes years to develop, pernicious anemia significantly depletes vitamin B_{12} and also possibly folic acid.

Strict vegetarians are susceptible to pernicious anemia because vitamin B_{12} is contained primarily in animal foods; others at risk are alcoholics, elderly patients, and patients of Scandinavian descent.

It's crucial to the treatment plan to determine the underlying cause of the pernicious anemia. For example, treating the patient with folic acid supplements if there's a primary vitamin B_{12} deficiency will correct only part of the condition. The more progressive complications, such as nervous tissue degeneration, would be overlooked and untreated. Early intervention with an appropriate diet or supplementation is critical to the treatment of pernicious anemia.

Iron-deficiency anemia

Iron-deficiency anemia is the classic form of microcytic anemia. This type is commonly seen in pregnancy and with large menstrual losses. A common sign of this form of anemia is thin, flat fingernails that eventually take on a "spoon" shape. Supplementation of an elemental form of iron is usually effective in treating the deficiency. Patients also should be encouraged to take iron supplements with vitamin C or citrus fruits and juices to enhance absorption. Heme synthesis is stimulated rapidly; therefore, close monitoring and proper dosing is important. Excessive amounts of iron are toxic, especially in children.

Complications

The treatment of anemia isn't as simple as taking an elemental iron supplement. Long-term complications of this type of management could be very dangerous because excessive amounts of iron can cause metabolic acidosis and cirrhosis. The tissues cannot store such elevated amounts, which eventually cause parenchymal cell damage. Supplementing iron intake in addition to receiving multiple blood transfusions will likely increase the body's iron stores to toxic levels. For these reasons, anemias should be properly diagnosed, treated, and professionally monitored.

Nursing considerations

• Anemia results from a disorder or disease.
• Anemia is a general term encompassing many forms of deficiency states. The patient's medical and diet histories may help determine which form of anemia he may have and its contributing factors.
• Review all drugs and nutritional supplements.
• Assess the patient for physical signs and symptoms of anemia.
• Realize the potential for toxicity that results from taking nutritional supplements.

Patient teaching

• Explain the danger of self-treatment of anemia without proper diagnosis.
• Educate the patient about the various kinds of anemia.
• Offer dietary alternatives for deficiencies, where appropriate.
• Teach the patient about the serious nature of over-supplementation of iron.
• Encourage regular professional monitoring.

Beriberi

Beriberi is the result of a vitamin B deficiency, particularly vitamin B_1 (thiamine). Thiamine is found in most foods and is added to many commercial breads and cereals. Thiamine deficiency occurs primarily in Asian countries, where consumption of polished rice, which contains very little thiamine, is a staple in the diet. In the United States and other developed countries, chronic alcoholism, malabsorption syndrome, hypothyroidism, and infections are the main causes of beriberi. Prolonged nausea and vomiting from a difficult pregnancy can also lead to a deficiency.

Thiamine pyrophosphate is important for key reactions in energy metabolism. Thiamine is necessary for the metabolism of proteins, nucleic acids, fats, and especially carbohydrates. This water-soluble vitamin plays an important role in carbohydrate metabolism; requirements for thiamine greatly increase when carbohydrate intake is increased.

Signs and symptoms

Signs and symptoms of thiamine deficiency vary with age. In adults, the symptoms include diarrhea, fatigue, weight loss, edema, and heart failure. In children, symptoms include impaired growth, muscle wasting, mental confusion, seizures, and GI problems such as nausea, vomiting, diarrhea, and constipation. Infants commonly have abdominal distension and tenderness, colicky pain, vomiting, and anorexia.

Serious conditions

Improper treatment of beriberi can prolong its symptoms. In particular, untreated beriberi can cause severe peripheral neuropathy and, eventually, paralysis. Other serious consequences include cardiac failure, subacute necrotizing encephalomyelopathy, cerebellar signs, and Wernicke's encephalopathy.

Complications

The typical treatment for beriberi is to replete the B vitamins, particularly vitamin B_1. A pure thiamine deficiency is rare; patients most often are deficient in other B vitamins and other nutrients. Thiamine toxicity is rarely a problem.

Nursing considerations

- Interview the patient about dietary intake.
- Inquire about alcohol use and the likelihood of alcoholism.
- Assess medical history, specifically for hypothyroidism, pregnancy, malabsorption syndrome, and GI conditions.
- Review medications and nutritional supplements.

Patient teaching

• Encourage the patient to consume thiamine-rich foods such as brown rice, legumes, lean meat, raw fruits and vegetables, seeds and nuts, whole grains, and yogurt.
• Tell the patient to avoid alcohol.
• Advise the patient to seek appropriate counseling for alcoholism.
• Instruct the patient about proper dosing of thiamine supplements and B vitamins.

Copper deficiency

More than 30% of the body's copper is stored in the liver. Large amounts can also be found in the tissues of the spleen, kidney, heart, and brain. Newborns have three times the adult level in their liver, but this is rapidly depleted as excretion mechanisms mature.

Copper is an essential trace mineral. It helps white blood cells fight infection. It's also needed for the body to properly absorb iron from the diet. Insufficient amounts of copper cause a reduction in hemoglobin, and copper-deficiency anemia can result. Besides oxygen transport, copper is necessary as a catalyst in protein reactions, as a cross-linking agent for elastin and collagen, and in the metabolism of essential fatty acids and ascorbic acid (vitamin C). Copper is also needed in various enzyme reactions.

Copper is best measured in a blood component known as ceruloplasmin. This is the copper-protein compound in which 95% of the body's circulating copper can be found. Testing for ceruloplasmin can be part of any routine blood work.

Finally, copper is part of taste sensitivity; part of the formation of melanin; and an essential factor in superoxide dismutase (an antioxidant that fights free radicals).

Signs and symptoms

Signs and symptoms of copper deficiency aren't exclusive, thereby making self-diagnosis of copper deficiency very difficult. Prolonged deficiency yields problems including diarrhea, inefficient use of iron and protein, and stunted growth. Other signs and symptoms are skeletal defects, degeneration of the nervous system, defects in the pigmentation and structure of the hair (Menkes' kinky hair syndrome), reproductive problems, and mild cardiac abnormalities. With an elevated zinc level, also monitor for high serum cholesterol, which can be present. Infants usually have impaired lung, bone, or nerve tissue.

Serious conditions

The body requires a delicate balance between copper and zinc to function properly. An imbalance can lead to thyroid disorders, mental disorders, and emotional problems. High-risk groups for copper-zinc imbalance are pregnant women, because of greater demands by the tissues; patients with sprue or celiac disease, because of malabsorption; patients with kidney failure; people who take megadoses of zinc; and premature infants fed only cow's milk, which is low in copper. Copper deficiency can also occur in patients receiving long-term total parenteral nutrition, if not supplemented properly. Taking supplements for a suspected copper deficiency is dangerous because of the need for a proper zinc-to-copper ratio. A recommended ratio is about 10 or 15 zinc to 1 copper.

Oral contraceptives also have been shown to increase serum levels of copper.

Complications

Copper toxicity occurs with over-supplementation of copper or improper balance of the zinc-to-copper ratio. It's rare for copper toxicity to occur by dietary means alone. Wilson's disease is a hereditary disorder in which the body can't metabolize copper, so copper accumulates in the body. If a patient with this rare disorder takes copper supplements, it could be fatal.

Too much copper can cause diarrhea, eczema, hemolytic anemia, high blood pressure, kidney disease, nausea, stomach pain, weakness, and severe CNS damage. High levels of copper are consistent with mental and emotional disorders such as hyperactivity, schizophrenia, clinical depression, insomnia, mood swings, stuttering, and senile dementia.

Nursing considerations

- Ask the patient about his supplement intake and assess his dietary habits.
- Assess the patient's oral contraceptive use, pregnancy history, and signs and symptoms of Wilson's disease, including cirrhotic liver, degenerative neurological problems, and a characteristic golden-brown or green ring around the cornea.

Patient teaching

- Instruct the patient about the zinc-to-copper ratio.

• Tell the patient about the signs and symptoms of copper toxicity.

• Encourage the patient to eat foods rich in copper such as legumes (especially soybeans), nuts, cocoa, black pepper, seafood, raisins, molasses, avocados, whole grains, and cauliflower.

Osteoporosis

Osteoporosis literally means porous bones. It's a progressive disease in which bones become weaker and more susceptible to fracture. Peak bone mass is normally achieved between ages 30 and 35. Between ages 55 and 70, women typically experience a 30% to 40% bone loss. Therefore, the healthier the bone density before age 35, the less likely a significant loss will occur in later years.

Although women primarily are affected by this debilitating disease, men are afflicted as well. Many women mistakenly believe that osteoporosis is something to be concerned with only after menopause. Although it's true that the decline in estrogen during menopause contributes to bone loss, research clearly shows that osteoporosis begins in the premenopausal years.

Risk factors include a small frame, late puberty, early menopause (naturally or artificially induced), family history of osteoporosis, hyperthyroidism, chronic kidney or liver disease, long-term use of certain drugs (corticosteroids, anticonvulsants, anticoagulants), a history of heavy smoking, and being of northern European or Asian descent. A diet high in animal protein, salt, sugar, caffeine, alcohol, and magnesium or phosphorus (found in most sodas and processed foods) may rob the bones of calcium to fulfill the body's requirement. Also, sufficient stomach acid is needed to absorb calcium. Elderly people commonly lack adequate hydrochloric acid to absorb calcium.

Signs and symptoms

Unfortunately, bone loss causes no symptoms while it's occurring. Not until a fracture takes place do most people become aware of the disease. As bone loss advances, the vertebrae are subject to compression fractures. This puts pressure on the nerves of the spine and various body systems; it eventually affects height, and it can be very painful. Compression fractures are responsible for the dowager's hump seen in many elderly people. Osteoporosis is also a contributing factor for tooth loss in aging. It causes the jawbone to weaken and no longer hold the teeth in place.

Serious conditions
The problem with self-treating osteoporosis is that it's more complex than a mere calcium deficiency. Calcium supplementation is appropriate in most cases, but other factors need to be addressed as well. Vitamins C, D, E, and K and protein each play an important role in the development and treatment of osteoporosis. Mineral intake also affects calcium levels. This involves regulation of magnesium, phosphorus, silicon, boron, zinc, manganese, and copper.

Complications
An extremely high intake of elemental calcium over a long period can contribute to the formation of kidney stones. Other conditions may be masked with random supplementation for osteoporosis, such as Paget's disease, bone cancer, fibrous dysplasia, and multiple myeloma.

Nursing considerations
• Interview the patient about dietary intake.
• Screen both men and women for this disorder.

• Specifically inquire about the patient's intake of foods high in calcium and vitamin D (other than dairy products), such as broccoli, chestnuts, clams, dandelion greens, most dark-green leafy vegetables, flounder, hazelnuts, kale, kelp, molasses, oats, oysters, salmon, sardines (with the bones), sea vegetables, sesame seeds, shrimp, soybeans, tahini (sesame butter), tofu, turnip greens, and wheat germ.
• Review the patient's use of drugs that may cause osteoporosis, such as corticosteroids, anticonvulsants, and anticoagulants.
• Screen the patient for obscure or questionable practices, such as use of sodium fluoride (once thought to help build bone), dehydroepiandrosterone (commonly called DHEA), and chondroitin.
• Accurately measure the patient's height and inquire about his previous height.
• Ask about the patient's bone fracture history and whether he has bone pain.

Patient teaching
• Instruct patient to consume whole-grain and high-fiber foods separately from taking calcium supplements, to increase absorption of calcium.

• Tell the patient to limit intake of almonds, asparagus, beet greens, cashews, chard, rhubarb, and spinach. These foods are high in oxalic acid and may inhibit calcium absorption.

• Advise the patient to avoid high-phosphate foods (soft drinks), processed foods, excessive protein, and caffeine and urge him to control alcohol intake.

• Encourage the patient to perform weight-bearing exercise to aid in bone mineralization.

• Tell the patient to consume high-calcium foods or supplements, as appropriate. If the patient is lactose intolerant, tell him to try lactose-free products, lactase enzyme pills, or nondairy sources of calcium.

Pellagra

Pellagra is a vitamin deficiency, particularly of vitamin B_3 (niacin). It's rare in the United States except in patients with alcoholism, chronic GI disturbances, or long-term treatment with the antibiotic isoniazid (INH). Pellagra is more common in populations where corn is the primary source of nutrition because corn has no niacin. Pellagra is usually coupled with other B-vitamin deficiencies.

Niacin, or nicotinic acid, is an essential component of certain coenzymes that function to carry hydrogen from a substrate through the mitochondrial electron transport system. Its oxidative products are used in metabolic processes, such as fatty acid synthesis. Nicotinic acid is produced from tryptophan in the liver by a series of enzymes. Its pharmacologic properties include peripheral vasodilation and the lowering of cholesterol.

Signs and symptoms

Classic signs and symptoms of pellagra include skin, GI, and CNS changes. Itchy dermatitis is common on exposed areas such as the hands, neck, and face. Trauma increases the dermatitis, which is usually symmetrical. Cracking and crusting can occur over thickened skin areas. Other effects include mouth soreness and red, swollen, and painful tongue and mucous membranes. Diarrhea usually results as a reaction to mucosal atrophy. Headache, sleep disturbances, anxiety, depression, thought disorders, hallucinations, and agitation are typical of pellagra. Advanced deficiency leads to seizures and catatonia, alternating with periods of lucidity. These subclinical signs and symptoms are sometimes mistaken for mental illness.

Serious conditions

Niacin and tryptophan deficiencies commonly are compounded by vitamin B_6 deficiency (pyridoxine) because vitamin B_6 converts tryptophan to nicotinic acid. Long-term use of INH for tuberculosis treatment can lead to pellagra if vitamin B_6 and tryptophan aren't available to the body. Therefore, supplementation with vitamin B_6 is necessary with INH therapy to enable the conversion of tryptophan. It's not safe or appropriate to supplement with tryptophan.

Complications

Because vitamin B_3 is water-soluble, it's often thought to be safe. However, large doses can still be toxic. With more recent research linking niacin supplementation to reduction of cholesterol levels, many people are megadosing to achieve the documented results. This is very dangerous without proper medical monitoring. Niacin toxicity can occur with as little as 1 g per day, which induces flushing and burning of the hands and face. This irritating effect is usually temporary until the dose is discontinued. At 3 g per day or more, complications include nausea, vomiting, diarrhea, and arrhythmias. Evidence of diabetes and hepatic injury may appear in serum values, and peptic ulcer symptoms may be aggravated.

Nursing considerations

- Review the patient's medical history for tuberculosis, CV problems, diabetes, liver disorders, and lipid levels.
- Observe the patient's skin and mouth for signs of pellagra.
- Ask the patient about GI symptoms.
- Assess the patient for dizziness or signs of dementia, anxiety, or depression.
- Assess the patient's dietary intake of niacin.
- Ask the patient about nutritional supplements he's taking, particularly vitamin B_3, vitamin B_6, and tryptophan.

Patient teaching

- Warn the patient about toxic effects of niacin replacement and megadosing.
- Explain to the patient the connection between vitamin B_3, vitamin B_6, and tryptophan.
- Educate the patient about dietary sources of niacin, such as liver, meat, fish, legumes (dried beans), whole-grain enriched cereals, avocados, bananas, broccoli, collards, figs, nuts and seeds, peanut butter, potatoes, prunes, and tomatoes.

- Recommend foods high in tryptophan, including halibut, salmon, swordfish, tuna, sunflower seeds, chicken, and turkey.

Rickets and osteomalacia

Rickets and osteomalacia are terms that describe a vitamin D deficiency. Rickets malformation of bones occurs primarily in children, and osteomalacia is seen in adults. Vitamin D is responsible for the absorption and maintenance of calcium and phosphate levels in the blood. Plasma becomes supersaturated by both of these minerals, and they are then sent to the bone for mineralization. Vitamin D also mobilizes these minerals out of the bone for renal reabsorption of calcium.

Dietary vitamin D is transported by chylomicrons and is taken up by the liver, where it becomes 25-hydroxyvitamin D_3. The kidney adds the hydroxyl group to make 1,25-dihydroxyvitamin D_3. Both are excreted in bile. Deficiency of either calcium or phosphorus increases the formation of 1,25-dihydroxyvitamin D_3.

Muscle weakness and bone pain are symptoms of vitamin D deficiency. Vitamin D replacement improves muscle function and corrects de-

creased phosphate levels. 25-Hydroxyvitamin D_3 may have a direct effect on bone to improve calcium deposition.

Vitamin D deficiencies are most likely to occur in chronic malabsorption, pregnancy, breast-feeding women, people who don't get adequate dietary vitamin D, and people who don't get enough exposure to sunlight (sunshine aids in the conversion of vitamin D). Because vitamin D is fat-soluble, it's also possible to develop a deficiency when the diet is so low in fat that adequate bile can't be manufactured and vitamin D isn't absorbed. People with long-term anorexia nervosa are at particular risk for this deficiency. Other at-risk populations include elderly people, postmenopausal women, patients with renal or hepatic disease, and those recuperating from intestinal resection or gastric surgery.

Signs and symptoms

Early signs and symptoms include nervousness, painful muscle spasms, leg cramps, and numbness of the arms and legs. Advanced vitamin D deficiency causes malformations from softening of the bones—bowed legs, knock-knees, scoliosis, narrow rib cage, protruding breast bone, or beading at the ends of the ribs—as well as tooth decay, delayed walking in children, irritability, restlessness, and profuse sweating. Osteomalacia causes pain in the bones of the shoulders, hips, and spine.

Serious conditions

Rickets in children is easy to identify because of the severe bone deformities that occur during a rapid growth period. However, osteomalacia (softening of the bones) commonly is misdiagnosed as osteoporosis (an increase in porosity of bone). Subclinical bone disease occurs with normal blood calcium levels. By the time severe bone disease is present, hypocalcemia and hypophosphatemia are found.

Complications

Because osteomalacia may go unrecognized and undiagnosed in adults, it's unwise for patients to take nutritional supplements for what appears to be osteoporosis, without receiving a full medical workup. Although calcium supplements usually contain some absorbable form of vitamin D, they aren't likely to provide proper amounts to promote repletion or prevent further loss.

Another major concern with self-treatment of a potential vitamin D deficiency is toxicity. Hypervitaminosis D occurs because the body's ability to absorb 25-hydroxyvitamin D_3 is unlimited. Acute hypercalcemia and hypercalciuria can result from excessive intake. This leads to nausea, anorexia, itching, polyuria, diarrhea, abdominal pain, and dehydration. Consistent, long-term abuse of vitamin D supplements can cause nephrocalcinosis, metastatic calcification, renal failure, and the development of kidney stones.

Nursing considerations

• Observe the patient for bony malformations.
• Ask the patient about muscle and leg cramps and peripheral numbness.
• Review the patient's dietary intake.
• Ask the patient about use of dietary supplements.
• Screen the patient for evidence of toxicity caused by vitamin D supplementation.
• Review the patient's medical record for a history of osteoporosis.

Patient teaching

• Explain to the patient the danger of taking vitamin D supplements without a proper medical workup.

• Encourage the patient to eat foods high in vitamin D, such as liver and fortified dairy products.

• Encourage the patient to get adequate exposure to the sun; about 10 to 15 minutes every day should be enough for the conversion of vitamin D to take place.

• Tell patient to limit intake of high-phosphate foods.

beta-carotene
biotin
calcium carbonate
calcium citrate
calcium glubionate
calcium gluconate
calcium lactate
calcium phosphate, tribasic
choline
chromium
cyanocobalamin (vitamin B_{12})
ferrous fumarate
ferrous gluconate
ferrous sulfate
folic acid (vitamin B_9)
inositol
lactobacillus
levocarnitine
lysine
magnesium chloride
magnesium gluconate
magnesium oxide
medium chain triglycerides
niacin (nicotinic acid, vitamin B_3)
niacinamide (nicotinamide)
omega-3 polyunsaturated fatty acids (fish oils)
pantothenic acid (vitamin B_5, calcium pantothenate)
phosphorus-replacement products
polysaccharide-iron complex
pyridoxine hydrochloride (vitamin B_6)
riboflavin (vitamin B_2)
selenium
thiamine hydrochloride (vitamin B_1)
vitamin A (retinol)
vitamin C (ascorbic acid)
vitamin D
vitamin E (tocopherols)
zinc gluconate
zinc sulfate

beta-carotene
Betatene, Lumitene, Max-Caro

Pregnancy Risk Category C

HOW SUPPLIED
Capsules: 5,000 IU, 10,000 IU, 25,000 IU; 15 mg, 60 mg

ACTION
Vitamin A precursor.

Route	Onset	Peak	Duration
P.O.	Unknown	4-6 wk	2-6 wk

INDICATIONS & DOSAGES
Dietary supplement—
Adults: 6 to 15 mg (equivalent to 10,000 to 25,000 IU of vitamin A) P.O. daily.
Children: 3 to 6 mg of beta-carotene (equivalent of 5,000 to 10,000 IU of vitamin A) P.O. daily.

Because potency of different supplement forms varies, follow manufacturer's label rec-

*Liquid contains alcohol. **May contain tartrazine. †Canada ‡Australia §U.K.

ommendations for specific products.

ADVERSE REACTIONS
GI: loose stools.
Musculoskeletal: arthralgia.
Skin: carotenodermia (yellow palms, soles and, to a lesser extent, face), ecchymosis.

INTERACTIONS
Drug-drug
Orlistat: may interfere with beta-carotene absorption. Tell patient to separate administration of drugs by 2 hours.

CONTRAINDICATIONS
Contraindicated in patients who are hypersensitive to the drug.

OVERDOSE & TREATMENT
Overdose may result in carotenodermia, which is usually reversible.

Patient should consult local poison control center.

NURSING CONSIDERATIONS
●Beta-carotene should be used cautiously by patients with impaired renal or hepatic function because safe use of the drug with these conditions hasn't been established.
●Beta-carotene is used as a dietary supplement and to reduce the severity of photosensitivity reactions in patients with erythropoietic protoporphyria.

Beta-carotene has also been used with variable success in the management of polymorphous light eruption and photosensitivity caused by other diseases.
●A patient taking beta-carotene should avoid supplemental vitamin A preparations because beta-carotene fulfills normal vitamin A requirements.
●Contents of beta-carotene capsules may be mixed with orange or tomato juice if children won't swallow capsules.

PATIENT TEACHING
●Advise patient older than age 60 who has renal or hepatic dysfunction to consult a doctor before starting beta-carotene therapy.
●Caution patient that large quantities of green or yellow vegetables or their juices or extracts aren't suitable substitutes for crystalline beta-carotene. Consumption of large amounts of these vegetables may cause adverse effects such as leukopenia or menstrual disorders.
●Inform parent or caregiver to consult doctor before giving drug to child.
●Inform patient that beta-carotene isn't effective as a sunscreen and shouldn't be used for that purpose.

Reactions may be *common*, uncommon, **_life-threatening_**, or **COMMON AND LIFE-THREATENING**.

• Advise parent or caregiver to keep medication away from children and pets.
• Tell breast-feeding patient that it isn't known if beta-carotene appears in breast milk; advise her to consult doctor before taking this drug.

---

biotin
Biotin, Biotin 5000, Vitamin H

Pregnancy Risk Category NR

HOW SUPPLIED
Capsules: 300 mcg, 1,000 mcg, 5,000 mcg
Lozenges: 1,000 mcg
Tablets: 300 mcg, 600 mcg

ACTION
Biotin plays a role in metabolizing fats and carbohydrates and converting proteins to carbohydrates. Biotin is critically involved in maintaining normal growth, nervous tissue, skin, hair, blood cells, and sex organs. The intestine manufactures part of the body's requirement for biotin.

Route	Onset	Peak	Duration
P.O.	Unknown	Unknown	Unknown

INDICATIONS & DOSAGES
Adequate intake—
Infants up to age 6 months: 5 mcg/day.

Infants ages 7 to 12 months: 6 mcg/day.
Children ages 1 to 3: 8 mcg/day.
Children ages 4 to 8: 12 mcg/day.
Children ages 9 to 13: 20 mcg/day.
Adolescents ages 14 to 18: 25 mcg/day.
Adults: 30 mcg/day.
Pregnant women: 30 mcg/day.
Breast-feeding women: 35 mcg/day.

Dietary supplement—
Adults and adolescents: 30 to 100 mcg P.O. daily.
Children ages 7 to 10: 30 mcg P.O. daily.
Children ages 4 to 6: 25 mcg P.O. daily.
Children from birth to age 3: 10 to 20 mcg P.O. daily.

Because potency of different supplement forms varies, patient should follow manufacturer's label recommendations for specific products.

ADVERSE REACTIONS
None reported.

INTERACTIONS
None reported.

CONTRAINDICATIONS
Contraindicated in patients who are hypersensitive to the supplement.

OVERDOSE & TREATMENT
No information available.

NURSING CONSIDERATIONS
● Estimated dietary intake is 100 to 200 mcg per day. Lack of biotin in a healthy diet is rare.
● A patient who consumes large amounts of raw egg whites may have a biotin deficiency. A protein in raw egg whites blocks biotin absorption.
● Biotin deficiency has been documented in patients receiving long-term parenteral nutritional support without proper vitamin supplementation, genetic disorders, seborrheic dermatitis in infants, and surgical removal of the stomach.
● Signs and symptoms of biotin deficiency include skin rash, hair loss, increased serum cholesterol levels, and cardiac problems.
● No specific requirement for biotin intake has been set, because of the intestine's role in manufacturing biotin.
● Because no information is available regarding safety of biotin use in pregnancy, pregnant women should avoid using it, unless directed by their doctor.
● Monitor patient's response to drug therapy.

PATIENT TEACHING
● Instruct patient to report adverse effects promptly to doctor.
● Instruct pregnant and breast-feeding patient to consult doctor before taking this supplement.
● Tell patient that dietary sources of biotin include liver, cauliflower, salmon, carrots, bananas, soy flour, cereals, and yeast.
● Instruct patient to keep all medication away from children and pets.

---

calcium carbonate
Apo-Cal†, Cal Carb-HD, Calci-Chew, Calciday-667, Calci-Mix, Calcite 500†, Calcium-600, Calglycine, Cal-Plus, Calsan†, Caltrate 600, Chooz, Dicarbosil, Gencalc 600, Mallamint, Nephro-Calci, Nu-Cal†, Os-Cal†, Os-Cal 500, Os-Cal Chewable†, Oysco, Oysco 500 Chewable, Oyst-Cal 500, Oystercal 500, Oyster Shell Calcium-500, Rolaids Calcium Rich, Super Calcium '1200', Titralac, Tums, Tums E-X

calcium citrate
Citracal, Citracal Liquitab†

calcium glubionate
Calcium-Sandoz Forte†, Neo-Calglucon

Reactions may be *common*, uncommon, *life-threatening*, or COMMON AND LIFE-THREATENING.

calcium gluconate

calcium lactate
Calphosan

calcium phosphate, tribasic
Posture

Pregnancy Risk Category C

HOW SUPPLIED
calcium carbonate
Contains 400 mg or 20 mEq of elemental calcium/g
Capsules: 600 mg, 1.25 g
Oral suspension: 1 g/5 ml, 1.25 g/5 ml
Powder packets: 6.5 g (2,400 mg calcium) per packet
Tablets: 650 mg, 1.25 g, 1.5 g
Tablets (chewable): 350 mg, 420 mg, 500 mg, 550 mg, 625 mg†, 750 mg, 835 mg, 850 mg, 1 g, 1.25 g

calcium citrate
Contains 211 mg or 10.6 mEq of elemental calcium/g
Tablets: 950 mg, 1.04 g
Tablets (effervescent): 2.376 g

calcium glubionate
Contains 64 mg or 3.2 mEq elemental calcium/g
Syrup: 1.8 g/5 ml

calcium gluconate
Contains 90 mg or 4.5 mEq of elemental calcium/g
Tablets: 500 mg, 650 mg, 1 g

calcium lactate
Contains 130 mg or 6.5 mEq of elemental calcium/g
Tablets: 325 mg, 650 mg

calcium phosphate, tribasic
Contains 400 mg or 20 mEq of elemental calcium/g
Tablets: 300 mg, 600 mg

ACTION
Replaces calcium and maintains calcium level.

Route	Onset	Peak	Duration
P.O.	Unknown	Unknown	Unknown

INDICATIONS & DOSAGES
Dietary supplement—
Adults: 500 mg to 2 g P.O. daily.
  Because potency of different supplement forms varies, patient should follow manufacturer's label recommendations for specific products.

ADVERSE REACTIONS
GI: abdominal pain, constipation, chalky taste, hemorrhage, irritation, nausea, thirst, vomiting.
GU: polyuria, renal calculi.
Metabolic: hypercalcemia.

INTERACTIONS
Drug-drug
Atenolol, fluoroquinolones, tetracyclines: decreases bioavailability of these drugs and calcium when taken together.

---

*Liquid contains alcohol.   **May contain tartrazine.   †Canada   ‡Australia   §U.K.

Tell patient to separate administration times by 2 to 4 hours.
Calcium channel blockers: decreases calcium effectiveness. Tell patient not to use together.
Cardiac glycosides: increases digitalis toxicity. Tell patients taking digitalis to use calcium cautiously, if at all.
Phenytoin: decreases absorption of both drugs. Advise patient to avoid using together or to have serum levels monitored.
Sodium polystyrene sulfonate: risk of metabolic acidosis in patients with renal disease. Tell patient not to use together.
Thiazide diuretics: risk of hypercalcemia. Have patient consult a doctor before using calcium.

Drug-food
Foods containing oxalic acid (rhubarb, spinach), phytic acid (bran, whole cereals), phosphorus (dairy products, milk): may interfere with calcium absorption. Tell patient not to use together.

Drug-lifestyle
Alcohol use: increases risk of osteoporosis. Advise patient to avoid using alcohol.
Smoking: increases risk of osteoporosis. Advise patient to avoid smoking.

CONTRAINDICATIONS
Contraindicated in patients with ventricular fibrillation, hypercalcemia, hypophosphatemia, or renal calculi; also contraindicated in cancer patients with bone metastases.

OVERDOSE & TREATMENT
Acute hypercalcemia syndrome is characterized by a markedly elevated plasma calcium level, lethargy, weakness, nausea, vomiting, and coma; it may lead to sudden death.

In case of overdose, calcium should be discontinued immediately. Treatment includes removal by emesis or gastric lavage, followed by supportive therapy, as needed.

NURSING CONSIDERATIONS
• Use all calcium products with extreme caution in patients with sarcoidosis, patients with renal or cardiac disease, and digitalized patients.
• Calcium is poorly absorbed. No more than 500 mg of elemental calcium should be given per dose.
• When determining the amount of calcium in a product, look at the amount of elemental calcium rather than the amount of calcium salt.
• Monitor blood calcium levels, as needed. Hypercalcemia may result after large doses in

chronic renal failure. Report abnormalities.

• With oral calcium, patient may need laxatives or stool softeners to manage constipation.

PATIENT TEACHING

• Tell patient to take oral calcium 1 to 1½ hours after meals if GI upset occurs.

• Tell patient to drink 8 ounces of water with each dose.

• Warn patient to avoid oxalic acid (in rhubarb and spinach), phytic acid (in bran and whole cereals), and phosphorus (in dairy products) in the meal preceding calcium consumption; these substances may interfere with calcium absorption.

• Warn elderly patient that calcium absorption may be decreased.

• Inform breast-feeding patient that calcium may pass into breast milk. Although quantities of calcium are not usually large, patient should consult doctor before taking this drug.

• Instruct patient to keep medications away from children and pets.

• Inform patient that coadministration with some medications may decrease their effectiveness.

---

choline
Intrachol, Lecithin, Lipotropic factor, PhosChol, Phosphatidyl Choline

Pregnancy Risk Category NR

HOW SUPPLIED
Capsules: 350 mg, 420 mg, 1,200 mg lecithin capsules (providing 58% to 60% soy phosphatides)
Powder: 375 mg/0.25 ml
Softgels: 440 mg, 565 mg, 900 mg, 1,200 mg lecithin softgels (providing 58% to 60% soy phosphatides)
Tablets: 250 mg, 300 mg, 500 mg, 650 mg

ACTION
Choline acts as a methyl donor in the body and is essential for liver function. It's required for the metabolism and excretion of fats. This is the major reason for using choline in patients with liver dysfunction or high cholesterol. Choline is also a precursor to the neurotransmitter, acetylcholine, in addition to being a key component of cell membranes. This is why choline is often used to enhance memory or as support in Alzheimer's patients.

Route	Onset	Peak	Duration
P.O.	Unknown	Unknown	Unknown

INDICATIONS & DOSAGES
Recommended intake—
Infants up to age 6 months: 125 mg/day.
Infants ages 7 to 12 months: 150 mg/day.
Children ages 1 to 3: 200 mg/day.
Children ages 4 to 8: 250 mg/day.
Children ages 9 to 13: 375 mg/day.
Boys ages 14 to 18: 550 mg/day.
Girls ages 14 to 18: 400 mg/day.
Adult men: 550 mg/day.
Adult women: 425 mg/day.
Pregnant women: 450 mg/day.
Breast-feeding women: 550 mg/day.

Dietary supplement—
Adults: less than 1 g P.O. daily. A typical diet provides 500 to 900 mg/day.
  Because potency of different supplement forms varies, patient should follow manufacturer's label recommendations for specific products.

ADVERSE REACTIONS
CNS: depression.
GI: nausea, decreased appetite, bloating, diarrhea, and abdominal pain.
Skin: diaphoresis.

INTERACTIONS
Drug-drug
Carnitine: increases intracellular carnitine levels by lowering urinary excretion of carnitine. Tell patient to use together only at recommended dosages.
Folic acid: promotes the conservation of folic acid. Tell patient to use together only at recommended dosages.
Nicotinic acid: increased levels of niacin may decrease choline levels. Monitor patient.

CONTRAINDICATIONS
Contraindicated in patients who are hypersensitive to choline or soy; these patients should avoid using lecithin, phosphatidylcholine, or choline products.

OVERDOSE & TREATMENT
Sustained megadosing (above 6,000 mg per day) may result in dizziness, nausea, and vomiting.
  Stop medication and consult doctor and poison control center.

NURSING CONSIDERATIONS
• Choline deficiency is rare but can lead to internal bleeding in the kidneys, excessively high blood pressure, heart disease, and degeneration in the liver.
• It has been theorized that supplementing with choline during pregnancy will enhance brain

function in newborns. Some prenatal vitamin preparations contain choline. It's controversial whether supplementing with choline during pregnancy is harmful or beneficial. Advise patient to consult doctor.

• Choline is well tolerated at recommended dosages.

• Choline supplements can be taken with meals to avoid adverse GI effects.

• If patient takes L-carnitine or folic acid with choline, monitor folic acid and carnitine levels at least weekly.

• At high dosages, choline may cause an unpleasant breath and body odor.

• Choline is generally available in a salt form, such as choline bitartrate, or as phosphatidylcholine present in lecithin.

PATIENT TEACHING

• Instruct patient to take choline supplements with meals to decrease stomach upset.

• Inform patient that higher dosages of choline may have a fishy odor.

• Advise patient not to exceed maximum recommended dosage.

• Discuss with patient (and parent, if appropriate) correct choline dosing and intake to avoid adverse effects.

• Instruct patient to avoid consumption of greater amounts than those found in food or prenatal vitamins.

• Dietary sources of choline include cabbage, cauliflower, chickpeas, green beans, lentils, soybeans, split peas, calf's liver, eggs, rice, and soy lecithin.

• Advise patient to keep all medication away from children and pets.

• Inform pregnant and breastfeeding patients that choline supplementation during pregnancy and lactation isn't recommended.

• Instruct pregnant and breastfeeding patients to consult doctor before taking any supplements or alternative medicines.

---

chromium
Chromemate, Chromium-Enriched Yeast, Chromium Picolinate, Chromium Polynicotinate (niacin-bound GTF chromium), GTF Chromium, Ultrachrome

Pregnancy Risk Category C

HOW SUPPLIED
Capsules: 100 mcg, 200 mcg, 500 mcg
Tablets: 50 mcg, 100 mcg, 200 mcg

ACTION
It's thought that chromium's main benefit is in improving

---

glucose tolerance, although existing data are insufficient. Chromium is a component of glucose tolerance factor, which facilitates the binding of insulin to insulin receptors. Thus, it may increase insulin's effects on lipid and carbohydrate metabolism and may aid in weight loss.

Route	Onset	Peak	Duration
P.O.	Unknown	Unknown	Unknown

INDICATIONS & DOSAGES
RDAs—
Infants up to age 6 months: 10 to 40 mcg/day.
Infants ages 6 to 12 months: 20 to 60 mcg/day.
Children ages 1 to 3: 20 to 80 mcg/day.
Children ages 4 to 6: 30 to 120 mcg/day.
Adults and children ages 7 and older: 50 to 200 mcg/day.

Dietary supplement to prevent deficiency—
Adults and teenagers: 50 to 200 mcg P.O. daily.
Children ages 7 to 10 years: 50 to 200 mcg P.O. daily.
Children ages 4 to 6 years: 30 to 120 mcg P.O. daily.
Children up to age 3 years: 10 to 80 mcg P.O. daily.

Because potency of different supplement forms varies, patient should follow manufacturer's label recommendations for specific products.

ADVERSE REACTIONS
CNS: cognitive, perceptual, and motor dysfunction; *seizures, coma.*
EENT: nasal mucosal ulceration, perforation of the nasal septum.
GI: nausea, vomiting, ulceration.
GU: *renal failure.*
Hematologic: anemia, *thrombocytopenia,* hemolysis.
Hepatic: hepatic dysfunction.
Respiratory: allergic asthma, *respiratory tract cancers.*

INTERACTIONS
Drug-drug
Insulin: may increase risk of hypoglycemia. Tell patient to monitor serum glucose levels closely.
Nicotinic acid: synergistic effect with chromium in improving glucose tolerance. Urge patient to use caution.
Vitamin B_3: use together may improve glucose tolerance. Urge patient to use caution.
Vitamin C: use together may increase chromium absorption. Urge patient to use caution.
Zinc: coadministration may decrease absorption of both chromium and zinc. Urge patient to use caution.

CONTRAINDICATIONS
Contraindicated in patients who are hypersensitive to chromium or any of its salt forms.

OVERDOSE & TREATMENT
Chromium toxicity may cause nausea and vomiting, GI ulceration, renal damage (acute tubular necrosis), hepatic damage, seizures, and coma. Severe eczematous dermatitis and ulceration may follow a topical overexposure to chromium.

Treatment includes ensuring the patient's airway patency, breathing, and circulation; symptomatic treatment; and chelation of chromium using dimercaprol.

NURSING CONSIDERATIONS
• *Alert:* Patients with renal insufficiency and patients who undergo dialysis should use chromium supplementation cautiously because the kidneys excrete chromium.
• Deficiency conditions result from inadequate nutrition, protein malnutrition, or intestinal malabsorption but don't occur in healthy individuals. Deficiency in chromium may affect glucose tolerance and cause peripheral or central neuropathy.
• *Alert:* It isn't known if chromium causes fetal harm or affects reproductive capacity.

• A deficiency in chromium may play a role in glucose intolerance during pregnancy. Women should avoid chromium supplements during pregnancy and breast-feeding.
• Chromium may interfere with dopamine, norepinephrine, and serotonin metabolism in the brain because of the picolinate salt.
• Advise diabetic patient about the potential of chromium to cause hypoglycemia.
• Oral chromium appears to be very well tolerated when given orally or intravenously.
• Toxicity rarely develops at recommended dosages.

PATIENT TEACHING
• Instruct patient with diabetes to carefully monitor serum glucose levels while using chromium and antidiabetics (such as insulin or a sulfonylurea) because the risk of hypoglycemia rises.
• Instruct patient with a history of renal insufficiency or end-stage renal disease that he should be closely monitored to determine chromium excretion. Daily serum chromium levels provide a valuable guideline to assess the kidney's ability to excrete chromium.
• Instruct parent or caregiver not to exceed the recommended dosages for daily chromium intake in infants and children.

---

*Liquid contains alcohol.   **May contain tartrazine.   †Canada   ‡Australia   §U.K.

• Inform breast-feeding patient that chromium appears in breast milk and will be absorbed into an infant's bloodstream. Patient should consult doctor before taking this drug.

• Instruct pregnant patient to consult doctor before taking this drug. Advise her that chromium is in most prenatal vitamin preparations.

• Discuss proper dietary habits. Inform patient that the best nutritional sources of chromium are brewer's yeast, calf's liver, American cheese, and wheat germ. Other sources are meats, fish, oysters, other dairy products, eggs, fresh fruit, potatoes with skin, whole grain products, and condiments such as black pepper and thyme.

• Advise patient to keep all medications away from children and pets.

• Remind patient to inform doctor of all medications and herbal supplements he's taking.

cyanocobalamin (vitamin B$_{12}$)
Crystamine, Crysti-12, Cyanocobalamin, Cyanoject, Cyomin, Rubesol-1000, Rubramin PC

Pregnancy Risk Category C (if doses exceed RDA)

HOW SUPPLIED
Tablets: 25 mcg, 50 mcg, 100 mcg, 250 mcg, 500 mcg, 1,000 mcg

ACTION
A coenzyme that stimulates metabolic function and is needed for cell replication, hematopoiesis, and nucleoprotein and myelin synthesis.

Route	Onset	Peak	Duration
P.O.	Unknown	8-12 hr	Unknown

INDICATIONS & DOSAGES
RDA—
Children ages 1 to 3: 0.9 mcg/day.
Children ages 4 to 8: 1.2 mcg/day.
Children ages 9 to 13: 1.8 mcg/day.
Adults and children ages 14 and older: 2.4 mcg/day.
Pregnant women: 2.6 mcg/day.
Breast-feeding women: 2.8 mcg/day.

Adequate intake—
Infants up to age 6 months: 0.4 mcg (0.06 mcg/kg)/day.
Infants ages 6 months to 1 year: 0.5 mcg (0.06 mcg/kg)/day.

Dietary supplement—
Adults and children: 1 to 25 mcg P.O. daily.

Cyanocobalamin deficiency—
Adults: 25 to 250 mcg P.O. daily.

Because potency of different supplement forms varies, patient should follow manufacturer's label recommendations for specific products.

ADVERSE REACTIONS
CV: peripheral vascular thrombosis, pulmonary edema, *heart failure.*
GI: transient diarrhea.
Skin: itching, transitory exanthema, urticaria.
Other: *anaphylaxis.*

INTERACTIONS
Drug-drug
Aminoglycosides, aminosalicylic acid and salts, anticonvulsants, colchicine, extended-release potassium products: malabsorption of vitamin B_{12}. Advise patient not to use together.

Drug-lifestyle
Alcohol use: malabsorption of vitamin B_{12}. Tell patient not to use together.
Smoking: increases requirement for vitamin B_{12}. Advise patient to avoid smoking during use.

CONTRAINDICATIONS
Contraindicated in patients who are hypersensitive to vitamin B_{12} or cobalt and in those with early Leber's disease.

OVERDOSE & TREATMENT
Even in large doses, vitamin B_{12} is usually nontoxic.

NURSING CONSIDERATIONS
• Use cautiously in anemic patients with coexisting cardiac, pulmonary, or hypertensive disease and in patients with severe vitamin B_{12}-dependent deficiencies.
• Determine reticulocyte count, hematocrit, vitamin B_{12}, iron, and folate levels before patient begins cyanocobalamin, as ordered.
• Don't give large oral doses of vitamin B_{12} routinely; drug is lost through excretion.
• Infection, tumors, or renal, hepatic, and other debilitating diseases may reduce therapeutic response.
• Deficiencies are more common in patients who are strict vegetarians and in their breast-fed infants.
• Vitamin B_{12} deficiency may suppress signs and symptoms of polycythemia vera.
• Vitamin B_{12} may cause false-positive results for intrinsic factor antibodies, which are present in the blood of half of all patients with pernicious anemia. Methotrexate, pyrimethamine, and most anti-infectives invalidate diagnostic blood assays for vitamin B_{12}.

- Patient should protect vitamin B_{12} from light and avoid refrigerating or freezing.

PATIENT TEACHING
- Teach patient healthy dietary habits. Explain that vitamin B_{12} is found in meat, fish, poultry, milk and milk drinks, and fortified ready-to-eat cereals.
- Instruct patient to report adverse effects promptly.

---

ferrous fumarate
Femiron, Feostat, Feostat Drops, Fersamal§, Hemocyte, Ircon, Nephro-Fer, Novofumar†, Palafer†, Palafer Pediatric Drops†, Span-FF

Pregnancy Risk Category A

HOW SUPPLIED
Each 100 mg of ferrous fumarate provides 33 mg of elemental iron.
Drops: 45 mg/0.6 ml
Oral suspension: 100 mg/5 ml
Tablets: 63 mg, 200 mg, 324 mg, 325 mg, 350 mg
Tablets (chewable): 100 mg

ACTION
Provides elemental iron, an essential component in the formation of hemoglobin.

Route	Onset	Peak	Duration
P.O.	4 days	7-10 days	2-4 mon

INDICATIONS & DOSAGES
RDA—
Infants up to age 6 months: 6 mg/day.
Children ages 6 months to 10 years: 10 mg/day.
Men ages 11 to 18 years: 12 mg/day.
Men ages 19 and older: 10 mg/day.
Women ages 11 and older: 15 mg/day.
Pregnant women: 30 mg/day.
Breast-feeding women: 15 mg/day.

Dietary supplement—
Because potency of different supplement forms varies, patient should follow manufacturer's label recommendations for specific products.

Iron deficiency—
Adults: 50 to 100 mg P.O. of elemental iron t.i.d.
Children: 3 to 6 mg/kg/day P.O. of elemental iron in three divided doses.

ADVERSE REACTIONS
GI: nausea, epigastric pain, vomiting, constipation, diarrhea, black stools, anorexia, abdominal cramps.

Other: temporarily stained teeth from suspension and drops.

INTERACTIONS
Drug-drug
Antacids, cholestyramine resin, cimetidine, vitamin E: decreases iron absorption. Tell patient to separate doses by at least 2 hours.
Chloramphenicol: delays response to iron therapy. Monitor patient.
Fluoroquinolones, penicillamine, tetracyclines: decreases GI absorption, possibly resulting in decreased serum levels or efficacy of antibiotic. Tell patient to separate doses by 2 to 4 hours.
Levodopa, methyldopa: decreases absorption and efficacy of levodopa and methyldopa. Monitor patient for decreased effect of these drugs.
L-thyroxine: decreases L-thyroxine absorption. Tell patient to separate doses by at least 2 hours. Monitor thyroid function.
Vitamin C: may increase iron absorption. Advise patient to take together.

Drug-herb
Oregano: may reduce iron absorption. Advise patient using oregano to wait at least 2 hours before taking iron supplements or iron-containing foods.

Drug-food
Cereals, cheese, coffee, eggs, milk, tea, whole-grain breads, yogurt: may impair oral iron absorption. Advise patient not to take together.

CONTRAINDICATIONS
Contraindicated in patients with primary hemochromatosis, hemosiderosis, hemolytic anemia unless iron deficiency anemia is also present, peptic ulcer disease, regional enteritis, or ulcerative colitis; also contraindicated in those receiving repeated blood transfusions.

OVERDOSE & TREATMENT
The lethal dose of iron is between 200 and 250 mg/kg; fatalities have occurred with lower doses. Signs and symptoms may follow ingestion of 20 to 60 mg/kg.

Between ½ and 8 hours after ingestion, patient may experience lethargy, nausea, vomiting, green or tarry stools, weak and rapid pulse, hypotension, dehydration, acidosis, and coma.

If death doesn't occur immediately, signs and symptoms may clear for about 24 hours. At 12 to 48 hours, they may return, accompanied by diffuse vascular congestion, pulmonary edema, shock, seizures, anuria, and hyperthermia. Death may follow.

Treatment requires immediate support of airway, respiration, and circulation. Induce emesis with ipecac in conscious patients with intact gag reflex; for unconscious patients, empty stomach by gastric lavage. Follow emesis with lavage, using 1% sodium bicarbonate solution, to convert iron to less irritating, poorly absorbed form. (Phosphate solutions have been used but carry risk of other adverse effects.) Use radiographic evaluation of abdomen to determine continued presence of excess iron; if serum iron levels exceed 350 mg/dl, deferoxamine may be used for systemic chelation.

Survivors are likely to sustain organ damage, including pyloric or antral stenosis, hepatic cirrhosis, CNS damage, and intestinal obstruction.

NURSING CONSIDERATIONS
• Urge patient to use cautiously on long-term basis.
• GI upset may be related to dose.
• Between-meal doses are preferable but drug may be taken with some foods, although absorption may be decreased. Enteric-coated products reduce GI upset but also reduce amount of iron absorbed.
• Check for constipation; record color and amount of stools.
• Oral iron may turn stools black. Although this unabsorbed iron is harmless, it could mask the presence of melena.
• Monitor hemoglobin levels and hematocrit and reticulocyte count during therapy, as ordered.
• Combination products such as Ferro-Sequels contain stool softeners that help to prevent constipation, a common adverse reaction.
• Because ferrous fumarate blackens feces, it may interfere with tests for occult blood in the stool; the guaiac test and orthotoluidine tests may yield false-positive results, but the benzidine test isn't usually affected.
• Iron overload may decrease uptake of technetium 99m and, thus, interfere with skeletal imaging.
• *Alert:* Don't confuse different iron salts; elemental content may vary.

PATIENT TEACHING
• Tell patient to take tablets with juice (preferably orange juice) or water, but not with milk or antacids.
• To avoid staining teeth, tell patient to take suspension with straw and place drops at back of throat.

- Instruct patient not to take large doses of iron for longer than 6 months without consulting doctor.
- Caution patient not to crush tablets or to chew extended-release iron preparations.
- Advise patient not to substitute one iron salt for another; the amount of elemental iron may vary.
- Tell patient that dietary sources of iron include fish, meat (especially liver), and fortified cereals and breads.
- *Alert:* Inform parents that as few as three tablets can cause serious poisoning and death in children.
- Inform elderly patient that iron-induced constipation is common; stress importance of proper diet.
- Tell breast-feeding patient to consult doctor. Iron supplements are often recommended and no adverse effects have been reported.

---

ferrous gluconate
Fergon*, Fertinic†, Novoferrogluc†

Pregnancy Risk Category A

HOW SUPPLIED
Each 100 mg of ferrous gluconate provides 11.6 mg of elemental iron.

Tablets: 240 mg, 325 mg

ACTION
Provides elemental iron, an essential component in the formation of hemoglobin.

Route	Onset	Peak	Duration
P.O.	4 days	7-10 days	2-4 mo

INDICATIONS & DOSAGES
RDA—
Infants up to age 6 months: 6 mg/day.
Children ages 6 months to 10 years: 10 mg/day.
Men ages 11 to 18: 12 mg/day.
Men ages 19 and older: 10 mg/day.
Women ages 11 and older: 15 mg/day.
Pregnant women: 30 mg/day.
Breast-feeding women: 15 mg/day.

Dietary supplement—
Because potency of different supplement forms varies, patient should follow manufacturer's label recommendations for specific products.

Iron deficiency—
Adults: 100 to 200 mg P.O. of elemental iron t.i.d.
Children: 3 to 6 mg/kg/day P.O. of elemental iron in three divided doses.

ADVERSE REACTIONS
GI: nausea, epigastric pain, vomiting, constipation, diarrhea, black stools, anorexia, abdominal pain.

INTERACTIONS
Drug-drug
Antacids, cholestyramine resin, cimetidine, vitamin E: decreases iron absorption. Tell patient to separate doses by at least 2 hours.
Chloramphenicol: delays response to iron therapy. Monitor patient.
Fluoroquinolones, penicillamine, tetracyclines: decreases GI absorption, possibly resulting in decreased serum levels or efficacy of antibiotic. Tell patient to separate doses by 2 to 4 hours.
Levodopa, methyldopa: decreases absorption and efficacy of levodopa and methyldopa. Monitor patient for decreased effect of these drugs.
L-thyroxine: decreases L-thyroxine absorption. Separate doses by at least 2 hours. Monitor thyroid function.
Vitamin C: may increase iron absorption. Tell patient to take together.

Drug-herb
Oregano: may reduce iron absorption. Advise patient taking oregano to wait at least 2 hours before taking iron supplements or iron-containing foods.

Drug-food
Cereals, cheese, coffee, eggs, milk, tea, whole-grain breads, yogurt: may impair oral iron absorption. Advise patient not to take together.

CONTRAINDICATIONS
Contraindicated in patients with peptic ulceration, regional enteritis, ulcerative colitis, hemosiderosis, primary hemochromatosis, or hemolytic anemia (unless an iron-deficiency anemia is also present); also contraindicated in those receiving repeated blood transfusions.

OVERDOSE & TREATMENT
The lethal dose of iron is between 200 and 250 mg/kg; deaths have occurred with lower doses. Signs and symptoms may follow ingestion of 20 to 60 mg/kg.

Between ½ and 8 hours after ingestion, patient may experience lethargy, nausea, vomiting, green or tarry stools, weak and rapid pulse, hypotension, dehydration, acidosis, and coma.

If death doesn't occur immediately, signs and symptoms may clear for about 24 hours. At 12 to 48 hours, they may return, accompanied by diffuse vascular congestion, pulmonary edema, shock, seizures, anuria, and hyperthermia. Death may follow.

Treatment requires immediate support of airway, respiration, and circulation. Induce emesis with ipecac in conscious patients with intact gag reflex; for unconscious patients, empty stomach by gastric lavage. Follow emesis with lavage, using 1% sodium bicarbonate solution, to convert iron to less irritating, poorly absorbed form. (Phosphate solutions have been used but carry risk of other adverse effects.) Use radiographic evaluation of abdomen to determine continued presence of excess iron; if serum iron levels exceed 350 mg/dl, deferoxamine may be used for systemic chelation.

Survivors are likely to sustain organ damage, including pyloric or antral stenosis, hepatic cirrhosis, CNS damage, and intestinal obstruction.

NURSING CONSIDERATIONS
• Urge patient to use cautiously on long-term basis.
• GI upset may be related to dose.
• Between-meal doses are preferable but drug may be taken with some foods, although absorption may be decreased. Enteric-coated products reduce GI upset but also reduce the amount of iron absorbed.
• Check for constipation; record color and amount of stools.
• Oral iron may turn stools black. Although this unabsorbed iron is harmless, it could mask melena.
• Monitor hemoglobin levels, hematocrit, and reticulocyte count, as ordered.
• Because ferrous gluconate blackens feces, it may interfere with test for occult blood in the stool; guaiac and orthotoluidine tests may yield false-positive results, but the benzidine test isn't usually affected.
• Iron overload may decrease uptake of technetium 99m and, thus, interfere with skeletal imaging.
• *Alert:* Don't confuse different iron salts; elemental content may vary.

PATIENT TEACHING
• To promote absorption, tell patient to take tablets with orange juice.
• Tell patient that dietary sources of iron include fish, meat (especially liver), and fortified cereals and bread.
• *Alert:* Inform parents that as few as three tablets can cause serious iron poisoning and death in children.
• Instruct patient not to take large doses of iron for longer

than 6 months without consulting doctor.

• Caution patient not to substitute one iron salt for another because the amounts of elemental iron vary.

• Inform elderly patient that iron-induced constipation is common; stress proper diet.

• Inform breast-feeding patient that iron supplements are often recommended and that no adverse effects have been reported; patient should consult doctor.

---

ferrous sulfate
Apo-Ferrous Sulfate†
Feosol*, Fer-In-Sol Drops*,
Fer-In-Sol Syrup*, Fer-Iron
Drops, Mol-Iron*

ferrous sulfate, exsiccated
Feosol, Feospan§,
Novoferrosulfa†, PMS-
Ferrous Sulfate†, Slow FE

Pregnancy Risk Category A

HOW SUPPLIED
Ferrous sulfate is 20% elemental iron; dried and powdered, about 32% elemental iron.
Capsules: 250 mg
Drops: 125 mg/ml
Elixir: 220 mg/5 ml*
Syrup: 90 mg/5 ml

Tablets: 200 mg (dried), 300 mg (dried), 325 mg
Tablets (extended-release): 160 mg (dried)

ACTION
Provides elemental iron, an essential component in the formation of hemoglobin.

Route	Onset	Peak	Duration
P.O.	4 days	7-10 days	2-4 mo

INDICATIONS & DOSAGES
RDA—
Infants up to age 6 months: 6 mg/day.
Children ages 6 months to 10 years: 10 mg/day.
Men ages 11 to 18: 12 mg/day.
Men ages 19 and older: 10 mg/day.
Women ages 11 and older: 15 mg/day.
Pregnant women: 30 mg/day.
Breast-feeding women: 15 mg/day.

Dietary supplement—
Because potency of different supplement forms varies, patient should follow manufacturer's label recommendations for specific products.

Iron deficiency—
Adults: 100 to 200 mg P.O. of elemental iron t.i.d.

Children: 3 to 6 mg/kg/day
P.O. of elemental iron in three
divided doses.

ADVERSE REACTIONS
GI: nausea, epigastric pain,
vomiting, constipation, black
stools, diarrhea, anorexia, abdominal pain.
Other: temporarily stained
teeth from liquid forms.

INTERACTIONS
Drug-drug
*Antacids, cholestyramine resin,
cimetidine, vitamin E:* decreases iron absorption. Tell patient
to separate doses, if possible.
Chloramphenicol: delays response to iron therapy. Monitor
patient.
*Fluoroquinolones, penicil-
lamine, tetracyclines:* decreases
GI absorption, possibly resulting in decreased serum levels or
efficacy of the antibiotic. Tell
patient to separate doses by 2 to
4 hours.
Levodopa, methyldopa: decreases absorption and efficacy
of levodopa and methyldopa.
Monitor patient for decreased
effect of these drugs.
L-thyroxine: decreases L-
thyroxine absorption. Tell patient to separate doses by at
least 2 hours. Monitor thyroid
function.

Vitamin C: may increase iron
absorption. Tell patient to take
together.

Drug-herb
Oregano: may reduce iron absorption. Tell patient to separate
from iron supplements or iron-
containing foods by at least 2
hours.

Drug-food
*Cereals, cheese, coffee, eggs,
milk, tea, whole-grain breads,
yogurt:* may impair oral iron
absorption. Tell patient not to
use together.

CONTRAINDICATIONS
Contraindicated in patients
with hemosiderosis, primary
hemochromatosis, hemolytic
anemia (unless iron deficiency
anemia is also present), peptic
ulceration, ulcerative colitis, or
regional enteritis. Also contraindicated in those receiving
repeated blood transfusions.

OVERDOSE & TREATMENT
The lethal dose of iron is between 200 and 250 mg/kg;
deaths have occurred with lower doses. Signs and symptoms
may follow ingestion of 20 to
60 mg/kg.
  Between ½ and 8 hours after
ingestion, patient may experience lethargy, nausea, vomiting,
green or tarry stools, weak and

rapid pulse, hypotension, dehydration, acidosis, and coma.

If death doesn't occur immediately, signs and symptoms may clear for about 24 hours. At 12 to 48 hours, signs and symptoms may return, accompanied by diffuse vascular congestion, pulmonary edema, shock, seizures, anuria, and hyperthermia. Death may follow.

Treatment requires immediate support of airway, respiration, and circulation. Induce emesis with ipecac in conscious patients with intact gag reflex; for unconscious patients, empty stomach by gastric lavage. Follow emesis with lavage, using 1% sodium bicarbonate solution, to convert iron to less irritating, poorly absorbed form. (Phosphate solutions have been used but carry risk of other adverse effects.) Use radiographic evaluation of abdomen to determine continued presence of excess iron; if serum iron levels exceed 350 mg/dl, deferoxamine may be used for systemic chelation.

Survivors are likely to sustain organ damage, including pyloric or antral stenosis, hepatic cirrhosis, CNS damage, and intestinal obstruction.

NURSING CONSIDERATIONS
• Tell patient to use cautiously on long-term basis.

• GI upset may be related to dose.
• Between-meal doses are preferable but drug may be taken with some foods, although absorption may be decreased. Enteric-coated products reduce GI upset but also reduce the amount of iron absorbed.
• Oral iron may turn stools black. Although this unabsorbed iron is harmless, it could mask melena.
• Monitor hemoglobin levels, hematocrit, and reticulocyte count during therapy, as ordered.
• Ferrous sulfate blackens feces and may interfere with tests for occult blood in the stool; guaiac and orthotoluidine tests may yield false-positive results, but the benzidine test isn't usually affected.
• Iron overload may decrease uptake of technetium 99m and, thus, interfere with skeletal imaging.
• *Alert:* Don't confuse different iron salts; elemental content may vary.

PATIENT TEACHING
• Tell patient to take with juice.
• Instruct patient not to crush or chew extended-release forms.
• *Alert:* Inform parents that as few as three tablets can cause serious iron poisoning and death in children.

Reactions may be *common*, uncommon, *life-threatening*, or COMMON AND LIFE-THREATENING.

• Instruct patient not to take large amounts of iron for longer than 6 months without checking with doctor.

• Caution patient not to substitute one iron salt for another because amounts of elemental iron vary.

• Advise patient to report constipation and change in stool color or consistency.

• Inform elderly patient that iron-induced constipation is common; stress proper diet.

• Tell patient that dietary sources of iron include fish, meat (especially liver), and fortified cereals and bread.

• Inform breast-feeding patient that iron supplements are often recommended and that no adverse effects have been reported; patient should consult doctor.

folic acid (vitamin B₉)
Folvite, Novo-Folacid†

Pregnancy Risk Category A

HOW SUPPLIED
Tablets: 0.4 mg, 0.8 mg

ACTION
Stimulates normal erythropoiesis and nucleoprotein synthesis.

Route	Onset	Peak	Duration
P.O.	Unknown	30-60 min	Unknown

INDICATIONS & DOSAGES
RDA—
Children ages 1 to 3: 150 mcg/day.
Children ages 4 to 8: 200 mcg/day.
Children ages 9 to 13: 300 mcg/day.
Children ages 14 to 18: 400 mcg/day.
Adults: 400 mcg/day.
Pregnant women: 600 mcg/day.
Breast-feeding women: 500 mcg/day.

Adequate intake—
Infants up to age 6 months: 65 mcg/day.
Infants ages 6 months to 1 year: 80 mcg/day.

Nutritional supplement—
Adults and children ages 4 and older: 400 mcg P.O. daily.
Children younger than age 4: up to 300 mcg P.O. daily.
Infants: 100 mcg P.O. daily.
Pregnant and lactating women: 800 mcg P.O. daily.

Because potency of different supplement forms varies, patient should follow manufacturer's label recommendations for specific products.

ADVERSE REACTIONS
CNS: altered sleep pattern, general malaise, difficulty concentrating, confusion, impaired judgment, irritability, overactivity.

GI: anorexia, nausea, flatulence, bitter taste.
Respiratory: *bronchospasm.*
Skin: allergic reactions including rash, pruritus, and erythema.

INTERACTIONS
Drug-drug
Aminosalicylic acid, chloramphenicol, methotrexate, oral contraceptives, sulfasalazine, trimethoprim: acts as antagonist of folic acid. Watch for decreased folic acid effect. Tell patient to use together cautiously.
Phenytoin: increases anticonvulsant metabolism causing decreased blood levels of the anticonvulsant. Monitor patient closely.

CONTRAINDICATIONS
Contraindicated in patients with vitamin B_{12} deficiency.

OVERDOSE & TREATMENT
Folic acid is relatively nontoxic. Adverse GI and CNS effects develop rarely in patients taking 15 mg of folic acid daily for 1 month.

NURSING CONSIDERATIONS
• *Alert:* Don't confuse folic acid with folinic acid.
• Patients undergoing renal dialysis are at risk for folate deficiency.
• The U.S. Public Health Service recommends use of folic acid during pregnancy to decrease neural tube defects.
• Drug alters serum and RBC folate levels; falsely low serum and RBC folate levels may occur with *Lactobacillus casei* assay in patients receiving anti-infectives, such as tetracycline, that suppress growth of this organism.
• Protect drug from light and heat; store at room temperature.

PATIENT TEACHING
• Teach patient about proper nutrition to prevent anemia.
• Stress importance of follow-up visits and laboratory studies.
• Teach patient about foods that contain folic acid, including liver, oranges, whole wheat, broccoli, and Brussels sprouts.
• Tell patient that folate is destroyed by overcooking and canning.

---

inositol
Cyclohexitol, Inose, Inosite, Inositol hexaphosphate, IP6, Myoinositol, Phytate, Phytic Acid

Pregnancy Risk Category C

HOW SUPPLIED
Capsules: 500 mg
Crystals: 600 mg/0.25 ml
Powder: 375 mg/0.25 ml, 500 mg/0.25 ml, 550 mg/1.25

---

ml, 600 mg/0.25 ml, 845 mg/
0.25 ml
Tablets: 250 mg, 500 mg,
600 mg, 650 mg

ACTION
Inositol is a key component of
cell membrane phospholipids
required for proper nerve,
brain, and muscle function. It
exerts a lipotropic effect, mean-
ing it promotes the export of fat
from liver and intestinal cells.
Inositol also has anti-cancer
properties; for example, it
boosts the natural killer cell
line. It also may reverse desen-
sitization of serotonin receptors.

Route	Onset	Peak	Duration
P.O.	Unknown	Unknown	Unknown

INDICATIONS & DOSAGES
Dietary supplement—
Adults: 500 to 1,000 mg P.O.
daily.

Because potency of different
supplement forms varies, patient should follow manufacturer's label recommendations for
specific products.

ADVERSE REACTIONS
None reported.

INTERACTIONS
Drug-drug
*Minerals (especially calcium,
zinc, and iron):* inositol may interfere with absorption of these
minerals. Tell patient not to use
together.

CONTRAINDICATIONS
Contraindicated in patients who
are hypersensitive to inositol or
any of its components.

OVERDOSE & TREATMENT
No information available.

NURSING CONSIDERATIONS
• Insufficient data exist on the
use of inositol in pregnancy.
• Inositol is found in some
prenatal vitamins.
• Inositol may interfere with
absorption of calcium, iron,
and zinc, so administration
times should be separated by at
least 2 hours.
• Monitor patient's response to
drug therapy.
• Monitor patient for adverse
signs and symptoms.

PATIENT TEACHING
• Discuss proper dosing
regimens with patient who is
taking inositol supplements.
• Instruct patient on dietary
sources of inositol, including
dried beans, chickpeas, lentils,
cantaloupe, citrus fruits (other
than lemons), calf's liver, pork,
veal, nuts, oats, rice, whole-
grain products, lecithin granules, and wheat germ.

- Inform patient that dividing the dose may provide steadier levels in the bloodstream.
- Instruct patient not to take inositol if he's allergic to it.
- Supplementation in children usually isn't necessary; advise parent or caregiver to consult doctor.
- Inform breast-feeding patient that little data exists on use of inositol during breast-feeding; urge patient to consult doctor.
- Advise pregnant and breast-feeding patient that breast milk is rich in endogenous inositol.
- Advise parent or caregiver to keep all medication away from children and pets.
- Urge patient to report adverse effects promptly.

---

lactobacillus
Acidophilus, Bacid, DDS-Acidophilus, Fermalac†, FLORAjen, Intestinex, Kala, Kyo-Dophilus, Lactinex, *Lactobacillus acidophilus,* More-Dophilus, Pro-Bionate, Probiotic, Superdophilus, Ultra-Flora DF

Pregnancy Risk Category NR

HOW SUPPLIED
Capsules: 500 million or more *Lactobacillus acidophilus* per capsule, 1 billion *L. acidophilus* per capsule, 2 billion *L. aci-dophilus* per capsule, 5 billion *L. acidophilus* (NCFM strain) per capsule
Granules: mixed culture of *L. acidophilus* and *L. bulgaricus*
Powder: more than 2 billion *L. acidophilus* per ¼ tsp, 2 billion *L. acidophilus* (NAS strain) per 1g, 4 billion U acidophilus -carrot derivative per 1 g, 5 billion *L. acidophilus* (NCFM strain) per ¼ tsp
Tablets: mixed culture of *L. acidophilus* and *L. bulgaricus* (chewable), 200 million *L. acidophilus* soy-based per tablet

ACTION
L. acidophilus, a normal component of the body's intestinal flora, inhibits the overgrowth of pathogenic fungi and bacteria by producing lactic acid, hydrogen peroxide, and bacteriocins. Bacteriocins are proteins that exert a lethal effect on pathogenic bacteria. *L. acidophilus* also competes for nutrients that pathogenic bacteria and fungi live on and alters oxygen tension levels in the surrounding environment. Bacteria inhibited by *L. acidophilus* include *Bacillus cereus, B. stearothermophilus, B. subtilis, Candida albicans, Clostridium perfringens, Escherichia coli, Klebsiella pneumoniae, L. bulgaricus, L. fermenti, L. helveticus, L. lactis, L. leichmanii, L. plantarum,*

Proteus vulgaris, Pseudomonas aeruginosa, P. fluorescens, Salmonella schottmuelleri, S. typhosa, Shigella dysenteriae, S. paradysenteriae, Serratia marcescens, Staphylococcus aureus, Streptococcus faecalis, S. lactis, and *Vibrio comma.* The antimicrobial activity of *L. acidophilus* result from immune system stimulation.

Route	Onset	Peak	Duration
P.O.	Unknown	Unknown	Unknown

INDICATIONS & DOSAGES

Uncomplicated diarrhea, antibiotic-induced diarrhea—
Adults: 1 to 10 billion live *L. acidophilus* P.O. daily, in divided doses with food or drink. Specific product dosing is as follows: 2 capsules (Bacid) b.i.d. to q.i.d. Or, 1 packet Lactinex granules with food or liquid t.i.d. or q.i.d. Or, 4 Lactinex tablets t.i.d. or q.i.d. with small amount of food or liquid. Or, 1 Pro-Bionate capsule q.d. to t.i.d. Or, ¼ to 1 tsp Pro-Bionate powder q.d. to t.i.d.
Children older than age 3:
1 to 5 billion live *L. acidophilus* P.O. daily, in divided doses with food or drink.

Urinary tract and yeast infections—
Adults: 1 to 10 billion live *L. acidophilus* P.O. daily, in divided doses with food or drink.
Children older than age 3:
1 to 5 billion live *L. acidophilus* P.O. daily, in divided doses with food or drink.

ADVERSE REACTIONS
GI: flatulence.

INTERACTIONS
Drug-drug
Antibiotics (all classes): destroys the live *L. acidophilus.* Tell patient to separate administration by at least 2 hours.
Chloramphenicol, sulfasalazine: affects the metabolism of these antibiotics. Tell patient not to use together and to wait until antibiotic therapy is completed before taking an *L. acidophilus* supplement.

Drug-herb
Berberine, oregano, plant tannins, uva-ursi: may destroy some living *L. acidophilus.* Tell patients taking any of these herbs to wait at least 2 hours before taking lactobacillus.

Drug-lifestyle
Alcohol use: negatively affects *L. acidophilus.* Tell patient to avoid using together or to separate by at least 4 hours.

CONTRAINDICATIONS

Contraindicated in patients who are allergic to lactose; also contraindicated in children younger than age 3.

OVERDOSE & TREATMENT

No information available.

NURSING CONSIDERATIONS

• Upsetting the normal flora balance of the GI tract can cause GI stress and diarrhea.

• *Alert:* Patient should separate the administration of antibiotics, natural or synthetic, and *L. acidophilus* supplements by at least 2 hours, to make sure the antibiotic doesn't destroy the *L. acidophilus*.

• *Alert:* Warn parents not to give *L. acidophilus* supplements to infants and children younger than age 3.

• For patients with lactose intolerance, *L. acidophilus* may be unsafe; tell these patients to use a dairy-free *L. acidophilus* supplement.

• *L. acidophilus* inhibits a wide range of pathogenic bacteria; tell patient to consider its use during and after certain antibiotic therapy.

• Supplement is usually well tolerated.

• Several strains of *L. acidophilus* are available. The two most researched strains are the DDS-1 and NCFM strains,

which exert benefits far greater than all other strains of *L. acidophilus*.

• Most brands must be refrigerated, to ensure that the *L. acidophilus* remain viable. However, the NCFM strain is stable at room temperature for 7 days, provided the temperature doesn't exceed 90° F (32° C).

• Fructo-oligosaccharides (FOS) are sometimes added to *L. acidophilus* supplements to feed beneficial bacteria, but FOS also feeds pathogenic fungi, mainly *C. albicans*. Avoid *L. acidophilus* supplements containing FOS when using as support for a yeast infection.

• *Bifidobacterium bifidum* is often combined with *L. acidophilus* to ensure benefit throughout both the small and large intestines (acidophilus works in the small intestine and bifidus works in the large intestine).

PATIENT TEACHING

• Instruct patient to avoid alcohol while taking an *L. acidophilus* supplement.

• Instruct patient with a history of lactose intolerance to use a dairy-free *L. acidophilus* supplement.

• Tell patient not to use this supplement if fever is present or if diarrhea worsens or persists for longer than 2 days, unless directed by doctor.

• Advise patient to separate the administration of antibiotics, natural or synthetic, and *L. acidophilus* supplements by at least 2 hours.

• Advise patient to always use refrigerated *L. acidophilus* to ensure maximum potency.

• Advise patient to take *L. acidophilus* with food or drink.

• Inform parent or caregiver that infants and children younger than age 3 shouldn't be given *L. acidophilus* supplements.

• Tell breast-feeding patient to contact doctor before using this supplement because the safety of using *L. acidophilus* while breast-feeding hasn't been established.

• Advise patient to keep medication away from children and pets.

• Tell patient to report adverse effects or new signs and symptoms promptly to doctor.

---

levocarnitine
Big C liquid carnitine, Carnifuel, L-carnitine, Levocarnitine, Mega L-carnitine, VitaCarn

Pregnancy Risk Category B

HOW SUPPLIED
Caplets: 500 mg
Capsules: 250 mg, 300 mg, 500 mg, 1,000 mg
Liquid: 500 mg/5 ml, 500 mg/15 ml, 250 mg/30 ml, 600 mg/15 ml, 1,000 mg/5 ml, 1,000 mg/15 ml
Powder: 2,000 mg/tsp
Tablets: 250 mg, 500 mg, 1,000 mg

ACTION
L-carnitine plays a critical role in skeletal and cardiac muscle. Fatty acids are transported via the acyl CoA-carnitine pathway to the inner mitochondrial membrane where they are converted into energy. This is one of the mechanisms by which carnitine improves exercise tolerance and physical performance. As a result, carnitine aids in oxygen utilization in patients with angina, COPD, congestive heart failure, peripheral vascular disease, and MI. In Alzheimer's patients, acetyl-L-carnitine serves as a precursor for acetylcholine. In asymptomatic AIDS patients, daily infusions of carnitine appear to increase the rate and absolute count of CD4 lymphocytes and reduce the frequency of apoptotic CD4 and CD8 cells.

Route	Onset	Peak	Duration
P.O.	Unknown	2-4.5 hr	Unknown

INDICATIONS & DOSAGES
Dietary supplement—
Adults and adolescents: initially, 1 g (solution) P.O. daily with food. Or, 1 g (tablets) P.O. b.i.d. or t.i.d. with meals. Typical dosage is 1 to 3 g P.O. daily.
Children: dosage is based on body weight; usual initial dose is 50 mg/kg/day in divided doses with meals.

Enhancing physical performance—
Adults: 2 g P.O. b.i.d. or t.i.d.

ADVERSE REACTIONS
GI: nausea, vomiting, abdominal cramping, diarrhea.
Musculoskeletal: muscle pain, loss of muscle function.
Other: body odor.

INTERACTIONS
Drug-drug
Choline: results in lower urinary excretion of carnitine and may increase intracellular carnitine levels. Generally safe to use together at recommended dosages.
Heparin: interferes with free and total L-carnitine radioenzyme and long-chain acyl-L-carnitine assays, leading to inaccurate results. Advise patient not to use together.
Warfarin: may increase anticoagulant effects. Monitor PT and INR closely if must be used together.
Valproic acid: inhibits biosynthesis of carnitine and possibly decreases its tissue uptake.

Drug-herb
D-carnitine: may cause L-carnitine deficiency. Tell patient not to use together.

CONTRAINDICATIONS
Contraindicated in patients who are hypersensitive to carnitine or any of its related compounds, including L-acetylcarnitine or L-propionylcarnitine.

OVERDOSE & TREATMENT
No information available.

NURSING CONSIDERATIONS
• *Alert:* Only the L-fraction of carnitine and not the D-fraction should be consumed. The D-isomer may lead to muscle pain and loss of muscle function because it causes a deficiency of carnitine in skeletal and cardiac muscle.
• Tell patient to avoid using the D-isomer or D,L-isomer combination of L-carnitine if he has heart failure, COPD, heart disease, peripheral vascular disease, or angina; doing so may significantly decrease exercise tolerance and oxygen utilization.

• Avoid use in patients with a history of liver disease.

• Carnitine interacts with heparin and warfarin, so tell patient to use caution if he's receiving anticoagulant therapy.

• Urge patient to take L-carnitine cautiously if he has impaired renal function.

• Serum levels of L-carnitine decrease by 80% after hemodialysis.

• Carnitine supplementation may be used by patients taking valproic acid (Depakote) and phenytoin (Dilantin), as directed by doctor.

• In women with a suspected carnitine deficiency, supplementation may be needed to ensure adequate levels in mother and fetus, as directed by doctor.

• Carnitine supplement may be given to preterm infants to support weight gain and growth, as directed by doctor.

• Inadequate intake of lysine, methionine, vitamin C, iron, niacin, and vitamin B_6 can lead to carnitine deficiency without carnitine supplementation.

• Monitor patient for tolerance after first week of administration and after dosage increase.

• If overdose is suspected, treatment is based on signs and symptoms.

PATIENT TEACHING

• Instruct patient to drink GI solution slowly because GI reactions may result from too-rapid consumption.

• Tell patient that oral solution may be consumed alone or put in drinks or other liquids to mask taste.

• Instruct patient to space doses evenly throughout the day (every 3 to 4 hours or as directed) during or after meals to maximize tolerance.

• Instruct patient not to change brands or dosage forms of levocarnitine; they may not be interchangeable.

• Inform breast-feeding patient that L-carnitine appears in breast milk, but because carnitine supplementation promotes weight gain and growth in preterm infants, it's probably safe to breast-feed a child whose mother has been supplementing with L-carnitine. Instruct patient to consult doctor.

• Instruct patient to report adverse effects promptly to doctor.

• Instruct parent or caregiver to keep all medication away from children and pets.

lysine
L-lysine

Pregnancy Risk Category NR

HOW SUPPLIED
Capsules: 500 mg
Powder: 580 mg L-lysine monohydrochloride and 464 mg L-lysine per 1 level scoop
Tablets: 1,000 mg

ACTION
Lysine is an essential amino acid necessary for collagen synthesis, growth, and maintenance of nitrogen balance.

Route	Onset	Peak	Duration
P.O.	Unknown	Unknown	Unknown

INDICATIONS & DOSAGES
Dietary supplement—
The estimated adult RDA is 5.5 mg/lb; infants need 44 mg/lb and children need 22 mg/lb.

Because potency of different supplement forms varies, patient should follow manufacturer's label recommendations for specific products.

Recurrent herpes simplex infections—
Adults: 1,000 mg P.O. daily for 12 months; or 1,000 mg P.O. t.i.d. for 6 months.

ADVERSE REACTIONS
GI: diarrhea, abdominal pain.

INTERACTIONS
Drug-drug
Calcium: may increase supplemental calcium absorption and decrease urine calcium loss. May be taken together for this reason.

CONTRAINDICATIONS
Contraindicated in pregnant and breast-feeding patients because insufficient information is available.

OVERDOSE & TREATMENT
No information available.

NURSING CONSIDERATIONS
• Lysine is required for collagen synthesis and it may be important to bone health.
• Lysine appears to antagonize herpes simplex virus growth in vitro.
• Patients most likely to have a lysine deficiency are vegetarians who avoid dairy and eggs, patients involved in frequent vigorous exercise, and burn patients.
• Monitor patient's response to therapy.

PATIENT TEACHING
• Discuss with patient the reasons for taking this drug.

- Tell patient that sources of lysine include brewer's yeast, legumes, dairy products, wheat germ, fish, and meat.
- Discuss with patient other, more proven therapies for recurrent herpes simplex infection.
- Instruct parent or caregiver to keep all medication away from children and pets.
- Instruct breast-feeding and pregnant patients to avoid this product because safety and effectiveness haven't been established.
- Instruct patient to inform doctor of all drugs and herbal remedies he takes.

magnesium chloride (12% magnesium)
Slow-Mag

magnesium gluconate (5.4% magnesium)
Almora, Mag-G, Magonate, Magtrate

magnesium oxide (60.3% magnesium)
Mag-200, Mag-Ox 400, Uro-Mag

Pregnancy Risk Category NR

HOW SUPPLIED
magnesium chloride
Sustained-release tablets:
535 mg (64 mg magnesium)

magnesium gluconate
Liquid: 54 mg/5 ml (2.9 mg/5 ml magnesium)
Tablets: 500 mg (27 mg magnesium)

magnesium oxide
Capsules: 140 mg (84.5 mg magnesium)
Tablets: 400 mg (241.3 mg magnesium)

ACTION
Magnesium is an important cofactor in many enzymatic reactions. Adequate magnesium is necessary for maintaining serum potassium and calcium levels because of its effect on the renal tubule.

Route	Onset	Peak	Duration
P.O.	Unknown	4 hr	4-6 hr

INDICATIONS & DOSAGES
RDAs—
Children up to age 3: 40 to 80 mg/day.
Children ages 4 to 6: 120 mg/day.
Children ages 7 to 10: 170 mg/day.
Adolescents and adult men: 270 to 400 mg/day.
Adolescents and adult women: 280 to 300 mg/day.
Pregnant women: 320 mg/day.
Breast-feeding women: 340 to 35 mg/day.

Dietary supplement—
Adults: 54 to 483 mg P.O. daily
in divided doses.

Because potency of different
supplement forms varies, patient should follow manufacturer's label recommendations for
specific products.

ADVERSE REACTIONS
GI: diarrhea, GI irritation.

INTERACTIONS
Drug-drug
Aminoquinolines: decreases therapeutic effect of aminoquinolines. Advise patient to avoid taking together.
Cellulose sodium phosphate:
decreases effect of cellulose
sodium phosphate. Tell patient
to take magnesium supplements
at least 1 hour before or after
cellulose sodium phosphate.
Digoxin: magnesium salts may
adsorb digoxin in the GI tract,
decreasing its bioavailability.
Monitor serum digoxin levels.
Nitrofurantoin: magnesium
salts may adsorb to nitrofurantoin in the GI tract, decreasing
its bioavailability and possibly
its anti-infective effect. Tell patient to separate administration
times.
Penicillamine: may decrease GI
absorption of penicillamine,
therefore decreasing its effect.
Tell patient to use together cautiously.

Sodium polystyrene sulfonate:
decreases effect of magnesium
supplement. Advise patient to
avoid using together.
Tetracyclines: magnesium salts
may adsorb to tetracyclines in
the GI tract, decreasing their
bioavailability and possibly
their anti-infective effect. Tell
patient to separate administration times by taking magnesium
supplements at least 1 to 3
hours before or after tetracycline.

CONTRAINDICATIONS
None known.

OVERDOSE & TREATMENT
Hypermagnesemia after oral ingestion is unlikely; however, it
may occur with an overdose.
Signs and symptoms may include hypotension, nausea,
vomiting, urine retention, bradycardia, cutaneous vasodilation (3 to 9 mEq/L), ECG
changes, hyporeflexia secondary to CNS depression (5 to 10
mEq/L), respiratory changes,
coma (> 9 mEq/L), asystolic arrest (> 14 to 15 mEq/L). Treatment includes discontinuation
of magnesium-containing preparations. Reversal of toxicity
with calcium is immediate but
transient. Dialysis is the treatment of choice (both peritoneal
and hemodialysis).

NURSING CONSIDERATIONS
● Tell patient to use cautiously if he has renal disease because of potential for accumulation (because magnesium is eliminated by the kidneys).
● Lack of magnesium may lead to irritability, muscle weakness, and irregular heartbeat.
● Magnesium is used as a dietary supplement to prevent or treat magnesium deficiencies.
● Magnesium is also used to prevent deficiencies and is based on normal daily recommended intakes of elemental magnesium.
● Instruct patient to take with meals to reduce diarrhea.
● Treatment dose is individualized depending on severity of deficiency.
● One gram magnesium = 83.3 mEq (41.1 mmol).

PATIENT TEACHING
● Advise elderly patient that he may be at risk for developing a magnesium deficiency because of poor food selection, decreased absorption, diseases that cause magnesium depletion, or medications that may increase urinary loss of magnesium.
● Tell patient that dietary sources of magnesium include green leafy vegetables, nuts, peas, beans, and cereal grains with intact outer layers. Cook-

ing may decrease the magnesium content of food.
● Tell patient to take magnesium supplements with meals.
● Inform patient that excessive doses may cause diarrhea.
● Advise patient with significant renal impairment to consult doctor before taking this drug.
● Tell patient that magnesium-containing antacids may also be used as dietary supplements.
● Instruct patient not to crush or chew extended-release forms.
● Tell patient to report adverse effects promptly to doctor.

medium chain triglycerides
MCT Oil

Pregnancy Risk Category C

HOW SUPPLIED
Oil: 960 ml (115 calories/15 ml)

ACTION
Medium chain triglycerides are more rapidly hydrolyzed than conventional food fat, require less bile for digestion, are carried by the portal circulation, and aren't dependent on chylomicron formation or lymphatic transport. Medium chain triglycerides are a useful energy source in malabsorption pa-

tients but they don't provide essential fatty acids.

Route	Onset	Peak	Duration
P.O.	Unknown	Unknown	Unknown

INDICATIONS & DOSAGES
Inadequate digestion or absorption of food fats—
Adults: 15 ml P.O. t.i.d. or q.i.d. Maximum, 100 ml/day.

ADVERSE REACTIONS
CNS: reversible *coma* in susceptible patients (such as those with advanced hepatic cirrhosis).
GI: nausea, vomiting, diarrhea, abdominal distention, cramps.

INTERACTIONS
None reported.

CONTRAINDICATIONS
None reported.

OVERDOSE & TREATMENT
No information available.

NURSING CONSIDERATIONS
• Use cautiously in patient with hepatic cirrhosis and complications, such as portacaval shunts or a tendency toward encephalopathy.
• Medium chain triglycerides provide 7.7 calories/ml.
• To minimize adverse GI effects, suggest smaller, more frequent doses with meals, salad dressing, or chilled fruit juice.

• Patient should use metal, glass, or ceramic containers and utensils.
• Medium chain triglycerides do not provide essential fatty acids.
• Arrange for counseling with dietitian so patient can learn how to incorporate this substance into his diet.

PATIENT TEACHING
• Instruct patient when and how to take drug to minimize GI adverse effects.
• Tell patient to report persistent or severe adverse reactions promptly.
• Caution patient not to use plastic utensils or containers.
• Recommend that patient consult a dietitian to learn how to incorporate this substance into his diet.

niacin (nicotinic acid, vitamin B₃)
Nia-Bid, Niacor, Niaspan, Nico-400, Nicobid, Nicolar**, Nicotinex, Slo-Niacin

niacinamide (nicotinamide)

Pregnancy Risk Category C

HOW SUPPLIED
niacin
Capsules (timed-release):
125 mg, 250 mg, 300 mg, 400 mg, 500 mg

Elixir: 50 mg/5 ml
Tablets: 25 mg, 50 mg, 100 mg, 250 mg, 500 mg
Tablets (timed-release): 250 mg, 375 mg, 500 mg, 750 mg, 1,000 mg

niacinamide
Tablets: 50 mg, 100 mg, 125 mg, 250 mg, 500 mg

ACTION
Stimulate lipid metabolism, tissue respiration, and glycogenolysis. Niacin decreases synthesis of low-density lipoproteins and inhibits lipolysis in adipose tissue.

Route	Onset	Peak	Duration
P.O.	Unknown	45 min	Unknown

INDICATIONS & DOSAGES
RDA—
Children ages 1 to 3: 6 mg daily.
Children ages 4 to 8: 8 mg daily.
Children ages 9 to 13: 12 mg daily.
Men ages 14 and older: 16 mg daily.
Women ages 14 and older: 14 mg daily.
Pregnant women: 18 mg daily.
Breast-feeding women: 17 mg daily.

Adequate intake—
Neonates and infants up to age 6 months: 2 mg (0.3 mg/kg) daily.
Infants ages 6 months to 1 year: 4 mg (0.4 mg/kg) daily.

Dietary supplement—
Niacin is recommended at 6.6 mg/1,000 Kcal intake. A B-complex or multivitamin supplement containing 10 to 25 mg is adequate.

Because potency of different supplement forms varies, patient should follow manufacturer's label recommendations for specific products.

Niacin deficiency—
Adults: up to 100 mg P.O. daily.

ADVERSE REACTIONS
CV: excessive peripheral vasodilation, especially niacin; hypotension; atrial fibrillation; *arrhythmias;* flushing.
EENT: toxic amblyopia.
GI: nausea, vomiting, diarrhea, possible activation of peptic ulceration, epigastric or substernal pain.
Hepatic: elevated liver enzyme levels, hepatic dysfunction.
Metabolic: hyperglycemia, hyperuricemia.
Skin: pruritus, dryness, tingling.

INTERACTIONS
Drug-drug
Antihypertensives (ganglionic or sympathetic blockers): potential additive vasodilating effect, causing orthostatic hypotension. Tell patient to use together cautiously, and warn patient about orthostatic hypotension.

Lovastatin (statin class): may lead to rhabdomyolysis. Tell patient to avoid using together.

Sulfinpyrazone: uricosuric effects may be decreased by niacin. Tell patient to avoid using together.

Drug-lifestyle
Alcohol use: may increase flushing effect. Advise patient to avoid using together.

CONTRAINDICATIONS
Contraindicated in patients hypersensitive to drug and in those with hepatic dysfunction, active peptic ulcers, severe hypotension, or arterial hemorrhage.

OVERDOSE & TREATMENT
Niacin, a water-soluble vitamin, seldom causes toxicity in patients with normal renal function.

NURSING CONSIDERATIONS
- Use cautiously in patient with gallbladder disease, diabetes mellitus, unstable angina, a history of liver disease, peptic ulcer, allergy, gout, or alcohol abuse.
- Patient should begin with smallest possible dose and increase gradually; observe for efficacy and adverse effects.
- Most reactions are dose-dependent.
- After signs and symptoms of niacin deficiency subside, advise adequate nutrition and RDA supplements to prevent recurrence.
- Drug may cause dose-related rise in glucose intolerance; serum glucose levels should be monitored carefully by diabetic patients.
- Niacin should be taken with meals to minimize adverse GI effects.
- Recommend aspirin (325 mg P.O. 30 minutes before niacin dose), as ordered, to possibly reduce flushing response to niacin.
- Timed-release niacin or niacinamide may prevent excessive flushing that occurs with large doses. However, timed-release niacin is linked to hepatic dysfunction, even at low doses.
- Monitor hepatic function and serum glucose levels early in therapy, as ordered.
- Drug alters results of fluorometric test for urine catechol-

amines and urine glucose tests that use cupric sulfate (Benedict's reagent).

PATIENT TEACHING
• Tell patient that niacin is a potent drug, not just a vitamin, and that it may cause serious adverse effects. Explain importance of adhering to therapy.
• Advise patient who takes extended-release product to swallow it whole and not to break, crush, or chew it.
• Instruct patient to avoid sudden position changes if dizziness occurs when taking this drug.
• Tell patient that flushing and warmth may subside with continued use and that use of alcohol may increase flushing.
• Tell patient to take with food to minimize stomach upset.
• Advise patient against self-medicating for hyperlipidemia.

omega-3 polyunsaturated fatty acids (fish oils)
Cardio-Omega 3, Emulsified Super Omega-3, EPA, Marine Lipid Concentrate, Max EPA, Promega, Promega Pearls, Sea-Omega 30, Sea-Omega 50, SuperEPA 1200, SuperEPA 2000

Pregnancy Risk Category NR

HOW SUPPLIED
Capsules: 600 mg, 1,000 mg, 1,200 mg
Liquid: eicosapentaenoic acid (EPA) 1,080 mg, docosahexaenoic acid (DHA) 720 mg, alpha linoleic acid 480 mg
Softgels: 330 mg, 700 mg, 1,000 mg

ACTION
Diets high in omega-3 fatty acids may lower very low-density lipoprotein, triglyceride, and total cholesterol levels; increase high-density lipoprotein (HDL) levels; prolong bleeding times; and decrease platelet aggregation. Omega 3 supplements contain DHA and EPA.

Route	Onset	Peak	Duration
P.O.	Unknown	Unknown	Unknown

INDICATIONS & DOSAGES
Dietary supplementation for patients at early risk for coronary artery disease—
Adults: 4 to 13 g/day P.O. (typically 1 to 2 capsules t.i.d. with meals).

Because potency of different supplement forms varies, patient should follow manufacturer's label recommendations for specific products.

ADVERSE REACTIONS
GI: fishy taste, belching, nausea, loose stools, diarrhea.

INTERACTIONS
Drug-drug
Anticoagulants, antiplatelets: increases risk of bleeding. Monitor PT, INR, and patient closely.

Drug-herb
Herbs with anticoagulant or antiplatelet potential: theoretically, could increase risk of bleeding. Discourage patient from using together.

CONTRAINDICATIONS
Insufficient information is available regarding use in pregnancy and breast-feeding. Pregnant and breast-feeding patients shouldn't take fish oil in amounts greater than provided by dietary consumption of fish.

OVERDOSE & TREATMENT
No information available.

NURSING CONSIDERATIONS
• Drug has been used in patients at early risk for coronary artery disease, primarily because of its effects on platelets and lipids (especially to reduce triglyceride levels).
• EPA and DHA may lower lipid and triglyceride levels and increase HDL levels.
• Urge diabetic patients to use cautiously and monitor serum glucose levels; omega-3 fatty acids can interfere with serum glucose control.

PATIENT TEACHING
• Inform parent or caregiver that until further information is available, omega-3 fatty acids shouldn't be given to children.
• Tell patient that dietary sources of omega-3 fatty acids include cold water fish such as cod, tuna, salmon, halibut, shark, and mackerel.
• Instruct breast-feeding patient not to take this supplement.
• Instruct patient to report adverse effects promptly to doctor.
• Instruct parent or caregiver to keep medication away from children and pets.

---

pantothenic acid (vitamin B$_5$, calcium pantothenate)

Pregnancy Risk Category A

HOW SUPPLIED
Capsules: 100 mg, 250 mg, 500 mg, 550 mg
Liquid: 200 mg/tsp
Softgels: 450 mg
Tablets: 25 mg, 100 mg, 200 mg, 218 mg, 250 mg, 500 mg, 545 mg
Tablets (sustained-release): 1,000 mg

Reactions may be *common*, uncommon, *life-threatening*, or COMMON AND LIFE-THREATENING.

ACTION

Pantothenic acid is a precursor of coenzyme A, which is a cofactor for many enzyme-catalyzed reactions involving transfer of acetyl groups. It's associated with oxidative metabolism of carbohydrates, gluconeogenesis, and synthesis of fatty acids, sterols, steroid hormones, and porphyrins.

Route	Onset	Peak	Duration
P.O.	Unknown	Unknown	Unknown

INDICATIONS & DOSAGES

Adequate intake—
Infants up to age 6 months: 1.7 mg/day (0.24 mg/kg).
Infants ages 7 to 12 months: 1.8 mg/day (0.2 mg/kg).
Children ages 1 to 3: 2 mg/day.
Children ages 4 to 8: 3 mg/day.
Children ages 9 to 13: 4 mg/day.
Adults and children ages 14 and older: 5 mg/day.
Pregnant women: 6 mg/day.
Breast-feeding women: 7 mg/day.

Dietary supplement—
Adults and children: 5 to 10 mg P.O. daily.

Because potency of different supplement forms varies, patient should follow manufacturer's label recommendations for specific products.

ADVERSE REACTIONS

GI: diarrhea with large doses.
Skin: dermatitis.

INTERACTIONS

None reported.

CONTRAINDICATIONS

None known.

OVERDOSE & TREATMENT

Diarrhea and water retention may occur with doses of 10 to 20 g/day.

Treatment involves reducing dosage or discontinuing pantothenic acid to control signs and symptoms.

NURSING CONSIDERATIONS

• Pantothenic acid deficiency hasn't been recognized in people with a normal diet because this vitamin is in so many ordinary foods (chicken, tomatoes, potatoes, cereals, vegetable juice, and liver, for example).
• Monitor patient's response to drug therapy.
• Discuss dietary habits, and address patient's concerns.
• Obtain thorough allergy history from patient, parent, or caregiver.

PATIENT TEACHING
• Inform breast-feeding and pregnant patient that intake of normal daily recommended amounts seems to cause no problems; however, tell her to consult her doctor before taking this or any drug.
• Instruct patient to report adverse effects and new signs and symptoms promptly to doctor.
• Instruct parent or caregiver to keep medication away from children and pets.
• Discuss dietary habits with patient.
• Remind patient to inform doctor of all drugs and herbal supplements being taken.

---

phosphorus-replacement products
K-Phos Neutral, Neutra-Phos-K Powder, Neutra-Phos Powder, Uro-KP-Neutral

Pregnancy Risk Category C

HOW SUPPLIED
Powder: Neutra-Phos (250 mg phosphorus, 7 mEq potassium, 164 mg sodium); Neutra-Phos-K (250 mg phosphorus, 14.25 mEq potassium)
Tablets: 250 mg phosphorous, 49.4 mg potassium, 250.5 mg sodium (Uro-KP-Neutral); 250 mg phosphorous, 45 mg potassium, 298 mg sodium (K-Phos Neutral)

ACTION
Phosphorous appears in all cells of the body. About 80% of body phosphorous is in the skeletal system, and the remainder has intracellular functions.

Route	Onset	Peak	Duration
P.O.	Unknown	Unknown	Unknown

INDICATIONS & DOSAGES
RDA—
Infants up to age 6 months: 100 mg/day.
Infants ages 7 to 12 months: 275 mg/day.
Children ages 1 to 3: 460 mg/day.
Children ages 4 to 8: 500 mg/day.
Children ages 9 to 18: 1,250 mg/day.
Adults: 700 mg/day.
Pregnant and breast-feeding women: 700 mg/day.

As a dietary supplement (when diet is restricted or if needs are increased)—
Adults: 1 capsule or 1 powder packet reconstituted in 75 ml of water, q.i.d. Provides 250 mg phosphorus per dose (1 g daily).

Because potency of different supplement forms varies, patient should follow manufacturer's label recommendations for specific products.

Phosphate supplementation should only be used under the direction of a doctor.

ADVERSE REACTIONS
CNS: headache, dizziness, mental confusion, *seizures,* weakness or heaviness of legs, tiredness, weakness, numbness or tingling of lips.
CV: tachycardia, *bradycardia.*
GI: diarrhea, nausea, stomach pain, vomiting, flatulence, thirst.
GU: low urine output.
Metabolic: electrolyte abnormalities, unusual weight gain.
Musculoskeletal: tingling, pain, or weakness of hands or feet; bone and joint pain; extraskeletal calcification.
Respiratory: dyspnea.
Other: edema in feet or lower legs.

INTERACTIONS
Drug-drug
ACE inhibitors: may cause hyperkalemia. Monitor serum potassium levels.
Antacids containing magnesium, aluminum, or calcium: may bind to phosphate and prevent its absorption. Advise patient to avoid using together.
Calcium-containing products: may reduce phosphate absorption and increase risk of calcium deposition in soft tissues. Advise patient to avoid using together.
Potassium-sparing diuretics and potassium-containing products: may cause hyperkalemia. Monitor serum potassium levels.

CONTRAINDICATIONS
Contraindicated in patients with Addison's disease; hyperphosphatemia; severely impaired renal function (less than 30% of normal); hyperkalemia; acidified urine, in urinary stone disease; and infected urolithiasis or struvite stone formation.

OVERDOSE & TREATMENT
No information available.

NURSING CONSIDERATIONS
● Urge caution in patients on sodium- or potassium-restricted diet because these products provide significant amounts of sodium and potassium.
● Also urge caution in patients with cardiac disease, acute dehydration, significant renal disease or impairment, cirrhosis of liver, severe hepatic disease, peripheral and pulmonary edema, hypernatremia, hypertension, preeclampsia, hypoparathyroidism, osteomalacia, acute pancreatitis, and rickets.
● Patients with kidney stones may pass old stones when phos-

phate therapy is started and should be warned of this possibility.

• Phosphate administration lowers calcium levels and increases urine phosphate levels.

• Patients may experience a mild laxative effect for the first few days.

• Drug should be taken with food to minimize possible stomach upset or laxative action.

PATIENT TEACHING

• Inform pregnant patient that this product can cause fetal harm; she should consult her doctor.

• Inform breast-feeding patient that it's not known if this drug appears in breast milk; instruct patient to consult doctor.

• Inform patient that he may experience a mild laxative effect for the first few days; tell him to reduce intake or discontinue drug if this persists and contact doctor.

• Instruct patient to take drug with food to minimize GI upset or laxative action.

• Instruct patient to contact doctor if he experiences new or adverse signs and symptoms.

• Discuss dietary habits with patient.

• Instruct patient to keep drugs away from children and pets.

polysaccharide-iron complex
Hytinic, Niferex, Niferex-150, Nu-Iron, Nu-Iron 150

Pregnancy Risk Category NR

HOW SUPPLIED
Capsules: 150 mg
Solution: 100 mg/5 ml
Tablets (film-coated): 50 mg

ACTION
Provides elemental iron, an essential component in the formation of hemoglobin.

Route	Onset	Peak	Duration
P.O.	Few days	2-10 days	2 mo

INDICATIONS & DOSAGES
RDA—
Infants up to age 6 months: 6 mg/day.
Children ages 6 months to 10 years: 10 mg/day.
Men ages 11 to 18: 12 mg/day.
Men ages 19 and older: 10 mg/ day.
Women ages 11 and older: 15 mg/day.
Pregnant women: 30 mg/day.
Breast-feeding women: 15 mg/ day.

Dietary supplement—
Because potency of different supplement forms varies, pa-

tient should follow manufacturer's label recommendations for specific products.

Iron deficiency—
Adults: 50 to 100 mg P.O. of elemental iron t.i.d.
Children: 3 to 6 mg/kg/day P.O. of elemental iron in three divided doses.

ADVERSE REACTIONS
GI: nausea, constipation, black stools, epigastric pain.

INTERACTIONS
Drug-drug
Antacids, cholestyramine, cimetidine, vitamin E: decreases iron absorption. Tell patient to separate doses by 2 to 4 hours.
Chloramphenicol: delays response to iron therapy. Monitor patient.
Fluoroquinolones, penicillamine, tetracyclines: decreases GI absorption, possibly resulting in decreased serum levels or efficacy of the antibiotic. Tell patient to separate doses, if possible.
Levodopa, methyldopa: decreases absorption and efficacy of levodopa and methyldopa. Monitor patient for decreased effect of these drugs.
Vitamin C: may increase iron absorption. Tell patient to take together.

Drug-herb
Oregano: may reduce iron absorption. Advise patient taking oregano to wait at least 2 hours before taking iron supplements or iron-containing foods.

Drug-food
Cereals, cheese, coffee, eggs, milk, tea, whole-grain breads, yogurt: may impair oral iron absorption. Tell patient not to use together.

CONTRAINDICATIONS
Contraindicated in patients who are hypersensitive to drug or its components and in those with hemochromatosis or hemosiderosis.

OVERDOSE & TREATMENT
The lethal dose of iron is between 200 and 250 mg/kg; deaths have occurred with lower doses. Signs and symptoms may follow ingestion of 20 to 60 mg/kg.

Between ½ and 8 hours after ingestion, patient may experience lethargy, nausea, vomiting, green or tarry stools, weak and rapid pulse, hypotension, dehydration, acidosis, and coma.

If death doesn't occur immediately, signs and symptoms may clear for about 24 hours. At 12 to 48 hours, signs and symptoms may return, accompanied by diffuse vascular con-

---

gestion, pulmonary edema, shock, seizures, anuria, and hyperthermia. Death may follow.

Treatment requires immediate support of airway, respiration, and circulation. Induce emesis with ipecac in conscious patients with intact gag reflex; for unconscious patients, empty stomach by gastric lavage. Follow emesis with lavage, using 1% sodium bicarbonate solution, to convert iron to less irritating, poorly absorbed form. (Phosphate solutions have been used, but carry risk of other adverse effects.) Use radiographic evaluation of abdomen to determine continued presence of excess iron; if serum iron levels exceed 350 mg/dl, deferoxamine may be used for systemic chelation.

Survivors are likely to have organ damage, including pyloric or antral stenosis, hepatic cirrhosis, CNS damage, and intestinal obstruction.

NURSING CONSIDERATIONS
• Oral iron may turn stools black. Although this unabsorbed iron is harmless, it may mask melena.
• Few adverse effects occur with polysaccharide-iron complex.
• Patient may take iron with juice but not with milk or antacids.

• Monitor hemoglobin levels, hematocrit, and reticulocyte count, as ordered.
• Drug may interfere with tests for occult blood in stool; guaiac and orthotoluidine tests may yield false-positive results. Benzidine test isn't usually affected. Iron overload may decrease uptake of technetium 99m and thus interfere with skeletal imaging.

PATIENT TEACHING
• Tell patient to take with juice (preferably orange juice).
• Tell patient that dietary sources of iron include fish, meat (especially liver), and fortified cereals and bread.
• If patient misses a dose, tell him to take it as soon as possible but not to double the dose.
• Inform parents that as few as three tablets can cause serious iron poisoning and death in children.
• Caution patient not to substitute one iron salt for another because the amounts of elemental iron vary.
• Advise elderly patient that iron-induced constipation may occur; stress importance of proper diet.

pyridoxine hydrochloride (vitamin B₆)
Nestrex◇, Orovite Comploment B₆§, Rodex

Pregnancy Risk Category A

HOW SUPPLIED
Capsules: 500 mg
Capsules (timed-release): 100 mg
Tablets: 10 mg, 25 mg, 50 mg, 100 mg, 200 mg, 250 mg, 500 mg
Tablets (timed-release): 100 mg

ACTION
Acts as a coenzyme that stimulates various metabolic functions, including amino acid metabolism.

Route	Onset	Peak	Duration
P.O.	Unknown	Unknown	Unknown

INDICATIONS & DOSAGES
RDA—
Children ages 1 to 3: 0.5 mg daily.
Children ages 4 to 8: 0.6 mg daily.
Children ages 9 to 13: 1.0 mg daily.
Boys ages 14 to 18: 1.3 mg daily.
Girls ages 14 to 18: 1.2 mg daily.
Men and women ages 19 to 50: 1.3 mg daily.

Men ages 51 and older: 1.7 mg daily.
Women ages 51 and older: 1.5 mg daily.
Pregnant women: 1.9 mg daily.
Breast-feeding women: 2.0 mg daily.

Adequate intake—
Infants up to age 6 months: 0.1 mg (0.01 mg/kg) daily.
Infants ages 6 months to 1 year: 0.3 mg (0.03 mg/kg) daily.

Dietary supplement—
Because potency of different supplement forms varies, patient should follow manufacturer's label recommendations for specific products.

Dietary vitamin B₆ deficiency—
Adults: 10 to 20 mg P.O. daily for 3 weeks; then 2 to 5 mg daily as supplement to proper diet.

ADVERSE REACTIONS
CNS: paresthesia, unsteady gait, numbness, somnolence, *seizures,* headache.

INTERACTIONS
Drug-drug
Levodopa: decreases levodopa effect. Advise patient not to use together.
Phenobarbital, phenytoin: decreases anticonvulsant levels,

increasing risk of seizures. Tell patient to avoid using together.

Drug-lifestyle
Alcohol use: delirium and lactic acidosis may follow alcohol consumption. Tell patient not to use together.

CONTRAINDICATIONS
Contraindicated in patients who are hypersensitive to drug.

OVERDOSE & TREATMENT
Signs and symptoms of overdose include ataxia and severe sensory neuropathy after long-term consumption of high daily doses of pyridoxine (2 to 6 g). These neurologic deficits usually resolve after pyridoxine is discontinued.

NURSING CONSIDERATIONS
• Prepare a dietary history. A single vitamin deficiency is unusual; lack of one vitamin often indicates a deficiency of others.
• Patient taking high doses (2 to 6 g/day) may experience difficulty walking because of diminished proprioceptive and sensory function.
• Carefully monitor patient's diet. Excessive protein intake increases daily pyridoxine requirements.
• *Alert:* Don't confuse pyridoxine with pralidoxime or pyridium.

• Pyridoxine is sometimes useful to reduce nausea and vomiting in pregnancy. However, use of large doses during pregnancy has been implicated in pyridoxine-dependency seizures in neonates.
• Drug alters determinations of urobilinogen in spot test using Ehrlich's reagent, resulting in false-positive reaction.

PATIENT TEACHING
• Stress importance of compliance and good nutrition if drug is taken as maintenance therapy to prevent recurrence of deficiency.
• Teach patient about dietary sources of vitamin B_6, such as yeast, wheat germ, liver, whole grain cereals, bananas, and legumes.
• Advise patient taking levodopa alone to avoid multivitamins containing pyridoxine because of decreased levodopa effect.
• Advise breast-feeding patient that it's unknown if drug appears in breast milk; advise her to contact doctor before taking this drug.
• Inform breast-feeding patient that pyridoxine may inhibit lactation by suppression of prolactin.

Reactions may be *common*, uncommon, *life-threatening*, or COMMON AND LIFE-THREATENING.

riboflavin (vitamin B₂)

Pregnancy Risk Category A

HOW SUPPLIED
Tablets: 25 mg, 50 mg, 100 mg
Tablets (sugar-free): 50 mg,
100 mg

ACTION
Converts to two other coenzymes needed for normal tissue reparation. Drug is necessary for activation of pyridoxine.

Route	Onset	Peak	Duration
P.O.	Unknown	Unknown	Unknown

INDICATIONS & DOSAGES
RDA—
Children ages 1 to 3: 0.5 mg daily.
Children ages 4 to 8: 0.6 mg daily.
Children ages 9 to 13: 0.9 mg daily.
Boys ages 14 to 18: 1.3 mg daily.
Girls ages 14 to 18: 1.0 mg daily.
Men ages 19 and older: 1.3 mg daily.
Women ages 19 and older: 1.1 mg daily.
Pregnant women: 1.4 mg daily.
Breast-feeding women: 1.6 mg daily.

Adequate intake—
Neonates and infants up to age 6 months: 0.3 mg (0.4 mg/kg) daily.
Infants ages 6 months to 1 year: 0.4 mg (0.4 mg/kg) daily.

Dietary supplement—
Because potency of different supplement forms varies, patient should follow manufacturer's label recommendations for specific products. A B-complex or multivitamin supplement containing 20 to 25 mg of riboflavin serves as a more than adequate dietary supplement.

ADVERSE REACTIONS
GU: bright yellow or orange urine.

INTERACTIONS
Drug-drug
Probenecid: reduces urinary excretion of riboflavin. Tell patient to avoid using together.
Propantheline, other anticholinergics: decreases rate and extent of absorption. Tell patient to avoid using together.

Drug-lifestyle
Alcohol use: impairs intestinal absorption of riboflavin. Tell patient to avoid using together.

CONTRAINDICATIONS
None known.

OVERDOSE & TREATMENT
No information available.

NURSING CONSIDERATIONS
- Riboflavin deficiency usually accompanies other vitamin B complex deficiencies and may require multivitamin therapy.
- Patient should take riboflavin with food to increase absorption.
- Drug should be protected from air and light.
- **Alert:** Don't confuse riboflavin with ribavirin.
- Drug alters urinalysis based on spectrophotometry or color reactions. Large doses of drug result in bright yellow urine. Riboflavin produces fluorescent substances in urine and plasma, which can falsely elevate fluorometric determinations of catecholamines and urobilinogen.

PATIENT TEACHING
- Tell patient to take drug with meals; food increases absorption.
- Stress proper nutritional habits to prevent deficiency.
- Tell patient about good dietary sources of riboflavin, such as whole-grain cereals and green vegetables. Liver, kidney, heart, eggs, and dairy products are also dietary sources but may not be appropriate, based on patient's serum cholesterol and triglyceride levels.
- Tell patient to store riboflavin in a tight, light-resistant container.
- Inform patient that riboflavin usually causes bright yellow or orange discoloration of urine.
- Inform pregnant and breast-feeding patients that riboflavin crosses the placental barrier; during pregnancy and breast-feeding, riboflavin requirements may increase. Patient should consult doctor.

---

selenium
Selenate, Selenite

Pregnancy Risk Category NR

HOW SUPPLIED
Tablets: 50 mcg, 100 mcg, 200 mcg

ACTION
Selenium is necessary for the enzymes glutathione and peroxidase, which facilitate the lowering of tissue peroxide levels in the body by destroying hydrogen peroxide. There is an overlap in action of selenium and vitamin E in that both are responsible for lowering tissue peroxide levels.

Route	Onset	Peak	Duration
P.O.	Unknown	Unknown	Unknown

Reactions may be *common*, uncommon, *life-threatening*, or COMMON AND LIFE-THREATENING.

INDICATIONS & DOSAGES
RDA—
Children up to age 3: 10 to 20 mcg.
Children ages 4 to 10: 20 to 30 mcg.
Adolescent and adult men: 40 to 70 mcg.
Adolescent and adult women: 45 to 55 mcg.
Pregnant women: 65 mcg.
Breast-feeding women: 75 mcg.

Prevent deficiency—
Children up to age 3: 10 to 20 mcg P.O. daily.
Children ages 4 to 6: 20 mcg P.O. daily.
Children ages 7 to 10: 30 mcg P.O. daily.
Adolescent and adult men: 40 to 70 mcg P.O. daily.
Adolescent and adult women: 45 to 55 mcg P.O. daily.
Pregnant women: 65 mcg P.O. daily.
Breast-feeding women: 75 mcg P.O. daily.
Because potency of different supplement forms varies, patient should follow manufacturer's label recommendations for specific products.

ADVERSE REACTIONS
CNS: irritability, unusual tiredness and weakness.
GI: nausea, vomiting, diarrhea, metallic taste.
Skin: dermatitis, fingernail weakening.
Other: garlic odor to breath and sweat, hair loss.

INTERACTIONS
Drug-drug
Vitamin C (high doses), heavy metals: reduces selenium absorption. Advise patient to avoid using together.

CONTRAINDICATIONS
None known.

OVERDOSE & TREATMENT
Toxic effects and adverse reactions appear at doses of 750 to 1,000 mcg/day. Signs and symptoms of overdose include diarrhea, fingernail weakening, garlic odor to breath and sweat, hair loss, irritability, itching of skin, metallic taste, nausea and vomiting, and unusual tiredness or weakness.
  If overdose is suspected, patient should reduce dosage or discontinue selenium to control signs and symptoms.

NURSING CONSIDERATIONS
• People who live in regions where selenium is low in their diet (or depleted in their soils or crops) have much higher rates of cancer.
• Signs and symptoms of deficiency may include lightening in the color of fingernail beds,

muscle discomfort or weakness, cardiomyopathy, and increased occurrence of liver cancer.
• Treatment of selenium deficiency is individualized based on severity.
• Obtain accurate dietary history.
• Monitor patient's response to drug therapy.

PATIENT TEACHING
• Tell pregnant or breast-feeding patient to consult her doctor before using dietary supplements. However, there are no reports of problems when selenium is taken at recommended doses.
• Discuss dietary habits with patient or caregiver.
• Tell patient that dietary sources of selenium include seafood, liver, red meat, and grains grown in selenium-rich soil.
• Instruct patient to report adverse effects to doctor.

---

thiamine hydrochloride (vitamin B₁)
Betamin‡, Beta-Sol‡

Pregnancy Risk Category A

HOW SUPPLIED
Elixir†: 250 mcg/5 ml
Tablets: 25 mg, 50 mg, 100 mg, 250 mg, 500 mg
Tablets (enteric-coated): 20 mg

ACTION
Combines with adenosine triphosphate to form a coenzyme needed for carbohydrate metabolism.

Route	Onset	Peak	Duration
P.O.	Unknown	Unknown	Unknown

INDICATIONS & DOSAGES
RDA—
Children ages 1 to 3: 0.5 mg/day.
Children ages 4 to 8: 0.6 mg/day.
Children ages 9 to 13: 0.9 mg/day.
Boys ages 14 to 18: 1.2 mg/day.
Girls ages 14 to 18: 1.0 mg/day.
Men ages 19 and older: 1.2 mg/day.
Women ages 19 and older: 1.1 mg/day.
Pregnant women: 1.4 mg/day.
Breast-feeding women: 1.5 mg/day.

Adequate intake—
Infants up to age 6 months: 0.2 mg (0.03 mg/kg) daily.
Infants ages 6 months to 1 year: 0.3 mg (0.03 mg/kg) daily.

Dietary supplement—
Because potency of different supplement forms varies, patient should follow manufactur-

---

er's label recommendations for specific products. A B-complex or multivitamin supplement containing 20 to 25 mg is more than adequate to provide supplementation.

ADVERSE REACTIONS
CNS: restlessness, weakness.
CV: cyanosis, *CV collapse.*
EENT: tightness of throat.
GI: nausea, hemorrhage.
Respiratory: pulmonary edema.
Skin: feeling of warmth, pruritus, urticaria, diaphoresis.
Other: *angioedema.*

INTERACTIONS
None known.

CONTRAINDICATIONS
Contraindicated in patients hypersensitive to thiamine products.

OVERDOSE & TREATMENT
Very large doses of thiamine administered parenterally may produce neuromuscular and ganglionic blockade and neurologic signs and symptoms.
   Treatment is supportive.

NURSING CONSIDERATIONS
• Thiamine malabsorption is most likely in alcoholism, cirrhosis, or GI disease.

• Clinically significant deficiency can occur in about 3 weeks with a thiamine-free diet.
• Obtain accurate dietary history; thiamine deficiency usually requires concurrent treatment for multiple deficiencies.
• Dosages of more than 30 mg t.i.d. may not be fully used. After tissue saturation with thiamine, drug is excreted in urine as pyrimidine.
• *Alert:* Don't confuse thiamine with Thorazine.
• Thiamine may produce false-positive results in phosphotungstate method for determination of uric acid, and in urine spot tests with Ehrlich's reagent for urobilinogen. Large doses interfere with Schack and Waxler spectrophotometric determination of serum theophylline levels.
• Advise patient to store thiamine in a light-resistant, nonmetallic container.

PATIENT TEACHING
• Stress proper nutritional habits to prevent deficiency.
• Inform patient that thiamine deficiency usually occurs with other vitamin deficiencies.
• Inform patient of dietary sources of thiamine, such as yeast, pork, beef, liver, whole grains, peas, and bananas.
• Instruct patient to protect oral form from light.

---

*Liquid contains alcohol.   **May contain tartrazine.   †Canada   ‡Australia   §U.K.

• Advise patient to report adverse effects promptly to doctor.
• Tell parent or caregiver to keep all medications away from children and pets.

---

vitamin A (retinol)
Aquasol A, Del-Vi-A, Palmitate-A 5000

Pregnancy Risk Category C

HOW SUPPLIED
Capsules: 10,000 IU, 25,000 IU, 50,000 IU
Drops: 30 ml with dropper (5,000 IU/0.1 ml, 50,000 IU/1 ml)
Tablets: 5,000 IU, 10,000 IU

ACTION
A coenzyme that stimulates retinal function, bone growth, reproduction, and integrity of epithelial and mucosal tissues.

Route	Onset	Peak	Duration
P.O.	Unknown	3-5 hr	Unknown

INDICATIONS & DOSAGES
RDA—
RDAs have been converted to retinol equivalents (REs). One RE has the activity of 1 mcg all-trans retinol, 6 mcg beta-carotene.
Neonates and infants up to age 1: 375 mcg RE/day or 1,250 IU/day.
Children ages 1 to 3: 400 mcg RE/day or 1,330 IU/day.
Children ages 4 to 6: 500 mcg RE/day or 1,665 IU/day.
Children ages 7 to 10: 700 mcg RE/day or 2,330 IU/day.
Boys and men ages 11 and older: 1,000 mcg RE/day or 3,330 IU/day.
Girls and women ages 11 and older: 800 mcg RE/day or 2,665 IU/day.
Pregnant women: 800 mcg RE/day or 2,665 IU/day.
Breast-feeding women (first 6 months): 1,300 mcg RE/day or 4,330 IU/day.
Breast-feeding women (second 6 months): 1,200 mcg RE/day or 4,000 IU/day.

Dietary supplement—
Patient should maintain adequate dietary nutrition and RE vitamin A supplements. Because potency of different supplement forms varies, patient should follow manufacturer's label recommendations for specific products.

ADVERSE REACTIONS
CNS: irritability, headache, *increased intracranial pressure,* fatigue, lethargy, malaise.
EENT: papilledema, exophthalmos.
GI: anorexia, epigastric pain, vomiting, polydipsia.
GU: hypomenorrhea, polyuria.

Reactions may be *common*, uncommon, *life-threatening*, or COMMON AND LIFE-THREATENING.

Hepatic: jaundice, *hepato-megaly, cirrhosis,* elevated liver enzyme levels.

Metabolic: slow growth, decalcification, hypercalcemia, premature closure of epiphyses, cortical thickening over the radius and tibia.

Musculoskeletal: migratory arthralgia, periostitis.

Skin: alopecia; dry, cracked, scaly skin; pruritus; lip fissures; erythema; inflamed tongue, lips, and gums; massive desquamation; increased pigmentation; night sweats.

Other: splenomegaly, *anaphylactic shock.*

INTERACTIONS
Drug-drug

Cholestyramine resin, mineral oil: reduces GI absorption of fat-soluble vitamins. Tell patient to avoid using together.

Isotretinoin, multivitamins containing vitamin A: increases risk of toxicity. Tell patient to avoid using together.

Neomycin (oral): decreases vitamin A absorption. Tell patient to avoid using together.

Oral contraceptives: may increase plasma vitamin A levels. Monitor patient closely.

Warfarin: increases risk of bleeding. Monitor PT and INR closely.

CONTRAINDICATIONS
Oral route is contraindicated in patients with malabsorption syndrome; if malabsorption is caused by inadequate bile secretion, oral route may be used together with administration of bile salts (dehydrocholic acid). Also contraindicated in patients who are hypersensitive to any ingredient in product and in those with hypervitaminosis A.

OVERDOSE & TREATMENT
Signs and symptoms of overdose include nausea, vomiting, anorexia, malaise, dry and cracking skin and lips, irritability, hair loss, headache, visual disturbances, vertigo, and bulging fontanelles in infants.

In cases of acute toxicity, increased intracranial pressure develops within 8 to 12 hours; cutaneous desquamation follows in a few days. Toxicity can follow a single dose of 25,000 IU/kg, which in infants represents about 75,000 IU/kg and in adults more than 2 million IU.

Chronic toxicity results from administration of 4,000 IU/kg for 6 to 15 months. In infants (ages 3 to 6 months), this represents about 18,500 IU daily for 1 to 3 months; in adults, 1 million IU daily for 3 days, 50,000 IU daily for longer than 18 months, or 500,000 IU daily for 2 months.

To treat toxicity, discontinue vitamin A if hypercalcemia persists; administer I.V. saline solution, prednisone, and calcitonin, if indicated. Perform liver function tests to detect possible liver damage.

NURSING CONSIDERATIONS
● *Alert:* Don't confuse drug with retinoic acid or vitamin A acid.
● Use cautiously in pregnant patients, avoiding doses exceeding RE.
● Assess patient's vitamin A intake from all sources.
● Liquid products are available for NG route. They may be mixed with cereal or fruit juice.
● Adequate vitamin A absorption needs suitable dietary protein, fat, vitamin E, and zinc intake and bile secretion; Give supplemental salts, as ordered. Zinc supplements may be needed in patients receiving long-term total parenteral nutrition.
● Watch for adverse reactions if dosage is high.
● Watch for skin disorders; high dosages may induce chronic toxicity.
● Vitamin A therapy may falsely increase serum cholesterol levels by interfering with the Zlatkis-Zak reaction. It also may falsely elevate bilirubin determinations with Ehrlich's reagent.

PATIENT TEACHING
● Tell patient not to take megadoses of vitamins without specific indications to avoid toxicity.
● Stress that prescribed vitamins shouldn't be shared with others.
● Teach patient about good food sources of vitamin A, such as green and yellow vegetables, cantaloupe, and liver. (Note that liver is also high in saturated fat.)
● Advise patient that liquid product can be mixed with food, if desired.
● Instruct patient to protect drug from light.

---

vitamin C (ascorbic acid)
Ascorbicap, C-Complex, Cebid Timecelles, Cecon, Cevi-Bid, Ce-Vi-Sol, C-Gram, Chew-C, Dull-C, Flavorcee, Fruit-C, Life-Line C, N'ice w/Vitamin C Drops, One-A-Day Extra Vitamin C, Pan C-500, Redoxon†, Sunkist Vitamin C, Vicks-Vitamin C (contains tartrazine), Vita-C

Pregnancy Risk Category C

HOW SUPPLIED
Capsules (timed-release):
500 mg
Crystals: 1 g/tsp
Lozenges: 60 mg

Oral liquid: 50 ml (35 mg/ 0.6 ml)*
Oral solution: 100 mg/ml
Powder: 100 g (4 g/tsp), 500 g (4 g/tsp)
Syrup: 500 mg/5 ml
Tablets: 25 mg, 50 mg, 100 mg, 250 mg, 500 mg, 1,000 mg
Tablets (chewable): 100 mg, 250 mg, 500 mg, 1,000 mg
Tablets (timed-release): 500 mg, 1,000 mg, 1,500 mg

ACTION
Stimulates collagen formation and tissue repair; involved in oxidation-reduction reactions.

Route	Onset	Peak	Duration
P.O.	Unknown	Unknown	Unknown

INDICATIONS & DOSAGES
RDAs—
Neonates and infants up to age 6 months: 30 mg.
Infants ages 6 months to 1 year: 35 mg.
Children ages 1 to 3: 40 mg.
Children ages 4 to 10: 45 mg.
Children ages 11 to 14: 50 mg.
Adults and children ages 15 and older: 60 mg.
Pregnant women: 70 mg.
Breast-feeding women (first 6 months): 95 mg.
Breast-feeding women (second 6 months): 90 mg.
Smokers: 100 mg

Prevention of vitamin C deficiency in patients with poor nutritional habits or increased requirements—
Adults: 70 to 150 mg P.O. daily.
Pregnant and breast-feeding women: at least 70 to 150 mg P.O. daily.
Children: at least 40 mg P.O. daily.
Infants: at least 35 mg P.O. daily.

Because potency of different supplement forms varies, patient should follow manufacturer's label recommendations for specific products.

ADVERSE REACTIONS
CNS: faintness, dizziness.
GI: diarrhea, heartburn, nausea, vomiting.
GU: acid urine, oxaluria, renal calculi.

INTERACTIONS
Drug-drug
Aspirin (high doses): increases risk of salicylate toxicity and ascorbic acid deficiency. Monitor patient closely.
Contraceptives, estrogen: increases serum levels of estrogen. Tell patient to watch for adverse reactions.
Oral iron supplements: increases iron absorption. Encourage use together for this reason.

---

*Liquid contains alcohol.   **May contain tartrazine.   †Canada   ‡Australia   §U.K.

Warfarin: decreases anticoagulant effect. Monitor patient closely.

Drug-herb
Bearberry: inactivation of bearberry in urine. Tell patient to avoid using together.

Drug-lifestyle
Smoking: may decrease serum ascorbic acid levels. Increased doses of drug may be needed; monitor patient closely.

CONTRAINDICATIONS
Contraindicated in patients allergic to tartrazine or sulfites. Large doses are contraindicated during pregnancy.

OVERDOSE & TREATMENT
Excessively high doses of parenteral ascorbic acid are excreted renally after tissue saturation and rarely accumulate. Serious adverse effects or toxicity are uncommon. Severe effects require discontinuation of therapy.

NURSING CONSIDERATIONS
• Urge patients with renal insufficiency to use cautiously because vitamin is normally excreted in urine.
• Closely monitor patients at risk for deficiency, such as elderly and indigent patients, patients on restricted diets, those receiving long-term treatment with I.V. fluids or hemodialysis, and drug addicts or alcoholics.
• Conditions that elevate metabolic rate (such as fever, burns, infection, trauma) will significantly increase need for ascorbic acid supplements.
• Vitamin C is found in citrus fruits, tomatoes, potatoes, and leafy vegetables.
• Patient should take large dosages in divided doses because the body uses only a limited amount and excretes the rest in urine.
• Patient should take oral solutions of ascorbic acid directly into the mouth or mix with food.
• Monitor patient for signs and symptoms of ascorbic acid deficiency, including irritability, emotional disturbances, pallor, and anorexia.
• Ascorbic acid is a strong reducing agent; it alters results of tests based on oxidation-reduction reactions. Large doses (over 500 mg) may cause false-negative glucose determinations using glucose oxidase method or false-positive results using copper reduction method or Benedict's reagent. Ascorbic acid shouldn't be used for 48 to 72 hours before an amine-dependent test for occult blood in the stool is conducted; a false-negative result may occur. Depending on reagents used, it

may also interact with other diagnostic tests.

PATIENT TEACHING
- Stress proper nutritional habits to prevent recurrence of deficiency.
- Inform patient that vitamin C is readily absorbed from citrus fruits, tomatoes, potatoes, and leafy vegetables.
- Inform parent or caregiver that infants fed on cow's milk alone will require supplemental ascorbic acid.
- Advise pregnant patient that effects on fetus are unknown. Patient should contact doctor before taking this vitamin.
- Advise breast-feeding patients to use cautiously because ascorbic acid appears in breast milk.

---

vitamin D
cholecalciferol
(vitamin D₃)
Delta-D, Vitamin D

ergocalciferol
(vitamin D₂)
Calciferol, Drisdol, Radiostol†, Vitamin D₃

Pregnancy Risk Category C

HOW SUPPLIED
Capsules: 400 IU
Oral liquid: 8,000 IU/ml in 60-ml dropper bottle
Softgels: 400 IU, 1,000 IU
Tablets: 400 IU, 1,000 IU

ACTION
Promotes absorption and utilization of calcium and phosphate, helping to regulate calcium homeostasis.

Route	Onset	Peak	Duration
P.O.	2-14 hr	4-12 hr	2 days-6 mo

INDICATIONS & DOSAGES
Adequate intake—
Adults and children from birth to age 50: 5 mcg (200 IU) P.O. daily.
Adults ages 51 to 70: 10 mcg (400 IU) P.O. daily.
Adults ages 71 years and older: 15 mcg (600 IU) P.O. daily.

Because potency of different supplement forms varies, patient should follow manufacturer's label recommendations for specific products.

ADVERSE REACTIONS
CNS: headache, weakness, somnolence, overt psychosis, irritability.
CV: calcification of soft tissues, including the heart; hypertension; ***arrhythmias.***
EENT: rhinorrhea, conjunctivitis (calcific), photophobia.
GI: anorexia, nausea, vomiting, constipation, dry mouth, metallic taste, polydipsia.

GU: polyuria, albuminuria, hypercalciuria, nocturia, impaired renal function, reversible azotemia.
Hepatic: elevated AST and ALT levels.
Metabolic: hypercalcemia, hyperthermia, falsely increased serum cholesterol levels, weight loss.
Musculoskeletal: bone and muscle pain, bone demineralization.
Skin: pruritus.
Other: decreased libido.

INTERACTIONS
Drug-drug
Cardiac glycosides: increases risk of arrhythmias. Monitor serum calcium levels.
Cholestyramine, colestipol, mineral oil: inhibits GI absorption of oral vitamin D. Space doses. Tell patient to use together cautiously.
Corticosteroids: antagonizes effect of vitamin D. Monitor vitamin D levels closely.
Magnesium-containing antacids: possible hypermagnesemia, especially in patients with chronic renal failure. Monitor serum magnesium levels.
Phenobarbital, phenytoin: increases vitamin D metabolism and decreases effectiveness. Monitor patient closely.

Thiazide diuretics: may cause hypercalcemia in patients with hypoparathyroidism. Monitor patient closely.
Verapamil: atrial fibrillation has occurred from increased calcium. Monitor patient closely.

CONTRAINDICATIONS
Contraindicated in patients with hypercalcemia, hypervitaminosis D, malabsorption syndrome, decreased renal function, or renal osteodystrophy with hyperphosphatemia.

OVERDOSE & TREATMENT
Signs and symptoms of overdose include hypercalcemia, hypercalciuria, hyperphosphatemia, and in severe cases, death from cardiac or renal failure.
   Treatment of overdose includes stopping therapy, starting a low-calcium diet, and increasing fluid intake. A loop diuretic, such as furosemide, may be given with saline I.V. infusion to increase calcium excretion. Supportive measures should be provided. Calcitonin may decrease hypercalcemia.

NURSING CONSIDERATIONS
• Ergocalciferol should be used with extreme caution, if at all, by patients with heart disease, renal stones, or arteriosclerosis.

• Drug should be used cautiously by cardiac patients, especially those taking cardiac glycosides, and by patients with increased sensitivity.

• *Alert:* Monitor patient's eating and bowel habits; dry mouth, nausea, vomiting, metallic taste, and constipation may be early evidence of toxicity.

• Monitor serum and urine calcium, phosphorus, potassium, and urea levels when high therapeutic dosages are used.

• Doses of 60,000 IU/day can cause hypercalcemia. Hypercalcemia may require I.V. hydration and aggressive diuresis.

• Malabsorption from inadequate bile or hepatic dysfunction may require addition of exogenous bile salts to oral form.

• Patients with hyperphosphatemia need dietary phosphate restrictions and binding drugs to avoid metastatic calcifications and renal calculi.

• Mineral oil interferes with absorption of fat-soluble vitamins.

PATIENT TEACHING
• Teach patient that vitamin D is needed to absorb calcium. Instruct patient to read labels for vitamin D content.

• Advise patient that vitamin D is fat soluble and that mineral oil will interfere with absorption.

• Instruct patient to take only as directed, and stress the dangers of excessive doses of fat-soluble vitamins.

• Instruct patient to restrict intake of magnesium-containing antacids.

• Instruct patient to swallow tablet or capsule whole; don't crush or chew.

• Tell patient to notify doctor if signs and symptoms of toxicity occur, such as weakness, lethargy, headache, anorexia, weight loss, nausea, vomiting, abdominal cramps, diarrhea, constipation, vertigo, polydipsia, polyuria, dry mouth, or muscle or bone pain.

---

vitamin E (tocopherols)
Amino-Opti-E, Aquasol E, E-Complex-600, E-200 I.U. Softgels, E-400 I.U. in a Water Soluble Base, E-1000 I.U. Softgels, E-Vitamin Succinate, Vita-Plus E

Pregnancy Risk Category A

HOW SUPPLIED
Capsules: 100 IU, 200 IU, 400 IU, 500 IU, 600 IU, 1,000 IU, 73.5 mg, 147 mg, 165 mg, 330 mg
Oral solution: 50 mg/ml
Tablets (chewable): 200 IU, 400 IU

ACTION
Unknown. Thought to act as an antioxidant and protect RBC membranes against hemolysis.

Route	Onset	Peak	Duration
P.O.	Unknown	Unknown	Unknown

INDICATIONS & DOSAGES
RDA—
RDAs for vitamin E have been converted to α-tocopherol equivalents α-TE). One α-TE equals 1 mg of D-α-tocopherol or 1.49 IU.
Infants up to age 6 months: 3 α-TE/day or 4 IU/day.
Infants ages 6 months to 1 year: 4 α-TE/day or 6 IU/day.
Children ages 1 to 3: 6 α-TE/day or 9 IU/day.
Children ages 4 to 10: 7 α-TE/day or 10 IU/day.
Men ages 11 and older: 10 α-TE/day or 15 IU/day.
Women ages 11 and older: 8 α-TE/day or 12 IU/day.
Pregnant women: 10 α-TE/day or 15 IU/day.
Breast-feeding women (first 6 months): 12 α-TE/day or 18 IU/day.
Breast-feeding women (second 6 months): 11 α-TE/day or 16 IU/day.

Dietary supplement—
Adults: 30 IU P.O. daily in conjunction with other vitamins.

Because potency of different supplement forms varies, patient should follow manufacturer's label recommendations for specific products.

Vitamin E deficiency in patients with impaired fat absorption—
Adults: depending on severity, 60 to 75 IU P.O. daily.
Children: 1 IU/kg daily.

To reduce risk of coronary artery disease—
Adults: 100 to 800 mg P.O. daily based on doctor's recommendation.

ADVERSE REACTIONS
CNS: fatigue, weakness, headache, blurred vision.
GI: nausea, flatulence, diarrhea.

INTERACTIONS
Drug-drug
Anticoagulants (oral): hypoprothrombinemic effects may increase, possibly causing bleeding. Monitor patient closely.
Cholestyramine, colestipol, mineral oil: inhibits GI absorption of oral vitamin E. Tell patient to space doses and use together cautiously.
Iron: may catalyze oxidation and increase daily requirements. Tell patient to avoid using together.

Vitamin K: antagonized effects of vitamin K possible with large doses of vitamin E. Tell patient not to use together.

CONTRAINDICATIONS
None reported.

OVERDOSE & TREATMENT
Signs and symptoms of overdose include a possible increase in blood pressure.

Treatment is supportive.

NURSING CONSIDERATIONS
• Use cautiously in patients with liver or gallbladder disease.
• Monitor patient with liver or gallbladder disease for response to therapy. Adequate bile is essential for vitamin E absorption.
• Water-miscible forms are more completely absorbed in GI tract.
• Requirements increase with rise in dietary polyunsaturated acids.
• Hypervitaminosis E signs and symptoms include fatigue, weakness, nausea, headache, blurred vision, flatulence, diarrhea.

PATIENT TEACHING
• Tell patient not to crush tablets or open capsules. An oral solution and chewable tablets are commercially available.
• Warn patient against self-medicating with megadoses, which can cause thrombophlebitis. Vitamin E is fat soluble and may accumulate.
• Tell patient to store vitamin E in a tight, light-resistant container.
• Inform patient of dietary sources of vitamin E.

---

zinc gluconate (14.3% zinc)
zinc sulfate (23% zinc)
Orazinc, PMS Egozinc†, Verazinc, Zinc 15, Zinc-220

Pregnancy Risk Category NR

HOW SUPPLIED
zinc gluconate
Tablets: 10 mg (1.4 mg zinc), 15 mg (2 mg zinc), 50 mg (7 mg zinc), 78 mg (11 mg zinc)

zinc sulfate
Capsules: 220 mg (50 mg zinc)
Tablets: 66 mg (15 mg zinc), 110 mg (25 mg zinc), 200 mg (45 mg zinc)

ACTION
Normal growth and tissue repair depend on adequate zinc. Zinc acts as an integral part of several enzymes important to protein and carbohydrate metabolism.

Route	Onset	Peak	Duration
P.O.	Unknown	2 hr	Unknown

INDICATIONS & DOSAGES
RDA—
Infants up to age 1: 5 mg/day.
Children ages 1 to 10: 10 mg/day.
Boys and men ages 11 and older: 15 mg/day
Girls and women ages 11 and older: 12 mg/day.
Pregnant women: 15 mg/day.
Breast-feeding women (first 6 months): 19 mg/day.
Breast-feeding women (second 6 months): 16 mg/day.

Dietary supplement—
Infants up to age 1 year: 5 mg P.O. daily.
Children ages 1 to 10: 10 mg P.O. daily.
Adults and children older than age 11: 12 to 15 mg P.O. daily.

Because potency of different supplement forms varies, patient should follow manufacturer's label recommendations for specific products.

ADVERSE REACTIONS
CNS: restlessness, unusual fatigue.
CV: hypotension.
EENT: ulcers in mouth or throat, sore throat.
GI: nausea, vomiting, dyspepsia, dehydration.

Hematologic: *leukopenia, neutropenia,* and sideroblastic anemia (secondary to zinc-induced copper deficiency).
Hepatic: jaundice.
Respiratory: pulmonary edema.
Other: fever.

INTERACTIONS
Drug-drug
Amiloride: decreases zinc excretion and potential zinc toxicity. Tell patient not to use together.
AZT, captopril and other ACE inhibitors, H₂ blockers and other proton pump inhibitors, oral contraceptives, thiazide diuretics: decreases zinc absorption. Monitor patient.
Copper, iron, phosphorous supplements: decreases effects if taken together. Tell patient to separate administration times by 2 hours to obtain full benefit of each supplement.
Fluoroquinolones, tetracyclines: GI absorption and serum levels of some fluoroquinolones and tetracyclines may be decreased, possibly resulting in a decreased anti-infective response. Tell patient to separate administration times by taking zinc supplements 2 hours after fluoroquinolone or tetracycline.
Penicillamine: decreases penicillamine and zinc absorption.

Tell patient to separate administration times by 2 hours.
Thiazide diuretics: increases zinc loss in urine. Tell patient to avoid taking together.

Drug-food
Bran products, phytates, protein, some minerals: may decrease zinc absorption. Tell patient not to use together.

CONTRAINDICATIONS
Contraindicated in pregnant and breast-feeding patients and in patients with copper deficiency.

OVERDOSE & TREATMENT
Long-term zinc doses of 100 mg or more daily may result in severe copper deficiency, impaired immunity, heart problems, and anemia. Signs and symptoms of overdose include chest pain, dizziness, fainting, shortness of breath, vomiting, and jaundiced eyes or skin.

If overdose is suspected, reduce dosage or discontinue zinc to control signs and symptoms.

NURSING CONSIDERATIONS
• To avoid GI upset, patient should take zinc with food but avoid foods high in calcium, phosphorus, or phytate.
• Use as a dietary supplement to prevent or treat zinc deficiencies is based on normal daily recommended intakes of elemental zinc (see RDA).
• Treatment dose is individualized depending on severity of deficiency.
• Obtain accurate diet history from patient or caregiver.
• Zinc deficiency may result in poor night vision, decreased wound healing, a decreased sense of taste and smell, reduced immunity, and poor development of reproductive organs.
• Monitor patient's response to drug.

PATIENT TEACHING
• Inform elderly patient that he may be at risk for developing a zinc deficiency because of poor food selection, decreased absorption, diseases that cause magnesium depletion, or medications that may decrease absorption or increase urinary loss of zinc.
• Inform pregnant patient that routine use of zinc supplements during pregnancy isn't recommended. However, the RDA does increase during pregnancy to 15 mg per day compared to the basal recommendation of 12 mg per day for nonpregnant women.
• Inform breast-feeding patient that during the first 6 months of breast-feeding, the RDA for zinc is 19 mg per day, calculat-

---

*Liquid contains alcohol. **May contain tartrazine. †Canada ‡Australia §U.K.

ed to replace zinc lost in breast milk. After 6 months, the RDA falls to 16 mg per day, reflecting diminished average milk production in this period.

• Discuss dietary habits with patient or caregiver.

• Tell patient that dietary sources of zinc include oysters (very high), seeds, nuts, peas, whole wheat, rye, and oats.

• Instruct patient that supplement is most effective if taken 1 hour before or 2 hours after meals. Supplement may be taken with meals if stomach upset occurs, but doctor should be alerted.

• Instruct patient to report adverse effects promptly to doctor.

• Instruct parent or caregiver to keep medication away from children and pets.

10

Miscellaneous OTC drugs

This small group of unrelated OTC drugs includes ammonia, bismuth subgallate, diethyltoluamide, glucose, and insulin.

Ammonia

Ammonia is a colorless gas with a very sharp odor. The major compound in smelling salts, ammonia can be toxic if taken in more than just a sniff.

Ammonia has been used in medicine for many years. Its pungent odor stimulates or arouses a person who has fainted. Providing smelling salts commonly restores the person to consciousness. However, even though ammonia and smelling salts have a positive role in health care, they shouldn't be overused. A person who faints easily should be evaluated to determine the cause, and he shouldn't rely on smelling salts as a routine means of recovering consciousness.

Bismuth subgallate

Bismuth is widely used to soothe minor stomachaches and aid in the eradication of *Helicobacter pylori,* the bacteria thought to contribute to the development of peptic ulcers.

Various forms of bismuth are used for many other purposes as well. For example, bismuth subgallate has a deodorizing action useful to patients with colostomies, ileostomies, or fecal incontinence. Bismuth compounds are also used in dental fillings and bone implants. They can be used to enhance the visibility of catheters and surgical items on X-rays and scans. They can be used to treat diaper rash. And, when added to antiseptic powders or ointments, they can help to heal wounds and remove warts.

Although independent home use of bismuth compounds can be safe and beneficial, encourage patients to seek medical attention if the condition for which they're using a bismuth compound worsens or fails to respond.

Diethyltoluamide

Diethyltoluamide, commonly known as DEET, is an insect repellent effective against mosquitoes, biting flies (gnats, sandflies, deer flies, stable flies, black flies), ticks, harvest mites, and fleas. DEET is available without a prescription in liquid, aerosol, spray, or towelette forms. It is available in various concentrations and in many different brands of insect repellent.

Encourage patients who use this product to carefully read and follow any precautions on the label. Especially if the product contains high levels of DEET, instruct the patient to use just enough repellent to cover exposed skin areas. Applying the repellent to clothing also helps repel insects and may lessen the exposure of skin to DEET. Tell patients not to apply the product under their clothing and to wash treated clothing after use.

Urge patients to keep DEET products away from their eyes, lips, and the membranes inside the nose. If some repellent accidentally contacts one of these areas, tell the patient to immediately rinse it with plenty of water and to consult a doctor if irritation, especially of the eyes, continues.

Tell patients not to apply DEET to wounds or to irritated or broken skin because of the increased chance of absorption and adverse reactions. Urge the patient to apply repellent sparingly in skinfold areas because irritation is more likely there.

DEET hasn't been studied in pregnant women; tell women who might be pregnant or who intend to become pregnant that they should check with a doctor about use of this product. Children may have an increased risk of adverse effects because of increased absorption of the chemical through their skin. Only products with low levels of DEET should be used on a child's exposed skin, and the product should be used sparingly. Tell patients to notify a doctor about any unusual or allergic reaction to this chemical.

Advise patients to store this product out of the reach of children and away from heat and direct light. Tell them not to refrigerate it, and urge them to discard outdated repellent.

Glucose

People who use insulin to treat diabetes may develop hypoglycemia if they are more active than usual, don't eat enough food, delay their meals, or inject too much insulin. Hypoglycemia warrants prompt attention to prevent more serious problems such as seizures, unconsciousness or, in rare circumstances, brain damage.

If hypoglycemia develops, the patient must quickly ingest a fast-acting carbohydrate to raise blood glucose levels. The best way to ensure the availability of a fast-acting carbohydrate is for the patient to keep a commercially prepared form of glucose with him at all times. Commercial glucose preparations are convenient to carry and provide an amount of glucose appropriate for correcting hypoglycemia.

Insulin

In patients with diabetes mellitus, beta cells in the pancreas make little or no insulin (a hormone that allows cells to use ingested glucose for energy). When that happens, the affected person experiences hyperglycemia, glycosuria, and possibly ketoacidosis, in which the body attempts to use fat stores rather than glucose for energy.

To reverse these harmful conditions and restore the ability of cells to use glucose for energy, people with diabetes may need to be treated with human, synthetic, or animal insulin. The drug comes in fast-, intermediate-, and long-acting forms; all are given by S.C. injection.

Patients who use insulin need information about its onset, peak, and duration. They need to learn appropriate preparation and administration techniques. And they need to learn how to time their meals in relation to peak serum insulin levels. If hypoglycemia develops more than once daily or on two consecutive days despite adequate teaching, urge the patient to notify a doctor.

**ammonia spirit
bismuth subgallate
diethyltoluamide (DEET)
glucose
insulins**

---

ammonia spirit, aromatic

Pregnancy Risk Category NR

HOW SUPPLIED
Solution: 30 ml, 60 ml, 120 ml;
pints; gallons
Inhalant: 0.33 ml, 0.4 ml

ACTION
Irritates the sensory receptors
in the nasal membranes, producing reflex stimulation of the
respiratory centers.

Route	Onset	Peak	Duration
P.O., inhalation	Immediate	Unknown	Unknown

INDICATIONS & DOSAGES
*Treatment or prevention of
fainting—*
Adults and children: 1 broken
capsule inhaled until awake or
no longer faint; or 2 to 4 ml
P.O. diluted in at least 30 ml of
water.

ADVERSE REACTIONS
EENT: irritation.

INTERACTIONS
None reported.

CONTRAINDICATIONS
None reported.

OVERDOSE & TREATMENT
None reported.

NURSING CONSIDERATIONS
● Tell person administering ammonia to avoid inhaling vapors
and to monitor patient closely
for response.

PATIENT TEACHING
● Teach patient how to use drug.
● Tell patient to store drug in re-
frigerator.

---

bismuth subgallate
Devrom

Pregnancy Risk Category NR

HOW SUPPLIED
Tablets: 200 mg

ACTION
Decreases fecal odors because
it has antimicrobial properties.

Route	Onset	Peak	Duration
P.O.	Unknown	Unknown	Unknown

INDICATIONS & DOSAGES
*To control fecal odors in
colostomy, ileostomy, or fecal
incontinence—*
Adults: 1 or 2 tablets P.O. t.i.d.
with meals. May chew or swallow whole.

Reactions may be *common,* uncommon, *life-threatening*, or COMMON AND LIFE-THREATENING.

ADVERSE REACTIONS
GI: temporary darkening of the tongue or stool.

INTERACTIONS
None reported.

CONTRAINDICATIONS
None reported.

OVERDOSE & TREATMENT
Signs and symptoms of overdose are rare but may include encephalopathy, methemoglobinemia, and seizures.

To hasten patient's recovery from bismuth-induced encephalopathy, use chelation with dimercaprol in doses of 3 mg/kg or penicillamine 100 mg/kg/day for 5 days. For methemoglobinemia, give methylene blue 1 to 2 mg/kg in a 1% sterile aqueous solution I.V. push over 4 to 6 minutes. Repeat within 60 minutes if necessary, up to a total dose of 7 mg/kg. Use I.V. diazepam for seizure control.

NURSING CONSIDERATIONS
• Bismuth absorbs X-rays and may interfere with diagnostic procedures of the GI tract.

PATIENT TEACHING
• Instruct patient that bismuth subgallate can't reduce odor caused by faulty hygiene.
• Tell patient to keep the drug away from children and pets.

---

diethyltoluamide (DEET)
Cutter, Deep Woods OFF, Muskol, OFF, OFF Skintastic, Repel, Skedaddle

Pregnancy Risk Category NR

HOW SUPPLIED
Lotion (6.5% to 19%), *pump spray* (4.75% to 100%), *aerosol spray* (14.25% to 38%), *liquid* (19%)

ACTION
Repels insects and protects skin from insect bites.

Route	Onset	Peak	Duration
Topical	Unknown	Unknown	Unknown

INDICATIONS & DOSAGES
Insect repellent effective against mosquitoes, black flies, harvestbugs, chiggers, midges, ticks, and fleas—
Adults and children older than age 2: for liquid or lotion, apply enough repellent to cover the exposed areas of the skin; rub in gently and let dry. For topical aerosol or spray, hold the container 6 to 8 inches from skin or clothing and spray enough repellent to cover exposed skin. Spread evenly with hands over all exposed skin and allow to dry. For towelette, wipe over exposed skin and let dry. Reapply as needed.

ADVERSE REACTIONS
Skin: local skin reactions (itching, burning, swelling).

INTERACTIONS
None reported.

CONTRAINDICATIONS
Contraindicated in children younger than age 2 because of possible CNS toxicity.

OVERDOSE & TREATMENT
Toxic encephalopathy, seizures, manic psychosis, and CV toxicity (sinus bradycardia and or-thostatic hypotension) have been linked to topical application of DEET, especially in children who received liberal applications of this compound. Death has been reported after oral ingestion of large amounts of DEET-containing insect repellants.

Contact a poison control center if overdose occurs.

NURSING CONSIDERATIONS
• Safety information is lacking on the use of DEET during pregnancy.
• Systemic toxicity has been reported after application of large topical doses in children. Avoid use in children younger than age 2.
• DEET is for external use only.
• Patient should use products containing less than 30% DEET, and use sparingly. One

application will last about 4 to 8 hours.

PATIENT TEACHING
• Instruct patient to tell doctor about other prescription or OTC medication use.
• Tell patient to wear long sleeves and protective clothing, when possible, and to apply the product to clothing to enhance repellent action. Caution patient not to apply repellent under clothing.
• Instruct patient to avoid applying product to the eyes, lips, or inside of nose. If exposure occurs in these areas, tell patient to rinse with water and contact doctor if irritation persists.
• Tell patient not to spray product directly onto face but instead to spray onto hand and carefully apply to face.
• Tell patient to avoid eyes, mucous membranes, or broken skin.
• Urge patient to read product label carefully; if product contains alcohol, warn patient to avoid open flames and smoking after application.
• Instruct patient to wash treated skin with soap and water as soon as protection is no longer needed.
• Urge patient to seek medical attention if he develops altered facial skin color, clumsiness, unsteadiness, confusion, seizures, fast or irregular

breathing, loss of consciousness, mood or mental changes,
muscle cramping, puffy or
swollen eyes, red skin, shortness of breath, trouble breathing, tightness in chest, wheezing, skin blisters, rash, hives,
itching, slow heartbeat, slurred
speech, tremors, trouble sleeping, uncontrolled jerking, or
unusual tiredness or weakness.

glucose
Liquid glucose gel (40%
dextrose): Glutose, Insta-
Glucose, Insulin Reaction;
Dex4 Glucose; B-D Glucose

Pregnancy Risk Category C

HOW SUPPLIED
Liquid glucose gel: Glutose
45-g tube and 15-g tube; Insta-
Glucose 30.8-g unit dose tube
(cherry flavor); Insulin Reaction 25-g unit dose tube (lime
flavor)
Tablets: Dex4 Glucose (lemon,
orange, raspberry, and grape
flavors)
Tablets (chewable): B-D Glucose 5-g tablets

ACTION
Glucose (a monosaccharide) is
absorbed from the intestine and
causes a rapid increase in
serum glucose levels.

Route	Onset	Peak	Duration
P.O.	< 10 min	40 min	Unknown

INDICATIONS & DOSAGES
Management of hypoglycemia—
**Adults and children older
than age 2:** 10 to 20 g P.O. Response should occur within 10
minutes. Repeat in 10 to 20
minutes, p.r.n. until serum glucose level exceeds 70 mg/dl.

ADVERSE REACTIONS
GI: nausea.

INTERACTIONS
None reported.

CONTRAINDICATIONS
None reported.

OVERDOSE & TREATMENT
None reported.

NURSING CONSIDERATIONS
• Drug shouldn't be given to
children younger than age 2 unless directed.
• Each gram of 40% dextrose
gel provides 400 mg dextrose.
• Tablets and gel may be administered orally to conscious hypoglycemic patients. Direct
absorption from the intestine
results in a rapid increase in serum glucose levels and is effective in small doses.
• Glucose isn't absorbed from
the buccal cavity; it must be
swallowed to be effective. Al-

though an unconscious person may have a swallowing reflex, the lack of a normal gag reflex may lead to aspiration. When possible, use other methods of treating hypoglycemia in unconscious patients.

PATIENT TEACHING
• Tell patient that he may need another dose if his glucose levels rise by less than 20 mg/dl in 20 minutes and he continues to have signs and symptoms of hypoglycemia.
• Tell patient to eat a well-balanced meal after the hypoglycemic episode has resolved.
• Advise patient that an adjustment of insulin, oral antidiabetic, diet, or exercise may be needed after a hypoglycemic episode.

---

insulins
insulin injection (regular insulin, crystalline zinc insulin)
Humulin-R, Novolin R, Novolin R PenFill, Pork Regular Iletin II, Regular Purified Pork Insulin, Velosulin Human BR†

isophane insulin suspension (neutral protamine Hagedorn insulin, NPH)
Humulin N, Novolin N, Novolin N PenFill, NPH insulin, NPH Purified Pork, Purified Pork NPH Iletin II

isophane insulin suspension with insulin injection
Humulin 50/50, Humulin 70/30, Novolin 70/30, Novolin 70/30 PenFill

insulin zinc suspension (lente)
Humulin L, Lente Iletin II, Lente Insulin, Lente Purified Pork Insulin, Novolin L

insulin zinc suspension, extended (ultralente)
Humulin-U

Pregnancy Risk Category B

HOW SUPPLIED
insulin injection
Injection (human): 100 units/ml (Humulin-R, Novolin R); 100 units/ml in 1.5-ml cartridge system (Novolin R PenFill)
Injection (from pork): 100 units/ml
Injection (purified pork): 100 units/ml (Pork Regular Iletin II, Regular Purified Pork Insulin)
isophane insulin suspension
Injection (human, recombinant): 100 units/ml (Humulin N, Novolin N); 100 units/ml in 1.5-ml cartridge system (Novolin N PenFill)

Reactions may be *common*, uncommon, *life-threatening*, or COMMON AND LIFE-THREATENING.

Injection (purified pork): 100 units/ml (NPH Purified Pork, Purified Pork NPH Iletin II)

isophane insulin suspension 50% with insulin injection 50%
Injection (human): 100 units/ml (Humulin 50/50)

isophane insulin suspension 70% with insulin injection 30%
Injection (human): 100 units/ml (Humulin 70/30, Novolin 70/30); 100 units/ml in 1.5-ml cartridge system (Novolin 70/30 PenFill)

insulin zinc suspension
Injection (purified pork): 100 units/ml (Lente Iletin II, Lente Purified Pork Insulin)
Injection (human): 100 units/ml (Humulin L, Novolin L)

insulin zinc suspension, extended
Injection (human): 100 units/ml (Humulin-U)

ACTION
Increases glucose transport across muscle and fat cell membranes to reduce serum glucose level. Promotes conversion of glucose to its storage form, glycogen. Triggers amino acid uptake and conversion to protein in muscle cells and inhibits protein degradation. Stimulates triglyceride formation and inhibits release of free fatty acids from adipose tissue. Stimulates lipoprotein lipase activity, which converts circulating lipoproteins to fatty acids.

Route	Onset	Peak	Duration
S.C.			
rapid	0.5-1.5 hr	2-3 hr	5-7 hr
inter-mediate	1-2.5 hr	4-15 hr	12-24 hr
long-acting	4-8 hr	10-30 hr	36 hr

INDICATIONS & DOSAGES
Type 1 insulin-dependent diabetes, adjunct to type 2 non–insulin-dependent diabetes inadequately controlled by diet and oral antidiabetics—
Adults and children: 0.2 to 1 unit/kg/day. Adjust doses to achieve control based on individual guidelines prescribed by doctor.

ADVERSE REACTIONS
Metabolic: hypoglycemia; hyperglycemia (rebound, or Somogyi effect); decreased serum magnesium, potassium, or inorganic phosphate levels.
Skin: rash, urticaria, pruritus, swelling, redness, stinging, warmth at injection site.
Other: lipoatrophy, lipohypertrophy, *hypersensitivity reactions, anaphylaxis.*

INTERACTIONS
Drug-drug
ACE inhibitors, anabolic steroids, beta blockers, calcium, chloroquine, clofibrate, guanethidine, lithium carbonate, MAO inhibitors, mebendazole, pentamidine, pyridoxine, salicylates, sulfonamides, tetracycline: causes prolonged hypoglycemic effect. Tell patient to monitor serum glucoses level carefully.
Acetazolamide, asparaginase, calcitonin, corticosteroids, cyclophosphamide, dextrothyroxine, diltiazem, diuretics, dobutamine, epinephrine, estrogens, ethacrynic acid, isoniazid, lithium carbonate, morphine sulfate, niacin, nicotine, phenothiazines, thiazide diuretics, thyroid hormone: diminishes insulin response. Tell patient to watch for hyperglycemia.
Diazoxide, phenytoin (high doses): may inhibit endogenous insulin secretion and cause hypoglycemia in diabetic patients. Tell patient to carefully adjust insulin dosage.
Oral contraceptives: may decrease glucose tolerance in diabetic patients. Tell patient to monitor serum glucose levels and adjust insulin dosage carefully.

Drug-herb
Basil, bay, bee pollen, burdock, sage: may affect glycemic control. Advise patient to avoid using together.
Garlic dust, ginseng: may decrease glucose levels. Advise patient to avoid using together.

Drug-lifestyle
Alcohol use: causes hypoglycemic effect. Advise patient to avoid using together.
Marijuana use: may increase serum glucose levels. Advise patient not to use marijuana.
Smoking: may increase serum glucose levels and decrease response to insulin. Tell patient to monitor serum glucose levels.

CONTRAINDICATIONS
Contraindicated in patients with history of systemic allergic reaction to pork.

OVERDOSE & TREATMENT
Insulin overdose may produce signs and symptoms of hypoglycemia (tachycardia, palpitations, anxiety, hunger, nausea, diaphoresis, tremors, pallor, restlessness, headache, and speech and motor dysfunction).

Treatment is based on signs and symptoms. If patient is responsive, give 10 to 15 g of a fast-acting oral carbohydrate. If signs and symptoms persist after 15 minutes, give another

10 g of carbohydrate. If patient is unresponsive, an I.V. bolus of dextrose 50% solution should immediately increase serum glucose levels. Some prefer to use dextrose 25% in water because it's less irritating if extravasation occurs. A common infusion rate is based on glucose content: 10 to 20 mg/kg/minute. Parenteral glucagon or epinephrine S.C. may also be given; both drugs raise serum glucose levels in a few minutes by stimulating glycogenolysis. Fluid and electrolyte imbalance may require I.V. fluids and electrolyte (such as potassium) replacement.

NURSING CONSIDERATIONS
• Insulin is the drug of choice to treat diabetes during pregnancy. Insulin requirements increase in pregnant diabetic women and then decline immediately postpartum. Monitor patient closely.
• Dosage is always expressed in USP units. Remember to use only the syringes calibrated for the concentration of insulin administered. U-500 insulin must be administered with a U-100 syringe because no syringes are made for this strength.
• Some patients may develop insulin resistance and need large insulin doses to control signs and symptoms of diabetes. U-500 insulin is available as Reg-

ular (Concentrated) Iletin II for such patients. This concentration requires a prescription.
• To mix insulin suspension, swirl vial gently or rotate between palms or between palm and thigh. Don't shake vigorously—this causes bubbling and air in syringe.
• Lente, semilente, and ultralente insulins may be mixed in any proportion. Regular insulin may be mixed with NPH or lente insulins in any proportion. When mixing regular with intermediate or long-acting insulin, always draw up regular insulin into syringe first.
• Switching from separate injections to a prepared mixture may alter response. When mixing NPH or lente with regular insulin in a syringe, give immediately to avoid loss of potency.
• Don't use insulin that changes color or becomes clumped or granular in appearance.
• Check expiration date on vial before using contents.
• Usual administration route is S.C. For proper S.C. administration, pinch a fold of skin with fingers at least 3 inches (7.6 cm) apart, and insert needle at a 45- to 90-degree angle.
• Press but don't rub site after injection. Rotate and document injection sites to avoid overuse of one area. Diabetic patients may achieve better control if in-

jection site is rotated within same anatomic region.

• Store insulin in cool area. Refrigeration is desirable but not essential.

PATIENT TEACHING
• Inform patient that therapy only relieves signs and symptoms and doesn't cure disease.
• Instruct patient about nature of disease and importance of following therapeutic regimen; adhering to specific diet, weight reduction, exercise, and personal hygiene programs; and avoiding infection. Emphasize importance of timing injections and meals and the danger of missing meals.
• Stress that accuracy of measurement is important, especially with concentrated regular insulin. Aids, such as magnifying sleeve or dose magnifier, may improve accuracy. Show patient and caregivers how to measure and administer insulin.
• Advise patient not to alter order of mixing insulins or change model or brand of insulin, syringe, or needle.
• Emphasize the importance of monitoring blood glucose levels and performing urine ketone tests to assess dosage and confirm success of therapy. It's important for patient to recognize hyperglycemia and hypoglycemia. Insulin-induced hypo-

glycemia is hazardous and may cause brain damage if prolonged; most adverse effects are self-limiting and temporary. Instruct patient in insulin peak times and their importance.
• Instruct patient on proper use of equipment for monitoring blood glucose levels.
• Advise patient not to smoke within 30 minutes after insulin injection. Cigarette smoking decreases absorption of insulin administered S.C.
• Inform patient that marijuana use may increase insulin requirements.
• Advise patient to wear a medical identification bracelet at all times, to carry ample insulin and syringes on trips, to have carbohydrates (sugar, candy, or commercial glucose product) on hand for emergencies, and to note changes in time zones, which may alter dose schedule.
• Tell patient that room temperature insulin may be less painful when injected.
• Instruct patient to store unopened preparations in the refrigerator. Vials in use can be stored at room temperature. Insulin in unopened, prefilled plastic or glass syringes is stable for 1 month if refrigerated.

Ophthalmic lubricants

Ophthalmic lubricants provide symptomatic relief from dry eyes, allergic and viral conjunctivitis, minor eye irritation, and blepharitis (when irritation of the eye is also present). These products stabilize the tear film, preventing tears from evaporating. In addition to surface-active properties, povidone-containing products are thought to form a hydrophilic layer, resembling mucin, on the corneal surface. Therefore, mucin- and aqueous-deficient conditions may benefit from these products.

Ophthalmic ointments have enhanced retention time, which may augment the integrity of the tear film. Preservatives such as benzalkonium chloride, chlorhexidine, chlorobutanol, methylparaben, propylparaben, EDTA, sodium perborate, thimerosal, and purite destroy or inhibit reproduction of microorganisms that may be unintentionally introduced into the product during administration.

Adverse reactions
• Blurred vision (more significant with ointments).
• Hypersensitivity to preservatives. As daily dosage increases, toxicity caused by preservatives becomes more likely.

Interactions
• Polyvinyl alcohol, when given with other products (those containing sodium bicarbonate, sodium borate, and the sulfates of sodium, potassium, and zinc) may thicken the solutions that contain it.

Nursing considerations
• Dosage should be 1 to 2 drops b.i.d. initially, increased up to hourly, if needed.
• Ointments are usually used b.i.d. but may be instilled as often as every few hours.
• Because ointments may blur vision, patients commonly use drops during daytime hours and ointments at bedtime.
• If irritation lasts longer than 72 hours, evaluation by an ophthalmic practitioner is best.
• Preservative-free products are more expensive.
• Benzalkonium chloride may reduce the effectiveness of ophthalmic lubricants through its toxic effects on the tear film and the corneal epithelium.
• Thimerosal doesn't alter the tear film; however, eye irritation may result after several weeks.

Patient teaching
• Tell patient to avoid dry or dusty places that may increase evaporation of the tear film.
• Advise patient to wash hands thoroughly before and after using an ophthalmic lubricant.
• Warn patient not to touch the tip of bottle or tube to any surface, including the eye.
• Tell patient to discard single-use packages immediately after

use and to discard or replace multidose bottles 30 days after the safety seal is broken.
- If patient uses both a drop and an ointment, advise him to instill the drop at least 10 minutes before the ointment.
- If patient needs multiple drops, tell him to wait about 5 minutes between drops.
- Avoid activities requiring good visual acuity for several minutes after applying ointment.

Brand name	Active ingredients	Form
Accu-Tears	light mineral oil white petrolatum	Ointment
Accu-Tears PVA	benzalkonium chloride polyvinyl alcohol 1.4%	Solution
Adsorbotear	hydroxyethylcellulose 0.41% povidone 1.67% thimerosal 0.004%	Solution
Akwa Tears	benzalkonium chloride 0.01% polyvinyl alcohol 1.4%	Preservative-free solution
Akwa Tears	lanolin mineral oil white petrolatum	Ointment
AquaSite	dextran 70 0.1% polycarbophil sorbic acid 0.2%	Solution
AquaSite Preservative-free	dextran 70 0.1% polyethylene glycol 400 0.2%	Preservative-free solution
Bion Tears	dextran 70 0.1% hydroxypropyl methylcellulose 0.3%	Preservative-free solution
Celluvisc	carboxymethylcellulose sodium 1%	Preservative-free solution
Computer Eye Drops	benzalkonium chloride 0.01% glycerin 1%	Solution
Dakrina	busan 1507 0.001% polyvinyl alcohol 2.7% povidone 2%	Solution

Brand name	Active ingredients	Form
DuraTears Naturale	lanolin mineral oil petrolatum	Ointment
Dwelle	NPX 0.001% polyvinyl alcohol 2.7% povidone 2%	Solution
GenTeal Lubricant	hydroxypropyl methylcellulose 0.3% sodium perborate	Solution
GenTeal Lubricant Gel	hydroxypropyl methylcellulose 0.3% sodium perborate 0.028%	Gel
HypoTears	benzalkonium chloride 0.01% polyethylene glycol 400 1% polyvinyl alcohol 1%	Solution
HypoTears	mineral oil white petrolatum	Ointment
HypoTears PF	polyethylene glycol 400 polyvinyl alcohol 1%	Preservative-free solution
HypoTears Select	polyethylene glycol 400 1% polyvinyl alcohol 1% sodium perborate	Solution
Lacri-Lube NP	lanolin alcohols mineral oil 42.5% white petrolatum 57.3%	Preservative-free ointment
Lacri-Lube S.O.P.	chlorobutanol 0.5% lanolin alcohols mineral oil 42.5% white petrolatum 56.8%	Ointment
Liquifilm Tears	chlorobutanol 0.5% polyvinyl alcohol 1.4%	Solution
Moisture Eyes	benzalkonium chloride 0.01% glycerin 0.3% propylene glycol 1%	Solution
Moisture Eyes PM	mineral oil 20% white petrolatum 80%	Preservative-free ointment

(continued)

Brand name	Active ingredients	Form
Moisture Eyes Preservative Free	propylene glycol 0.95%	Preservative-free solution
Murine Tears Lubricant	benzalkonium chloride polyvinyl alcohol 0.5% povidone 0.6%	Solution
Murocel Lubricant Ophthalmic	methylcellulose 1% methylparaben 0.023% propylene glycol propylparaben 0.01%	Solution
Ocucoat	benzalkonium chloride 0.01% dextran 70 0.1% hydroxypropyl methylcellulose 0.8%	Solution
Ocucoat PF	dextran 70 0.1% hydroxypropyl methylcellulose 0.8%	Preservative-free solution
Puralube Tears	benzalkonium chloride polyethylene glycol 400 1% polyvinyl alcohol 1%	Solution
Refresh	polyvinyl alcohol 1.4% povidone 0.6%	Solution
Refresh Plus	carboxymethylcellulose 0.5%	Preservative-free solution
Refresh PM	lanolin alcohols mineral oil 41.5% white petrolatum 56.8%	Preservative-free ointment
Refresh Tears	carboxymethylcellulose sodium 0.5% purite (stabilized oxychloro complex)	Solution
Tearisol	benzalkonium chloride 0.01% hydroxypropyl methylcellulose 0.5%	Solution
Tears Naturale	benzalkonium chloride 0.01% dextran 70 0.1% hydroxypropyl methylcellulose 0.3%	Solution

Brand name	Active ingredients	Form
Tears Naturale Free	dextran 70 0.1% hydroxypropyl methylcellulose 0.3%	Preservative-free solution
Tears Naturale II	dextran 70 0.1% hydroxypropyl methylcellulose 0.3% polyquad 0.001%	Solution
Tears Plus	chlorobutanol 0.5% polyvinyl alcohol 1.4% povidone 0.6%	Solution
Tears Naturale P.M.	lanolin mineral oil white petrolatum	Ointment
Tears Renewed	light mineral oil white petrolatum	Ointment
Thera Tears	sodium carboxymethylcellulose 0.25% sodium perborate	Solution
Thera Tears	sodium carboxymethylcellulose 0.25%	Preservative-free solution
Ultra Tears	benzalkonium chloride 0.01% hydroxypropyl methylcellulose 1%	Solution
Visine Tears	benzalkonium chloride glycerin 0.2% hydroxypropyl methylcellulose 0.2% polyethylene glycol 400 1%	Solution
Visine Tears Preservative Free	glycerin 0.2% hydroxypropyl methylcellulose 0.2% polyethylene glycol 400 1%	Preservative-free solution
Viva-Drops	polysorbate 80	Preservative-free solution

Extraocular irrigating solutions

Extraocular irrigating solutions are used to cleanse the eye and remove unwanted substances from the ocular area.

Adverse reactions
Adverse effects are related to preservatives.

Interactions
None.

Nursing considerations
• These solutions aren't indicated for open wounds in or near the eyes.
• If the eye is exposed to chemicals or extreme heat, tell patient to flush it for 10 minutes and to then seek further evaluation from an ophthalmic practitioner.
• If symptoms don't resolve within 72 hours or if eye pain continues or vision changes, tell patient to seek evaluation.

Patient teaching
• Tell patient not to use while wearing contact lenses.
• Caution against using an eyecup because it may have bacterial or fungal contamination.
• To use drug, tell patient to bend over a sink, tilt his head to the side, and hold the bottle near the inner corner of the eye. Tell him to squeeze the bottle, allowing the solution to flow across the ocular surface toward the outer corner. Tell him to blot excess liquid from around the eye and repeat in the other eye, if necessary.
• Urge patient to discard ophthalmic products 30 days after breaking the safety seal.

Brand name	Active ingredients
Accu-Wash	benzalkonium chloride sodium chloride sodium phosphate
Bausch & Lomb Eye Wash	boric acid EDTA 0.025% sodium borate sodium chloride sorbic acid 0.1%
Collyrium for Fresh Eyes	benzalkonium chloride 0.01% boric acid sodium borate
Dacriose	benzalkonium chloride 0.01% EDTA 0.3% sodium chloride sodium phosphate

Brand name	Active ingredients
Eye Stream	benzalkonium chloride sodium acetate 0.39% sodium citrate 0.17% sodium hydroxide or hydrochloric acid
Lavoptik Eye Wash	benzalkonium chloride 0.005% sodium chloride 0.49% sodium phosphate

Eyelid scrubs

Eyelid scrubs are used to clean the eyelid and eyelid margins to prevent or treat blepharitis (inflammation of the eyelid margins). These cleansers remove oil, debris, and skin cells that may cause irritation or inflammation of the eyelid.

Adverse reactions
None reported.

Interactions
None.

Nursing considerations
• Blepharitis causes red, scaly, thickened eyelids with loss of eyelashes. It is commonly a chronic condition. Good eyelid hygiene is the cornerstone of prevention and treatment.
• If a patient's signs and symptoms persist, he should be referred to an ophthalmic practitioner. The patient may need an antibacterial product for resolution.
• Ocular lubricants may be used if the eye is also irritated.

Patient teaching
• Tell patient to use hot compresses for 15 to 20 minutes b.i.d. to q.i.d., followed by eyelid scrubs.
• Urge patient to wash hands thoroughly before and after use.
• Tell him to apply 3 to 4 drops of eyelid scrub to a cotton applicator or gauze pad, close the eye, and clean the upper lid using side-to-side strokes. Then he should open the eye, look up, and clean the lower eyelid using side-to-side strokes. Tell him to repeat on the other eye using a new applicator and then rinse the eyelids and eyelashes with clean, warm water.

Brand name	Active ingredients
Eye Scrub	benzyl alcohol cocamidopropylamine oxide disodium laureth sulfosuccinate EDTA polyethylene glycol 200 glyceryl monotallowate polyethylene glycol 78 glyceryl cocoate
Lid Wipes-SPF	cocoamidopropylamine oxide glycerin laureth-23 polyethylene glycol 80 glyceryl cocoate polyethylene glycol 200 glyceryl monotallowate sodium chloride

Brand name	Active ingredients
OcuSoft Solution and Pads	cocoamidopropyl hydroxysulftaine lauroamphocarboxyglycinate polyethylene glycol 15 tallow polyamine polyethylene glycol 80 polyethylene glycol 150 distearate quaternium-15 sodium laureth-13 carboxylate sodium trideceth sulfate sorbitan laurate

Mouth and throat lozenges and sprays

Mouth and throat lozenges and sprays provide temporary relief from sore throat pain, throat irritation, and sore mouth. Benzocaine and dyclonine, which are anesthetics, numb the mouth and throat to ease pain and discomfort. In addition, some products contain an antiseptic agent, such as cetylpyridinium chloride. However, these local antiseptics aren't effective for viral infections. Menthol and camphor, which are counterirritants, are found in some products and are thought to have a mild anesthetic effect and reduce discomfort by producing a sensation of warmth or cold.

Adverse reactions

Local allergic reactions and irritation.

Interactions

None reported.

Nursing considerations

• Patients with diabetes should select a sugar-free spray or lozenge.
• If sore throat is severe or persists for several days, patient should seek medical evaluation.
• Sore throats accompanied by fever, headache, nausea, or vomiting also need medical evaluation.
• Allergic reactions to benzocaine and other ingredients may occur.

Patient teaching

• Tell patient not to eat or drink while numbness (caused by the anesthetic) persists.
• Suggest such nondrug options as hard candy, warm saline gargles, and fruit juices.
• Most products can be used every 3 to 4 hours as needed. Warn against exceeding the recommended dosage.

Brand name	Active ingredients	Class
Celestial Seasonings Echinacea Complete Care	echinacea root extract 50 mg menthol 1 mg	Anesthetic Herbal medication
Celestial Seasonings Echinacea Cold Season	echinacea root extract 50 mg menthol 1.8 mg	Anesthetic Herbal medication
Cepacol Sore Throat Maximum Strength, Cherry (lozenge)	benzocaine 10 mg cetylpyridinium chloride menthol 3.6 mg	Anesthetic Antiseptic

Brand name	Active ingredients	Class
Cepacol Sore Throat Maximum Strength, Cherry (spray)	cetylpyridinium chloride dyclonine hydrochloride 0.1%	Anesthetic Antiseptic
Cepacol Sore Throat Maximum Strength, Cool Menthol (spray)	cetylpyridinium chloride dyclonine hydrochloride 0.1%	Anesthetic Antiseptic
Cepacol Sore Throat Maximum Strength, Mint (lozenge)	benzocaine 10 mg cetylpyridinium chloride menthol 2 mg	Anesthetic Antiseptic
Cepacol Sore Throat Maximum Strength, Sugar Free, Cherry (lozenge)	benzocaine 10 mg cetylpyridinium chloride menthol 4.5 mg	Anesthetic Antiseptic
Cepastat Extra Strength Sore Throat (lozenge)	eucalyptus oil menthol phenol 29 mg	Anesthetic
Cepastat Sore Throat, Cherry (lozenge)	menthol phenol 14.5 mg	Anesthetic
Fisherman's Friend, Extra Strong, Sugar Free (lozenge)	menthol 10 mg	Anesthetic
Fisherman's Friend Original, Extra Strong (lozenge)	menthol 10 mg	Anesthetic
Fisherman's Friend, Regular (lozenge)	menthol 6 mg	Anesthetic
Fisherman's Friend, Sugar Free (lozenge)	menthol 3 mg	Anesthetic
Halls Juniors Sugar Free Cough Drops	menthol 2.5 mg	Anesthetic
Halls Mentho-Lyptus Cough Suppressant Drops, Cherry (lozenge)	menthol 7.6 mg	Anesthetic
Halls Mentho-Lyptus Cough Suppressant Drops, Honey-Lemon (lozenge)	menthol 8.6 mg	Anesthetic *(continued)*

Brand name	Active ingredients	Class
Halls Mentho-Lyptus Cough Suppressant Drops, Mentho-Lyptus (lozenge)	menthol 7 mg	Anesthetic
Halls Mentho-Lyptus Cough Suppressant Drops, Spearmint (lozenge)	menthol 6 mg	Anesthetic
Halls Mentho-Lyptus Extra Strength Cough Suppressant Drops, Ice Blue (lozenge)	menthol 12 mg	Anesthetic
Halls Mentho-Lyptus Sugar Free Cough Supp Drops, Black Cherry (lozenge)	menthol 5 mg	Anesthetic
Halls Mentho-Lyptus Sugar Free Cough Supp Drops, Citrus Blend (lozenge)	menthol 5 mg	Anesthetic
Halls Mentho-Lyptus Sugar Free Cough Supp Drops, Menthol (lozenge)	menthol 5.8 mg	Anesthetic
Halls Plus Maximum Strength Cherry, Honey Lemon, Mentho-Lyptus (lozenge)	menthol 10 mg	Anesthetic
Herbal Quincers, Assorted Fruit	herbal extracts menthol 2.5 mg	Anesthetic Herbal extracts
Herbal Quincers, Original (lozenge)	herbal extracts menthol 4.5 mg	Anesthetic Herbal extracts
Luden's Honey Lemon (lozenge)	menthol 2 mg	Anesthetic
Luden's Honey Licorice	menthol 2 mg	Anesthetic
Luden's Maximum Strength Cherry (lozenge)	menthol 10 mg	Anesthetic
Luden's Original Menthol (lozenge)	menthol 2 mg	Anesthetic

Brand name	Active ingredients	Class
N'Ice Sore Throat & Cough, Assorted, Cherry, Citrus, Herbal Mint or Honey Lemon (lozenges)	menthol 5 mg	Anesthetic
Ricola Cough Drops	menthol 1.1 to 4.8 mg (varies with product flavor)	Anesthetic
Ricola Sugar Free Herb Throat Drops	menthol 1.1 to 4.8 mg (varies with product flavor)	Anesthetic
Ricola Throat Lozenges, Echinacea Honey Lemon, Echinacea Orange Spice	echinacea extract menthol 2.7 to 4.5 mg (varies with product flavor)	Anesthetic Herbal medicine
Robitussin Cough Drops, Cherry, Honey-Lemon, Menthol Eucalyptus (lozenge)	eucalyptus oil menthol 7.4 to 10 mg (varies with product flavor)	Anesthetic
Robitussin Honey Cough, Herbal with Natural Honey Center, Honey Lemon (lozenge)	menthol 5 mg	Anesthetic
Robitussin Honey Cough Herbal-Almond, Herbal Honey Grapefruit (lozenge)	menthol 2.5 mg	Anesthetic
Robitussin Liquid Center Cough Drops, Cherry with Honey-Lemon Center (lozenge)	eucalyptus oil menthol 8 mg	Anesthetic
Robitussin Liquid Center Cough Drops, Honey Lemon with Cherry Center (lozenge)	eucalyptus oil menthol 10 mg	Anesthetic
Robitussin Sugar Free Cough Drops, Cherry or Peppermint (lozenge)	menthol 10 mg	Anesthetic
Sucrets Children's Sore Throat, Cherry (lozenge)	dyclonine hydrochloride 1.2 mg	Anesthetic *(continued)*

Brand name	Active ingredients	Class
Sucrets Maximum Strength Sore Throat, Black Cherry & Wintergreen (lozenge)	dyclonine hydrochloride 3 mg	Anesthetic
Sucrets Sore Throat, Assorted Flavors (lozenge)	dyclonine hydrochloride 2 mg	Anesthetic
Sucrets Sore Throat, Original Mint (lozenge)	hexylresorcinol 2.4 mg	Antiseptic
Vicks Chloraseptic Sore Throat, Cherry or Menthol (spray)	phenol 1.4%	Anesthetic
Vicks Chloraseptic Sore Throat, Cherry or Menthol (lozenge)	benzocaine 6 mg menthol 10 mg	Anesthetic
Vicks Cough Drops, Cherry or Menthol (lozenge)	menthol 1.7 to 3.3 mg (varies with product flavor)	Anesthetic
Vicks Original Cough Drops, Cherry (lozenge)	menthol 3.1 mg	Anesthetic
Vicks Original Cough Drops, Menthol (lozenge)	menthol 6 mg	Anesthetic

Saliva substitutes

Saliva substitutes are used to ease the discomfort of xerostomia, a condition that results from little or no salivation. These products are formulated to resemble natural saliva, both chemically and physically.

Adverse reactions
None reported.

Interactions
None reported.

Nursing considerations
• These products can be used as often as needed.
• Evaluate patient for secondary causes, such as drug therapy that has anticholinergic actions (as with antihistamines or antidepressants) or that reduces fluid volume (as with diuretics or antihypertensives).
• Advise against self-treatment if the patient has any of the following problems: mouth soreness from ill-fitting dentures, fever, swelling, loose teeth, severe tooth pain, bleeding gums without evidence of trauma, or

signs and symptoms of dental caries, gingivitis, or periodontal disease.
• Some products may have a high sodium content. Patients on a low-sodium diet (such as those with hypertension or heart failure) should avoid these products.

Patient teaching
• Tell patient that good oral hygiene and regular visits to the dentist are essential to minimize the risk of tooth decay and other complications.
• Caution patient to avoid substances that may reduce salivation (such as tobacco products, alcohol, antihistamines, and oral decongestants).
• Warn patient to limit intake of sugary and acidic foods to prevent tooth decay.
• Inform patient that using a very soft toothbrush may decrease decay by reducing tissue abrasion.
• If dryness persists despite using a saliva substitute or if complications develop, urge patient to see a dentist.

Brand name	Active ingredients	Form
Glandosane Mouth Moisturizer Aerosol Spray	calcium chloride dihydrate 0.007 g dipotassium hydrogen phosphate 0.017 g magnesium chloride hexahydrate 0.003 g potassium chloride 0.061 g sodium carboxymethylcellulose 0.51 g	Aerosol spray

(continued)

Brand name	Active ingredients	Form
Glandosane Mouth Moisturizer Aerosol Spray *(continued)*	sodium chloride 0.043 g sorbitol 1.52 g	Liquid
Optimoist Liquid	calcium chloride citric acid hydroxyethyl cellulose malic acid polysorbate 20 sodium benzoate sodium hydroxide sodium monofluorophosphate sodium phosphate monobasic xylitol	Gel
Oralbalance Moisturizing Gel	glucose oxidase glycerate polyhydrate hydroxyethyl cellulose lactoperoxidase lysozyme lactoferrin xylitol	Solution
Salivart Synthetic Saliva Solution	calcium chloride magnesium chloride potassium chloride potassium phosphate sodium carboxymethylcellulose 1% sodium chloride sorbitol	Solution

Enemas and bowel evacuants

Enemas and bowel evacuant kits can be used to treat constipation but are more commonly used to empty the distal colon in preparation for surgery, child delivery, or endoscopic or radiologic procedures involving the GI tract.

Several types of laxatives are commonly included in enemas or bowel evacuant kits. Emollient laxatives, such as docusate sodium and calcium, are anionic surfactants that soften the stool. Glycerin, classified as a hyperosmotic laxative, promotes a bowel movement through two mechanisms—osmotic and local irritant effects. Mineral oil is a lubricant laxative that softens the fecal contents by coating them and preventing colonic absorption of water. Saline laxatives, such as magnesium citrate, monobasic and dibasic sodium phosphate, and sodium biphosphate, draw water into the intestinal tract, which increases intraluminal pressure and enhances intestinal motility. Bisacodyl, a stimulant laxative, increases intestinal peristaltic activity.

Adverse reactions
- *Emollients:* diarrhea, mild abdominal cramping.
- *Hyperosmotics:* rectal irritation.
- *Lubricants:* impaired absorption of fat-soluble vitamins, anal pruritus.
- *Saline laxatives:* abdominal cramping, nausea and vomiting, dehydration, fluid and electrolyte imbalances.
- *Stimulant laxatives:* severe cramping, excess electrolyte and fluid loss, enteric loss of protein, malabsorption and hypokalemia, cathartic colon (if used routinely for prolonged periods of time).

Interactions
- *Emollients:* enhanced systemic absorption of mineral oil.
- *Hyperosmotics:* None.
- *Lubricants:* absorption of medications (including oral anticoagulants, oral contraceptives, and digoxin) may be reduced. Mineral oil may reduce the absorption of fat-soluble vitamins (A, D, E, K).
- *Saline laxatives:* absorption of some medications (including oral anticoagulants, digoxin, and some phenothiazines) may be reduced.
- *Stimulant laxatives:* None.

Nursing considerations
- Advise against using emollient and lubricant laxatives in children younger than age 6. Rectally administered saline laxatives shouldn't be given to children younger than age 2.
- To prevent cathartic colon, stimulant laxatives shouldn't be used for longer than 1 week.

Patient teaching
• Tell the patient to lie on his left side with knees bent or in the knee-to-chest position. Advise him to let the enema solution flow into the rectum slowly and to retain it until definite lower abdominal cramping occurs.
• For suppositories, tell the patient to lie on his side and insert the suppository, pointed end first, high into the rectum. He should retain the enema for 15 to 20 minutes.

Brand name	Active ingredients	Form
Evac-Q-Kwik System	*Liquid:* magnesium citrate 25 mEq/30 ml *Suppository:* bisacodyl 10 mg *Tablets:* bisacodyl 15 mg/3 tabs	Bowel evacuant kit Saline laxative Stimulant laxative
Fleet Bisacodyl Enema	bisacodyl 10 mg glycerin	Enema Stimulant and hyperosmotic laxative
Fleet Mineral Oil Enema	mineral oil, 100%	Enema Lubricant laxative
Fleet Prep Kit 1	*Liquid:* sodium phosphate oral solution 45 ml *Suppository:* bisacodyl 10 mg *Tablets:* bisacodyl 20 mg/4 tabs	Bowel evacuant kit Saline laxative Stimulant laxative
Fleet Prep Kit 2	*Enema:* liquid castile soap 9 ml *Liquid:* sodium phosphate oral solution 45 ml *Tablets:* bisacodyl 20 mg/4 tabs	Bowel evacuant kit Saline laxative Stimulant laxative
Fleet Prep Kit 3	*Enema:* bisacodyl 10 mg, glycerin *Liquid:* sodium phosphate oral solution 45 ml *Tablets:* bisacodyl 20 mg/4 tabs	Bowel evacuant kit Saline laxative Stimulant laxative
Fleet Ready-to-Use Enema	dibasic sodium phosphate 7 g/118 ml monobasic sodium phosphate 19 g/118 ml (total sodium 4.4 g/118 ml)	Enema Saline laxative
Fleet Ready-to-Use Enema for Children	dibasic sodium phosphate 3.5 g/59 ml monobasic sodium phosphate 9.5 g/59 ml (total sodium 2.2 g/59 ml)	Enema Saline laxative

Brand name	Active ingredients	Form
Therevac Plus	benzocaine 20 mg docusate sodium 283 mg glycerin	Anesthetic Emollient and hyperos- motic laxative Enema
Therevac-SB	docusate sodium 283 mg glycerin	Emollient and hyperos- motic laxative Enema

Anorectal preparations

Anorectal products are used to temporarily ease the burning, itching, swelling, irritation, and discomfort of hemorrhoids. Hemorrhoid remedies usually contain one or more of the following: anesthetics, astringents, protectants, vasoconstrictors, and corticosteroids.

Local anesthetics (such as benzocaine, pramoxine, menthol, camphor, and benzyl alcohol) temporarily block the transmission of nerve impulses, which relieves itching, irritation, burning, and pain.

Zinc oxide and witch hazel, which are astringents, have a local drying effect that temporarily reduces irritation, discomfort, itching, and burning.

Several protectants are available and may be used alone or in combination to form a physical barrier on the skin. They protect the area from physical irritants and prevent water loss.

Phenylephrine and ephedrine are the primary vasoconstrictors used in anorectal preparations. By stimulating alpha-adrenergic receptors, arteriole vasoconstriction reduces swelling. Vasoconstrictors also relieve itching, discomfort, and irritation through an unknown mechanism.

Hydrocortisone, a corticosteroid, is used in anorectal products as a vasoconstrictor, anti-inflammatory, and antipruritic.

Adverse reactions
- *Anesthetics:* local (burning, itching) or systemic allergic reactions.
- *Astringents:* local reactions are rare.
- *Protectants:* minimal; lanolin alcohols may cause allergic reactions.
- *Vasoconstrictors:* nervousness, tremor, insomnia, nausea, or anorexia possible; increased blood pressure, cardiac arrhythmias, increased hyperthyroid or prostatic hyperplasia symptoms aren't likely with topical use of approved dosage regimen.
- *Corticosteroids:* may mask signs and symptoms of bacterial or fungal infection; skin atrophy.

Interactions
- *Vasoconstrictors:* antihypertensives, MAO inhibitors, tricyclic antidepressants.
- *Protectants:* aluminum hydroxide gel and kaolin won't adhere to the skin properly if petrolatum or greasy ointments are present.

Nursing considerations
- *Anesthetics:* avoid use if patient reports previous allergy. Pramoxine is structurally different from other anesthetics (benzocaine, lidocaine); thus, it has less cross-sensitivity and fewer adverse reactions.

• *Astringents:* witch hazel is for external use only. Zinc oxide and calamine may be used internally or externally.

• *Vasoconstrictors:* because of a slight chance of systemic absorption and adverse effects, patients with diabetes, hypertension, hyperthyroidism, or enlarged prostate should be monitored closely if using a product containing a vasoconstrictor.

• Pregnant and breast-feeding women should use only external products. Children younger than age 12 with hemorrhoids should be seen by a doctor.

Patient teaching

• Advise against using products more often than recommended.

• If symptoms don't improve within 7 days or if redness, irritation, pain, or other symptoms develop or increase, tell patient to stop drug and notify doctor.

• Tell patient to eat a high-fiber diet, increase fluid intake to prevent constipation, avoid straining during defecation, avoid prolonged sitting on the toilet, cleanse the anal area regularly and thoroughly after each bowel movement, and sit in warm water for 15 minutes two or three times daily.

• Tell patient to use anorectal preparations after bowel movements for maximum benefit.

• If patient uses a hemorrhoid product internally, tell him to apply with an applicator or finger. An applicator is preferred to place drug in a specific location or where a finger cannot reach. Urge patient to lubricate the applicator before insertion.

Brand name and active ingredients	Indications and dosages	Nursing considerations
Anusol Anti-Itch hydrocortisone acetate 1%	*Relieves pain, soreness, burning, and itching caused by hemorrhoids and other anorectal disorders; protects irritated tissue* **Adults:** apply to lower portion of anal canal t.i.d. to q.i.d.	• Tell patient to cleanse area with soap and water before use, and then blot or pat dry. • Urge patient to stop drug and notify doctor if symptoms persist longer than 7 days, if they worsen, or if bleeding occurs. • Advise against exceeding recommended dosage. • Warn against contact with eyes. • Tell patient not to insert into rectum with fingers or mechanical device. • Advise against using for diaper rash.

Brand name and active ingredients	Indications and dosages	Nursing considerations
Anusol Suppositories topical starch 51%	*Relieves itching, burning, and discomfort from hemorrhoids and other anorectal disorders; protects irritated tissue* **Adults:** insert suppository P.R. up to six times daily or after each bowel movement.	• Tell patient to cleanse area with soap and water before use, and then blot or pat dry. • Tell patient to stop using and notify doctor if symptoms persist longer than 7 days, if they worsen, or if bleeding occurs. • Caution against exceeding recommended dosage. • Warn patient to avoid contact with eyes. • Tell patient not to insert into rectum with fingers or mechanical device. • Advise against using for diaper rash.
Cortaid Intensive Therapy Cream hydrocortisone 1% **Nupercainal Ointment** dibucaine 1%	*Relieves external anal itching* **Adults and children ages 12 and older:** apply to affected area t.i.d. or q.i.d.	• Tell patient to cleanse area with soap and water before use, and then blot or pat dry. • Tell patient to stop using and notify doctor if symptoms persist longer than 7 days, if they worsen, or if bleeding occurs. • Caution against exceeding recommended dosage. • Warn patient to avoid contact with eyes. • Tell patient not to insert into rectum with fingers or mechanical device. • Advise against using for diaper rash.
Nupercainal Hemorrhoidal and Anesthetic Ointment dibucaine 1%	*Relieves pain, itching, and burning from hemorrhoids* **Adults:** instill into rectum using enclosed applicator in morning, evening, and after each bowel movement. Apply additional ointment to external anal tissue. Maximum 30 g daily.	• Tell patient to avoid contact with eyes. • Urge patient to stop using and notify doctor if symptoms persist longer than 7 days, if they worsen, or if bleeding, redness, irritation, or swelling occurs.

Brand name and active ingredients	Indications and dosages	Nursing considerations
Preparation H Cream glycerin 12% petrolatum 18% phenylephrine hydrochloride 0.25% shark liver oil 3% **Preparation H Ointment** mineral oil 14% petrolatum 71.9% phenylephrine hydrochloride 0.25% shark liver oil 3% **Preparation H Suppositories** cocoa butter 85.5% phenylephrine hydrochloride 0.25% shark liver oil 3%	*Relief from itching, burning, and discomfort from hemorrhoids; shrinks hemorrhoidal tissue; provides coating for relief from discomfort; protects inflamed tissue* **Adults and children ages 12 and older (cream, ointment):** apply externally to lower portion of anal canal up to q.i.d., in the morning, evening, and after each bowel movement. **Adults (suppositories):** insert 1 suppository into rectum as directed up to q.i.d., in the morning, evening, and after each bowel movement.	• Tell patient to cleanse affected area with soap and water before use, and then blot or pat dry. • Tell patient to stop using and notify doctor if symptoms persist longer than 7 days, if they worsen, or if bleeding occurs. • Caution against exceeding recommended dosage. • Caution against use if patient has heart disease, hypertension, thyroid disease, diabetes, or difficulty urinating because of enlarged prostate. • Warn patient not to use if he takes prescription drugs for hypertension or depression. • Explain that ointment can be used intrarectally with applicator provided. Advise against using fingers or mechanical devices to insert.
Preparation H Anti-Itch hydrocortisone 1%	**Adults and children ages 12 and older:** apply to affected area t.i.d. or q.i.d.	• Tell patient to cleanse affected area with soap and water before use, and then blot or pat dry. • Tell patient to stop using and notify doctor if symptoms persist longer than 7 days, if they worsen, or if bleeding occurs. • Caution against exceeding recommended dosage. • Tell patient to avoid contact with eyes. • Advise against inserting into rectum with fingers or mechanical device. • Tell patient not to use for diaper rash.

Vaginal preparations

Vaginal preparations come in many dosage forms. Among them are douches, towelettes, creams, ointments, and cleansing washes. Most products contain multiple ingredients to treat a combination of symptoms. They are used to cleanse, deodorize, relieve itching and irritation, alter vaginal pH, moisturize, or remove discharge. Ingredients include antiseptics, counterirritants, astringents, surfactants, pH agents, lubricants, antihistamines, anesthetics, and deodorants.

Antiseptics, which inhibit or destroy bacteria, include povidone-iodine, cetylpyridinium chloride, eucalyptol, menthol, oxyquinoline sulfate, phenol, sodium perborate, thymol, and chlorhexidine gluconate.

Counterirritants, known for anesthetic and antipruritic action, include povidone-iodine, eucalyptol, menthol, phenol, methyl salicylate, and thymol. Ammonium alum is an astringent, which helps protect the skin.

Surfactants help to distribute the drug over an area; these include docusate sodium, octoxynol 9, alkyl aryl sulfonate, sodium lauryl sulfate, and benzalkonium chloride.

Sodium perborate, sodium bicarbonate, lactic acid, sodium acetate, and citric acid are used for pH alteration. Lubricants, used to moisturize or replenish moisture, include propylene glycol, glycerin, and mineral oil. Tripelennamine is an antihistamine used to treat itching. Anesthetics include lidocaine and benzocaine. Many vaginal preparations also contain deodorants.

Adverse reactions
Local irritation, sensitivity, hypersensitivity.

Interactions
None reported.

Nursing considerations
• Drug should be applied only to affected area.
• Avoid products that contain povidone-iodine if patient is pregnant or has a thyroid disorder because of possible absorption through the skin.
• If symptoms persist, irritation develops, or area becomes infected, patient should stop using and notify a doctor.
• If patient complains of a discharge, tell her to see a doctor.
• Instruct patient to follow directions on package.
• Pregnant patients shouldn't douche.
• Douching doesn't protect from pregnancy or sexually transmitted diseases (STDs).
• Patient shouldn't douche more than twice a week.
• Douching may lead to pelvic

inflammatory disease (PID). Patient should notify doctor if she has abnormal discharge or bleeding, pain or tenderness in the lower abdomen or pelvis, nausea, and fever.

Patient teaching
• Tell patient to follow package instructions and to apply only to vaginal area.
• Caution against using a product that contains povidone-iodine if patient is pregnant or has a thyroid disorder.
• Tell patient to stop drug and notify doctor if symptoms wors-

en, abnormal discharge begins, or area becomes infected.
• Tell patient not to douche during pregnancy and to consult doctor before using any vaginal product.
• Stress that douching doesn't prevent pregnancy or STDs.
• Advise against douching more than twice a week.
• Douching has been linked to PID. Tell patient to notify doctor immediately if she has abnormal discharge, bleeding, fever, nausea, or pain and tenderness in the lower abdomen or pelvic area.

Brand name and active ingredients	Indications and dosages	Nursing considerations
Astroglide glycerin methylparaben polyquaternium propylene glycol propylparaben purified water	*Relief from vaginal dryness* **Adults:** apply a few drops to genital area or squeeze applicator contents into vagina.	• Tell patient to stop using if irritation occurs. • May be applied to inner and outer surfaces of condoms to enhance use. • Product isn't a spermicide or contraceptive.
Betadine Concentrated Medicated Douche povidone-iodine 10% **Betadine Disposable Douche** povidone-iodine 0.3%	*Relief from minor vaginal irritation and itching; cleanses and deodorizes* **Adults:** insert nozzle gently into vagina and let solution flow into and out of vagina. Use up to twice weekly for cleansing and deodorizing or q.d. for 5 days for irritation.	• Advise against using for longer than 7 days unless directed by doctor. • Caution against using drug to treat STDs. • Tell patient not to use when pregnant, breast-feeding, or experiencing abdominal or pelvic pain, vaginal discharge or bleeding, nausea, fever, frequent urination, genital sores, or ulcers. These may be symptoms of PID or an STD. • Tell iodine-sensitive patient not to use product.

(continued)

Brand name and active ingredients	Indications and dosages	Nursing considerations
H-R Lubricating Jelly carbomer 934P hydroxypropyl methylcellulose methylparaben propylene glycol propylparaben sodium hydroxide water **KY Jelly** chlorhexidine gluconate gluconodelta lactone glycerin hydroxyethylcellulose methylparaben purified water sodium hydroxide **Lubrin vaginal inserts** carylic-capric triglyceride glycerin polyethylene glycol-6-32 polyethylene glycol-20 polytheylene glycol-40 stearate polysorbate 80	*Vaginal dryness, lubrication; lubrication of condoms* **Adults:** apply 1- to 2-inch strip to vaginal area p.r.n. or place insert into vagina p.r.n.	• Don't use as a contraceptive; doesn't contain spermicide. • Tell patient to stop using drug if irritation occurs.
Massengill Disposable Douches cetylpyridinium chloride citric acid diazolidinyl urea edetate disodium octoxynol-9 purified water SD alcohol 40 sodium citrate **Massengill with Vinegar** cetylpyridinium chloride citric acid diazolidinyl urea edetate disodium octoxynol-9 purified water sodium citrate vinegar	*Vaginal cleansing* **Adults:** insert nozzle gently into vagina and let solution flow into and out of vagina. Use up to twice weekly.	• Tell patient not to use when pregnant, breast-feeding, or experiencing abdominal or pelvic pain, vaginal discharge or bleeding, nausea, fever, frequent urination, genital sores, or ulcers. These may be symptoms of PID or an STD. • Tell patient to stop using drug if dryness or irritation occurs.

Brand name and active ingredients	Indications and dosages	Nursing considerations
Massengill Clean Relief Towelettes hydrocortisone 0.5%	*Relief from external vaginal itching caused by irritation and rashes* **Adults and children ages 12 and older:** wipe with 1 towelette from front to back up to q.i.d.	• Tell patient to avoid contact with eyes. • Stop using and notify doctor if symptoms persist longer than 7 days, if they worsen, or if they recur within a few days. • Advise against using with other products that contain hydrocortisone. • Advise against use with vaginal discharge or for diaper rash.
Replens Vaginal Moisturizer Prefilled Applicators carbomer 934P glycerin hydrogenated palm oil glyceride mineral oil polycarbophil sorbic acid	*Vaginal dryness* **Adults:** apply 1 applicatorful for 2 to 3 days p.r.n.	• Tell patient product isn't a contraceptive.
Summer's Eve Disposable Douche citric acid decyl glucoside EDTA octoxynol 9 sodium benzoate **Summer's Eve Disposable Douche Extra Cleansing** benzoic acid purified water sodium chloride vinegar	*Vaginal cleansing* **Adults:** insert nozzle gently into vagina and let solution flow into and out of vagina. Use up to twice weekly.	• Tell patient not to use when pregnant, breast-feeding, or experiencing abdominal or pelvic pain, vaginal discharge or bleeding, nausea, fever, frequent urination, genital sores, or ulcers. These may be symptoms of PID or an STD. • Have patient stop using if dryness or irritation occurs.
Summer's Eve Medicated Disposable Douche povidone-iodine 0.3%	*Relief from vaginal irritation, itching, and soreness* **Adults:** insert nozzle gently into vagina and let solution flow into and out of	• Tell patient not to use to treat STDs. • Tell patient not to use when pregnant, breast-feeding, or experiencing abdominal or pelvic pain, vaginal discharge or

(continued)

Brand name and active ingredients	Indications and dosages	Nursing considerations
Summer's Eve Medicated Disposable Douche (continued)	vagina. Use daily for 7 days.	bleeding, nausea, fever, frequent urination, genital sores, or ulcers. These may be symptoms of PID or an STD. • Advise against use if patient is sensitive to iodine; if patient has pain, soreness, swelling, redness, itching, dryness, or irritation; or if symptoms last longer than 7 days.
Vagisil Powder aloe benzethonium chloride cornstarch magnesium stearate mineral oil silica	*Absorbs wetness, neutralizes odor, and fights odor-causing bacteria* **Adults:** apply daily to external vaginal area after bathing or showering.	• Patient may use as an all-over body powder.
Vagisil Intimate Moisturizer aloe callicrein chamomile methylparaben poloxamer 407 polyquaternium-32 propylene glycol propylparaben water	*Vaginal dryness* **Adults:** apply a few drops to vaginal opening and external area p.r.n.	• Patient shouldn't use as a contraceptive because product doesn't contain spermicide. • Tell patient to stop using if irritation occurs.
Vagisil Crème Maximum Strength benzocaine 20% resorcinol 3% **Vagisil Crème Regular Strength** benzocaine 5% resorcinol 2%	*Relief from vaginal itching* **Adults and children ages 12 and older:** apply a fingertip amount to affected area t.i.d. or q.i.d.	• Tell patient not to apply drug to large area or get it in eyes. • Tell patient to notify doctor if symptoms worsen, persist for longer than 7 days, or recur within a few days.

Analgesics for menstrual cramps

Brand name and active ingredients	Indications and dosages	Nursing considerations
Diurex PMS acetaminophen 500 mg pamabrom 25 mg pyrilamine maleate 15 mg	*Relief from menstrual cramps* **Adults and children ages 12 and older:** 2 caplets P.O. with water every 4 to 6 hours p.r.n. Maximum 8 caplets in 24 hours.	• Advise against taking for longer than 10 days. • Drug may turn urine a golden color. • Advise against exceeding recommended dosage. • Tell patient to consult doctor before taking drug if she also takes other drugs. • Tell patient to avoid hazardous activities. Drug may cause drowsiness.
Midol Maximum Strength PMS Formula acetaminophen 500 mg pamabrom 25 mg pyrilamine maleate 15 mg	*Relief from menstrual cramps* **Adults and children ages 12 and older:** 2 caplets or gelcaps P.O. with water every 4 hours p.r.n. Maximum 8 caplets or gelcaps in 24 hours.	• Tell patient not to take for longer than 10 days. • Urge patient to tell doctor if pain lasts longer than 10 days. • Patient should avoid alcohol, sedatives, and tranquilizers unless directed by doctor. Drug may cause drowsiness. • Caution patient to avoid hazardous activities. • Advise against giving to children because drug may cause excitability. • Drug contains caffeine equal to one cup of coffee. Patient should limit caffeine-containing drugs, food, or beverages. • Advise against taking drug if patient has emphysema, chronic bronchitis, or glaucoma, unless directed by a doctor. • Patients who drink more than three alcoholic beverages daily should notify doctor before taking drug.
Midol Maximum Strength Teen Formula	*Relief from menstrual cramps* **Adults and children ages 12 and older:**	• Tell patient not to take for longer than 10 days. • Advise patient to notify *(continued)*

Brand name and active ingredients	Indications and dosages	Nursing considerations
Midol Maximum Strength Teen Formula *(continued)* acetaminophen 500 mg pamabrom 25 mg	2 caplets P.O. with water every 4 hours p.r.n. Maximum 8 caplets in 24 hours.	doctor if pain lasts for longer than 10 days. • Tell patient who drinks more than three alcoholic drinks per day to consult doctor before taking.
Pamprin Maximum Strength acetaminophen 250 mg magnesium salicylate 250 mg pamabrom 25 mg	*Relief from menstrual cramps* **Adults and children ages 12 and older:** 2 caplets P.O. with water every 4 to 6 hours p.r.n. Maximum 8 caplets in 24 hours.	• Tell patient not to take for longer than 10 days. • Advise against taking for fever for longer than 3 days. • Urge patient to notify doctor about ringing in ears, hearing loss, persistent or worsening pain or fever, new symptoms, redness, or swelling. • Tell patient not to take with anticoagulants or if she has diabetes, gout, arthritis, or allergies to salicylates, unless directed by a doctor. • Advise against taking during last trimester of pregnancy.
Pamprin Maximum Strength Multi-Symptom Menstrual Relief acetaminophen 500 mg pamabrom 25 mg pyrilamine maleate 15 mg	*Relief from menstrual cramps* **Adults and children ages 12 and older:** 2 tablets or caplets P.O. with water every 4 to 6 hours p.r.n. Maximum 8 tablets or caplets in 24 hours.	• Tell patient not to take for longer than 10 days. • Tell patient to avoid alcohol, sedatives, and tranquilizers unless directed by doctor. Drug may cause drowsiness. • Caution patient to avoid hazardous activities. • Advise against giving drug to children because it may cause excitability. • Tell patient not to take if she has emphysema, chronic bronchitis, or glaucoma, unless directed by a doctor.

Brand name and active ingredients	Indications and dosages	Nursing considerations
Pamprin Maximum Strength Multi-Symptom Menstrual Relief *(continued)*		• Patients who drink more than three alcoholic beverages daily should notify doctor before taking this drug.
Premsyn PMS acetaminophen 500 mg pamabrom 25 mg pyrilamine maleate 15 mg	*Relief from menstrual cramps* **Adults and children ages 12 and older:** 2 caplets P.O. with water every 4 to 6 hours p.r.n. Maximum 8 caplets in 24 hours.	• Tell patient to continue use throughout menstrual cycle if needed but not to take longer than 10 days. • Tell patient to avoid alcohol, sedatives, and tranquilizers unless directed by doctor. Drug may cause drowsiness. • Urge patient to avoid hazardous activities. • Advise against use in children because drug may cause excitability. • Tell patient not to take drug if she has emphysema, chronic bronchitis, or glaucoma, unless directed by a doctor. • Patients who drink more than three alcoholic beverages daily should notify doctor before taking drug.
Tylenol Menstrual Relief acetaminophen 500 mg pamabrom 25 mg	*Relief from menstrual cramps* **Adults and children ages 12 and older:** 2 caplets P.O. with water every 4 to 6 hours p.r.n. Maximum 8 caplets in 24 hours.	• Tell patient not to take drug with other products that contain acetaminophen. • Urge patient to notify doctor if she has new or worsened symptoms, redness, or swelling.

Rubs and liniments

Brand name and active ingredients	Indications and dosages	Nursing considerations
Absorbine Jr. menthol 1.27%	*Minor aches and pains of muscles and joints caused by arthritis, strains, bruises, sprains, and backache* **Adults and children ages 2 and older:** apply generous amount to affected area and massage gently up to q.i.d.	• Tell patient not to apply to wounds. • Tell patient to notify doctor if symptoms worsen, persist for longer than 7 days, or recur. • Caution patient to avoid eyes. • Tell patient not to bandage affected area tightly.
Arthricare capsaicin 0.075% menthol 2%	*Relief from minor aches and pains caused by arthritis, backache, sprains, and strains* **Adults and children ages 2 and older:** apply to affected area t.i.d. or q.i.d.	• Warn patient to avoid eyes, mucous membranes, and broken or irritated skin. • Tell patient to notify doctor if symptoms worsen, persist for longer than 7 days, or recur. • Caution patient not to bandage affected area tightly or use with heating pad or after showering or bathing. • Tell patient to expect temporary redness.
Aspercreme trolamine salicylate 10% **Mobisyl crème** trolamine salicylate 10% **Myoflex crème** trolamine salicylate 10% **Sportscreme Cream** trolamine salicylate 10%	*Relief from mild joint or muscle pain* **Adults:** apply liberally and rub in gently b.i.d. to q.i.d.	• Patient should take one dose h.s. • Tell patient not to use for longer than 10 days. • Urge patient to notify doctor if condition worsens or persists. • Advise use in children only with medical supervision. • Tell patient to avoid eyes and mucous membranes. • Tell patient not to apply to inflamed, raw, or weeping skin.

Brand name and active ingredients	Indications and dosages	Nursing considerations
Banalg camphor 2% menthol 1% methyl salicylate 4.9%	*Relief from minor aches and pains of muscles and joints caused by backache, strains, bruises, and sprains; aches and pains caused by arthritis and rheumatism* **Adults:** apply to affected area t.i.d. or q.i.d.	• Warn patient against applying to wounds or to broken or irritated skin. • Caution patient not to use with a heating pad. • Tell patient not to bandage affected area tightly.
Ben-Gay menthol 10% methyl salicylate 15% **Ben-Gay Ultra Strength** camphor 4% menthol 10% methyl salicylate 30%	*Relief from minor aches and pains of muscles and joints caused by backache, arthritis, strains, and sprains* **Adults:** apply generous amount to affected area and massage until disappears t.i.d. or q.i.d.	• Caution against use with a heating pad. • Warn patient not to bandage affected area tightly. • Tell patient to notify doctor if skin redness or irritation occurs, or if pain lasts longer than 10 days. • Tell patient to avoid eyes, mucous membranes, and broken or irritated skin.
Ben-Gay Arthritis Formula menthol 8% methyl salicylate 30%	*Relief from minor aches and pains, stiffness of muscles and joints caused by arthritis* **Adults:** apply generous amount to affected area and massage until disappears t.i.d. or q.i.d.	• Caution against use with a heating pad. • Warn patient not to bandage affected area tightly. • Tell patient to notify doctor if skin redness or irritation occurs, or if pain lasts longer than 10 days. • Tell patient to avoid eyes, mucous membranes, and broken or irritated skin.
Deep Heating menthol 8% methyl salicylate 30%	*Relief from minor aches and pains of muscles and joints caused by backache, strains, bruises, sprains, and arthritis* **Adults and children ages 2 and older:** apply to affected area t.i.d. or q.i.d.	• Tell patient to avoid eyes and mucous membranes. • Tell patient not to bandage affected area tightly, apply to wounds or damaged skin, or use with a heating pad. • Tell patient to notify doctor if skin irritation occurs or if symptoms worsen, persist for longer than 7 days, or recur.

Brand name and active ingredients	Indications and dosages	Nursing considerations
Flexall 454 camphor 3.1% menthol 16% methyl salicylate 10%	*Relief from arthritis pain, backache, bursitis, tendinitis, muscle strains and sprains, bruises, and cramps* **Adults:** apply generous amount to affected area and massage until it disappears, p.r.n.	• Caution against use with a heating pad. • Warn patient not to bandage affected area tightly. • Tell patient to notify doctor if skin redness or irritation occurs, or if pain lasts longer than 10 days. • Tell patient to avoid eyes, mucous membranes, and broken or irritated skin.
Heet camphor 3.6 % capsicum oleoresin 0.025% methyl salicylate 15%	*Relief from minor aches and pains of muscles and joints caused by backache, strains, bruises, sprains, and arthritis* **Adults and children ages 2 and older:** apply to affected area t.i.d. or q.i.d.	• Tell patient not to bandage area tightly or use with heating pad. • Urge patient to notify doctor if symptoms worsen, persist for longer than 7 days, or recur. • Tell patient to avoid eyes, mucous membranes, broken or irritated skin, and wounds. • Caution patient to consult doctor before use if skin is red or irritated, or if he has impaired circulation or diabetes. • Warn patient to keep away from fire or flame and to avoid smoking until product dries. • Remind patient to let product dry before contacting clothing.
Icy Hot Balm menthol 7.6% methyl salicylate 29% **Icy Hot Cream** menthol 10% methyl salicylate 30%	*Relief from arthritis, sore muscles, backache, bursitis, body aches, and leg cramps* **Adults:** apply generous amount to affected area and massage until it disappears p.r.n.	• Caution against use with a heating pad. • Warn patient not to bandage tightly. • Tell patient to notify doctor if skin redness or irritation occurs, or if pain lasts longer than 10 days. • Tell patient to avoid eyes, mucous membranes, and broken or irritated skin.

Brand name and active ingredients	Indications and dosages	Nursing considerations
Mineral Ice menthol 2%	*Relief from minor aches and pains of muscles and joints caused by arthritis, sports injuries, backache, strains, sprains, and bruises* **Adults and children ages 2 and older:** apply to affected area t.i.d. or q.i.d.	• Tell patient that product may be used with wet or dry bandage or ice pack. • Warn against bandaging area tightly or using with topical drugs or a heating pad. • Warn patient not to apply to wounds or broken skin. • Tell patient to notify doctor if symptoms worsen, persist for longer than 7 days, or recur.
Sundown Osteo-Bi-Flex camphor 6% menthol 12% methyl salicylate 30%	*Relief from aches and pains of muscles and joints caused by arthritis* **Adults and children ages 2 and older:** apply to affected area t.i.d. or q.i.d.	• Caution patient to avoid eyes. • Warn patient not to apply to wounds or broken skin. • Tell patient to notify doctor if symptoms worsen, persist for longer than 7 days, or recur. • Caution against use with a heating pad. • Warn patient not to bandage area tightly. • Tell patient to notify doctor if arthritis symptoms occur in children younger than age 12.
Zostrix Sports capsaicin 0.075%	*Relief from minor aches and pains of muscles and joints caused by sprains, backache, strains, bruises, and arthritis* **Adults and children ages 2 and older:** apply thin film to affected area t.i.d. or q.i.d.	• Tell patient that temporary burning sensation may last several days. • Urge patient to apply after exercise or showering and to wash hands afterward. • Avoid eyes and broken skin. • Warn patient not to bandage area tightly. • Tell patient to notify doctor if symptoms worsen, persist for longer than 7 days, or recur.

Topical antibiotics

Brand name and active ingredients	Indications and dosages	Nursing considerations
Bactine First Aid Antibiotic Plus Anesthetic, Campho-Phenique First Aid Antibiotic Plus Pain Reliever Maximum Strength, Mycitracin Plus Pain Reliever, Spectrocin Plus, Triple Antibiotic Extra bacitracin 500 units/g lidocaine 4% neomycin 0.5% polymyxin B sulfate 10,000 units/g **Betadine First Aid Antibiotic + Pain Reliever** bacitracin 500 units/g polymyxin B sulfate 10,000 units/g pramoxine 1% **Mycitracin Triple Antibiotic First Aid Maximum Strength** bacitracin 500 units/g neomycin 0.5% polymyxin B sulfate 10,000 units/g **Neosporin Plus Maximum Strength First Aid** bacitracin 500 units/g neomycin 0.5% polymyxin B sulfate 10,000 units/g pramoxine 1%	*To treat or prevent superficial skin infections* **Adults and children:** apply to affected area q.d. to t.i.d.	• Tell patient not to get drug in his eyes. • Caution patient not to apply drug over large areas of body. • Urge patient to consult doctor for use in deep or puncture wounds, animal bites, or serious burns. • Tell patient to notify doctor if symptoms worsen or persist. • Warn patient not to use for longer than 7 days.

Components of oral rehydration solutions

Diarrhea and dehydration are common problems among children. To help correct the fluid loss and electrolyte imbalance that can result, you may administer an oral rehydration solution. The American Academy of Pediatrics recommends that oral rehydration solutions contain 75 to 90 mEq/L of sodium, 20 to 30 mEq/L of potassium, 30 mEq/L of bicarbonate, enough chloride to provide electroneutrality, and 2% to 3% glucose.

Osmolality should be about 300 mOsm/L. Maintenance solutions are similar but contain 40 to 60 mEq/L of sodium. The World Health Organization (WHO) has developed an oral rehydration solution to manage diarrhea caused by cholera in developing countries. It differs somewhat from American guidelines, as you'll see in this comparison of common oral rehydration solutions and home remedies for managing diarrhea.

Solution	Osmolality (mOsm/L)	Carbo-hydrates (g/L)	Sodium (mEq/L)	Potassium (mEq/L)	Chloride (mEq/L)	Bicar-bonate (mEq/L)
Rehydration						
WHO solution	310-333	20-25	90	20	80	30-80
Rehydrate	305	25	75	20	65	30 (citrate)
Maintenance						
Ricelyte	200	30	50	25	45	34 (citrate)
Resol	270	20	50	20	50	34 (citrate)
Pedialyte	249	25	45	20	35	30 (citrate)
Infalyte	200-290	20-30	50	25	45	34
Clear liquids						
Gatorade	330	46	20	3	17	3
Apple juice	650-734	120	0.1-3.5	24-32	30	-
Jello water	570-640	100-150	15-27	0.1-20	-	-
Ginger ale	520-560	53	0.8-5.5	0.1-1.5	2	-
Pedialyte Freezer Pops	-	25	45	20	35	30 (citrate)
Chicken broth	380-500	0	140-251	1.5-8.2	250	-

Sunscreens and sunblocks

Patients should avoid UV radiation if they have light skin, a history of one or more serious sunburns, blonde or red hair, a history of freckling, growths on lips or skin from sun exposure, or a need for therapy with a photosensitizing drug. If such a patient can't or won't stay indoors or wear protective clothing, the best choice is to use a sunscreen.

Sun protection factor
When selecting a product, the patient must consider sun protection factor (SPF), UVA/UVB protection, sunscreen base, and substantivity. (See *SPF product categories*.) The higher the SPF, the more effective the product is in preventing sunburn. If it normally takes 60 minutes for a patient to experience a bright erythematous sunburn, a sunscreen of SPF 6 will allow the patient to stay in the sun six times longer before receiving the same sunburn. An SPF of 15 blocks out 93% of UVB, an SPF of 30 blocks out 96.7%, an SPF of 40 blocks out 97.5%, and an SPF of 70 blocks out 98.6%. Because such small benefit is gained as SPF is increased beyond 30, the FDA publicizes that an SPF of 30 provides adequate protection for all skin types, including patients with UV-induced skin disorders.

Sunscreens primarily target UVB radiation (290 to 320 nm), which is responsible for causing skin cancer, nonmalignant skin tumors, and sunburn. During the past few years, focus has been placed on UVA radiation (320 to 400 nm) as well because it may be the cause of photoaging. Because the effect of UVA is still debatable, not all products contain UVA protection.

Base and skin type
A patient should also take into account the sunscreen base and his skin type. (See *Understanding skin types*.) Foams and sprays may contain substantial amounts of alcohol, which can cause contact dermatitis, photosensitivity, stinging, and drying of the skin. Oil bases may clog pores, leading to possible comedone formation. For patients with oily skin, an alcohol base

SPF product categories

SPF	Description
2-12	Minimal sunburn protection
12-30	Moderate sunburn protection
30+	High sunburn protection

SPF: Sun protection factor

may be preferred, whereas patients with dry or sensitive skin may choose a cream or lotion with a moisturizer that doesn't clog pores.

The efficacy of the sunscreen also depends on its ability to remain effective during prolonged exposure to sweat and water. If the product is labeled water and sweat resistant, it retains its SPF for at least 40 minutes. If the product is labeled very water and sweat resistant, it retains its SPF for at least 80 minutes. Some products may be labeled waterproof or sweat proof even though the FDA replaced these terms with very water and sweat resistant in 1998.

Sunscreens should be applied at least 30 minutes before sun exposure and reapplied as directed on the label. They should be applied liberally to all exposed areas.

Understanding skin types

Skin type	Sunburn and tanning profile
I	Always burns easily; never tans (sensitive)
II	Always burns easily; tans minimally (sensitive)
III	Burns moderately; tans gradually (normal)
IV	Burns minimally; always tans well (normal)
V	Rarely burns; tans profusely (insensitive)
VI	Never burns; deeply pigmented (insensitive)

OTC multivitamin ingredients

Product and manufacturer	Iron (mg)	A (IU)	D (IU)	E (IU)	B_1 (mg)
ADEKS Tablets (Scandipharm)		4,000	400	150	1.2
Advanced Formula Centrum Liquid (Lederle)	9	2,500	400	30	1.5
Albee C-800 (Robins)				45	15
Albee with C (Robins)					15
Albee-T Tablets (Robins)					15.5
Bounty Bears Plus Iron (NBTY)	15	2,500	400	15	1.05
Bugs Bunny Complete (Bayer)	18	5,000	400	30	1.5
Bugs Bunny Plus Iron (Bayer)	15	2,500	400	15	1.05
Bugs Bunny with Extra C (Bayer)		2,500	400	15	1.05
Centrum Tablets (Lederle)	18	5,000	400	30	1.5
Centrum Jr. & Extra Calcium (Lederle)	18	5,000	400	30	4.5
Centrum Silver (Lederle)		5,000	400	45	1.5
Children's Sunkist Multivitamin Complete (Ciba)	18	5,000	400	30	1.5

B_2 (mg)	B_3 (mg)	B_5 (mg)	B_6 (mg)	B_{12} (mcg)	C (mg)	Other contents
1.2	10	10	1.5	12	60	beta carotene (3 mg), biotin (50 mcg), fructose, vitamin K, zinc (1.1 mg)
1.7	20	10	2	6	60	biotin (300 mcg), chromium, iodine, manganese, selenium, zinc (15 mg)
17	100	25	25	12	800	
10.2	50	10	5		300	
10	100	23	8.2	5	500	
1.2	13.5		1.05	4.5	60	folic acid (0.3 mg)
1.7	20	10	2	6	60	aspartame, biotin (40 mcg), calcium (100 mg), copper, folic acid (400 mcg), iodine, magnesium, phenylalanine, zinc (3.3 mg)
1.2	13.5		1.05	4.5	60	
1.2	13.5		1.05	4.5	250	folic acid (0.3 mg)
1.7	20	10	2.0	6	60	calcium (162 mg), chromium, folic acid (400 mcg), iodine, leutin, magnesium (100 mg), nickel, phosphorus, potassium, selenium (20 mg), silicon, vanadium, zinc (15 mg)
1.7	20	10	2	6	60	biotin (45 mcg), calcium (108 mg), chromium, copper, folic acid (0.4 mg), iodine, manganese, molybdenum, phosphorus, vitamin K, zinc (15 mg)
1.7	20	10	3	25	60	biotin (30 mcg), boron, chlorine, chromium, copper, folic acid (400 mg), iodine, magnesium, manganese, molybdenum, nickel, phosphorus, potassium, selenium, silicon, vanadium, vitamin K, zinc (15 mg)
1.7	20	10	2	6	60	aspartame, biotin (40 mcg), folic acid (0.4 mg), phenylalanine, trace minerals, zinc (10 mg) *(continued)*

Product and manufacturer	Iron (mg)	A (IU)	D (IU)	E (IU)	B$_1$ (mg)
Dayalets Filmtabs (Abbott)		5,000	400	30	1.5
Flintstone's Children's (Bayer)		2,500	400	15	1.05
Flintstone's Complete Tablets (Bayer)	18	5,000	400	30	1.5
Flintstones Plus Calcium (Bayer)		2,500	400	15	1.05
Flintstones Plus Iron (Bayer)	15	2,500	400	15	1.05
Fosfree (Mission)	14.5	5,000	150		4.5
Fosfree Tablets (Mission)	28	3,000	300		9
Garfield Complete with Minerals (Menley & James)	18	5,000	400	30	1.5
Garfield Plus Extra C Chewable (Menley & James)		2,500	400	15	1.05
Geritol Extend Caplets (GlaxoSmithKline)	10	3,333	200	15	1.2
Gerivite Liquid (Goldline)					0.8
Hair Booster Vitamins (NBTY)	18				
ICAPS Plus Tablets (Ciba Vision)		6.000		60	
ICAPS Time Release (Ciba Vision)		7.000		100	
Lipogen Tablets (Goldline)		1.667		10	1.5
Multi-Day Tablets (NBTY)		5,000	400	30	1.5
Multi-Day Plus Minerals (NBTY)	18	6,500	400	30	1.7
Myadec Tablets (Parke Davis)	18	5,000	400	30	1.5

B$_2$ (mg)	B$_3$ (mg)	B$_5$ (mg)	B$_6$ (mg)	B$_{12}$ (mcg)	C (mg)	Other contents
1.7	20		2	6	60	folic acid (0.4 mg)
1.2	13.5		1.05	4.5	60	folic acid (0.3 mg), sucrose
1.7	20	10	2	6	60	biotin (40 mcg), folic acid (0.4 mg), trace minerals, zinc (15 mg)
1.2	13.5		1.05	4.5	60	calcium (200 mg), folic acid (0.3 mg)
1.2	13.5		1.05	4.5	60	folic acid (0.3 mg)
2	10.5	14	2.5	2	50	calcium (175.5 mg)
4	21	2	5	4	100	calcium (351 mg)
1.7	20	10	2	6	60	aspartame, biotin (40 mcg), folic acid (0.4 mg), phenylalanine, sorbitol, trace minerals, zinc (15 mg)
1.2	13.5		1.05	4.5	250	folic acid (0.3 mg)
1.4	15		2	2	60	calcium, folic acid (0.2 mg), selenium, trace minerals, vitamin K, zinc (15 mg)
0.4	8.3	1.7	0.2	0.2		alcohol (18%), choline, iodine, magnesium, manganese, sugar
	35	100		6		choline, copper, folic acid (0.4 mg), inositol, iodine, manganese, PABA, protein, zinc (15 mg)
20					200	copper, manganese, selenium, zinc (40 mg)
20					200	copper, strontium, zinc (40 mg)
0.33	0.33	3.3	1.7	0.33	100	choline (111 mg), copper, inositol (111 mg), selenium, zinc (10 mg)
1.7	20	10	2	6	60	
1.7	20	10	2	6	60	biotin (40 mcg), folic acid (0.4 mg), trace minerals, zinc (15 mg)
2	20	10	3	6	60	biotin (30 mcg), trace minerals, vitamin K, zinc (15 mg) *(continued)*

Product and manufacturer	Iron (mg)	A (IU)	D (IU)	E (IU)	B$_1$ (mg)
Natalins Tablets (Meade Johnson)	30	4,000	400	15	1.5
Nephro-Vite Vitamin B Complex (R&D)					1.5
Ocuvite Tablets (Lederle)		5,000		30	
Oncivite (Mission)		10,000	400	200	0.37
One-A-Day Essentials (Bayer)		5,000	400	30	1.5
One-A-Day Extra Antioxidant Softgels (Bayer)		5,000		200	
One-A-Day 55 Plus Tablets (Bayer)		6,000	400	60	4.5
One-A-Day Maximum Formula (Bayer)	18	5,000	400	30	1.5
Opticare PMS Tablets (Standard Drug)	2.5	2,083	17	14	4.2
Optilets-M-500 (Abbott)	20	5,000	400	30	15
Optilets-500 Filmtabs (Abbott)		5,000	400	30	15
Optivite PMT (Optimox)	2.5	2,083		16.6	4.2
Poly-Vi-Sol Tablets (Meade Johnson)		2,500	400	15	1.05
Poly-Vi-Sol with Iron (Meade Johnson)	12	2,500	400	15	1.05
Poly-V-Sol with Iron Drops (Meade Johnson)	10	1,500	400	5	0.5
Poly-Vitamin Drops (Schein)		1,500	400	5	0.5
Prenatal -S (Goldline)	60	4,000	400	11	1.5
Prenavite Tablets (Rugby)	60	4,000	400	11	1.5

B₂ (mg)	B₃ (mg)	B₅ (mg)	B₆ (mg)	B₁₂ (mcg)	C (mg)	Other contents
1.6	1.7		2.6	2.5	70	
1.7	20	10	10	6	60	biotin (300 mg), folic acid (0.8 mg)
					60	copper, selenium (40 mg), zinc (40 mg)
0.5	5	2.5	25	1.5	500	folic acid (0.4 mg)
1.7	20	10	2	6	60	folic acid (0.4 mg)
					250	copper, manganese, selenium, zinc (7.5 mg)
3.4	20	20	6	25	120	biotin (30 mcg), calcium (220 mg), trace minerals, vitamin K, zinc (15 mg)
1.7	20	10	2	6	60	biotin (30 mcg), folic acid (0.4 mg), trace minerals, zinc (15 mg)
4.2	4.2	4.2	50	10.4	250	amylase, protease, and lipase activity; bioflavonoids; biotin (10.4 mg); choline; folic acid (0.03 mg); inositol; PABA; rutin; trace minerals
10	100	20	5	12	500	copper, iodine, magnesium, manganese
10	100	20	5	12	500	
4.2	4.2	4.2	50	10.4	250	betaine, biotin, choline, folic acid (0.03 mg), inositol, PABA, pancreatin, rutin, trace minerals
1.2	13.5		1.05	4.5	60	folic acid (0.3 mg), sugar
1.2	13.5		1.05	4.5	60	copper, folic acid (0.3 mg), sugar, zinc (8 mg)
0.6	8		0.4		35	(Contents listed are per 1 ml.)
0.6	8		0.4	2	35	
1.7	18		2.6	4	100	calcium (200 mg), folic acid (0.8 mg), zinc (25 mg)
1.7	18		2.6	4	100	calcium (200 mg), folic acid (0.8 mg), zinc (25 mg) *(continued)*

Product and manufacturer	Iron (mg)	A (IU)	D (IU)	E (IU)	B₁ (mg)
Protegra Softgels		5,000	200		
Sesame Street Complete (McNeil-CPC)	10	2,750	200	10	0.75
Sesame Street Plus Extra C Tablets (McNeil-CPC)		2,750	200	10	0.75
Sesame Street Plus Iron (McNeil-CPC)	10	2,750	200	10	0.75
Stresstabs Tablets (Lederle)				30	10
Stress Formula 600 (Vanguard)				30	15
Stress-600 with Zinc (Nion)				45	20
Stresstabs + Zinc (Lederle)				30	10
Stuart Formula Tablets (J&J-Merck)	5	5,000	400	10	1.5
Stuart Prenatal Tablets (Wyeth-Ayerst)	60	4,000	400	11	1.8
Therabid Tablets (Mission)		5,000	200	30	15
Theragran Tablets (Mead Johnson)		5,000	400	30	3
Theragran Antioxidants (Mead Johnson)		5,000		200	
Theragran-M Caps (Mead Johnson)	27	5,000	400	30	3
Theravite Liquid (Barre-National)		10,000	400		10
Tri-Vi-Sol with Iron Drops (Mead-Johnson)	10	1,500	400		
Unicap Tablets (Upjohn)		5,000	400	30	1.5
Unicap Plus Iron Tablets (Upjohn)	22.5	5,000	400	30	1.5
Unicap Sr. Tablets (Upjohn)	10	5,000	200	15	1.2

B_2 (mg)	B_3 (mg)	B_5 (mg)	B_6 (mg)	B_{12} (mcg)	C (mg)	Other contents
		5			250	copper, manganese, selenium, zinc
0.85	10		0.7	3	40	biotin (15 mg), calcium (80 mg), copper, folic acid (0.2 mg), iodine, magnesium, sucrose, zinc (8 mg)
0.85	10	5	0.7	3	80	folic aid (0.2 mg), sucrose
0.85	10	5	0.7	3	40	folic acid (0.2 mg)
10	100	20	5	12	500	biotin (45 mcg), folic acid (0.4 mg)
10	100	20	5	12	500	folic acid (0.4 mg)
10	100	25	10	25	600	biotin (45 mcg), copper, folic acid (0.4 mg), zinc (5.5 mg)
10	100	20	5	12	500	biotin (45 mcg), copper, folic acid (0.4 mg), zinc (23.9 mg)
1.7	20		1	3	50	calcium, copper, folic acid (0.1 mg), iodine
1.7	18		2.6	4	100	calcium (200 mg), folic acid (0.8 mg), zinc (25 mg)
10	100	20	10	5	500	
3.4	20	10	3	9	90	biotin (30 mcg), folic acid (0.4 mg), lactose
					250	copper, manganese, selenium, zinc
3.4	20	10	3	9	90	biotin (30 mcg), calcium (40 mg), folate (400 mcg), lactose, sucrose, trace minerals, zinc (15 mg)
10	100	21	4.1	5	200	sugar (Contents listed are per 5 ml.)
					35	fruit flavor (Contents listed are per 1 ml.)
1.7	20		2	6	60	
1.7	20	10	2	6	60	calcium, folic acid (0.4 mg)
1.4	16	10	2.2	3	60	folic acid (0.4 mg), trace minerals, zinc (15 mg) *(continued)*

Product and manufacturer	Iron (mg)	A (IU)	D (IU)	E (IU)	B_1 (mg)
Unicap T Tablets (Upjohn)	18	5,000	400	30	10
Vi-Daylin Tablets (Ross)		2,500	400	15	1.05
Vi-Daylin Multivitamin + Iron (Ross)	10	1,500	400	5	0.5
Vita Bee with C (Rugby)					15
Vicon-C Capsules (Whitby)					20
Vicon Plus (Whitby)		4,000		50	10
Vitalets (Freeda)	10	5,000	400	5	2.5
Z-Bec Tablets (Robins)				45	15
Z-Gen Tablets (Goldline)				45	15

B$_2$ (mg)	B$_3$ (mg)	B$_5$ (mg)	B$_6$ (mg)	B$_{12}$ (mcg)	C (mg)	Other contents
10	100	25	6	18	500	copper, folic acid (0.4 mg), iodine, manganese, potassium, selenium, zinc (15 mg)
1.2	13.5		1.05	4.5	60	folic acid (0.3 mg), sucrose
0.6	8		0.4		35	alcohol (< 0.5%), fruit flavor (Contents listed are per 1 ml.)
10.2	50	10	5		300	
10	100	20	5		300	magnesium, zinc sulfate (80 mg)
5	25	10	2		150	magnesium, manganese, zinc (18 mg)
0.9	20	3	2	5	60	biotin (25 mcg), calcium, manganese
10.2	100	25	10	6	600	zinc (22.5 mg)
10.2	100	25	10	6	600	zinc (5.2 mg)

Selected sugar-free OTC drugs

Patients with diabetes should choose sugar-free OTC drugs if possible, such as those listed here. But keep in mind that sugar-free drugs may contain other sources of carbohydrates, such as fructose, sorbitol, or alcohol. Advise patients to carefully read each product's ingredients to look for carbohydrates.

Drug	Manufacturer
Analgesics	
Children's Myapap Elixir	My-K Labs
Infant's Panadol Drops	Bayer Consumer
Children's Tylenol Oral Suspension Liquid	McNeil Consumer
Children's Tylenol Allergy-D	McNeil Consumer
Infant's Tylenol Drops	McNeil Consumer
Infant's Tylenol Suspension Drops	McNeil Consumer
Tempra 1 Drops	Bristol-Myers
Tempra 2 Syrup	Bristol-Myers
Antacids and antigas medications	
Alka-Mints	Bayer Consumer
Amphojel Suspension	Wyeth-Ayerst
Amphojel Tablets	Wyeth-Ayerst
Di-Gel Liquid	Schering-Plough
Gaviscon Liquid	GlaxoSmithKline
Gelusil Liquid	Warner-Lambert
Pepto-Bismol Liquid	Proctor & Gamble
Pepto-Bismol Tablets	Proctor & Gamble
Riopan Plus Suspension	Whitehall-Robins
Riopan Suspension	Whitehall-Robins
Tagamet HB Tablets	GlaxoSmithKline
Titralac Plus Liquid	3M
Titralac Plus Tablets	3M
Titralac Tablets	3M
Tums E-X Chewable Tablet	GlaxoSmithKline
Antidiarrheals	
Donnagel Chewable Tablets	Wyeth-Ayerst
Donnagel Liquid	Wyeth-Ayerst
Pepto-Bismol Liquid	Proctor & Gamble
Pepto-Bismol Tablets	Proctor & Gamble

Drug	Manufacturer
Calcium supplements	
Caltrate 600 Tablets	Lederle
Cough and cold medications	
Cepacol Sore Throat Children's Liquid	J.B. Williams
Diabetic Tussin Allergy Relief Medication	Health Care Products
Diabetic Tussin C Expectorant Liquid	Health Care Products
Diabetic Tussin DM Liquid	Health Care Products
Diabetic Tussin DM Maximum Strength Liquid	Health Care Products
Dimetane D-C Oral Syrup	Whitehall-Robins
Dimetapp Allergy Children's Elixir	Whitehall-Robins
Phanatuss Syrup	Pharmakon
Scot-Tussin DM Cough Chasers Lozenge	Scot-Tussin
Scot-Tussin DM	Scot-Tussin
Scot-Tussin Expectorant	Scot-Tussin
Scot-Tussin Senior Clear	Scot-Tussin
Laxatives	
Citrucel	GlaxoSmithKline
Metamucil Smooth Texture Sugar Free	Proctor & Gamble
Mouth and sore throat medications	
Anbesol Oral Gel	Whitehall-Robins
Baby Orajel Liquid	Del Pharmaceuticals
Cepacol Maximum Strength Spray	J.B. Williams
Cepacol Sore Throat Lozenge	J.B. Williams
Cheracol Sore Throat	Lee Pharm
Diabetic Tussin Cough Drops Lozenge	Health Care Products
N'Ice	Heritage Consumer
Robitussin Lozenge	Whitehall-Robins
Sucrets Throat Spray	GlaxoSmithKline
Vitamin and mineral supplements	
Bugs Bunny Complete	Bayer Consumer
Bugs Bunny with Extra C Children's	Bayer Consumer
Bugs Bunny Vitamins Plus Iron	Bayer Consumer
Tri-Vi-Sol	Mead Johnson
Vi-Daylin	Ross
Vi-Daylin Plus Iron ADC Drops	Ross

Patient-teaching aids

The following pages contain six patient-teaching aids that you can use to augment your verbal teaching about OTC medications. These aids explain in clear and simple terms how to take all common medication types safely and effectively. Feel free to photocopy the appropriate aid and give it to your patient as part of your usual teaching plan.

❏ Taking tablets or capsules
❏ Taking liquid drugs
❏ Giving an oral drug to a child
❏ Using eyedrops
❏ Using eardrops
❏ Using a vaginal medication

Taking tablets or capsules

❏ First, wash your hands. Then gather everything you need, such as the drug, a glass of water or juice and, if you plan to crush a tablet, a commercial pill crusher. If you need to divide a scored tablet, get a knife or a pill-splitter.

❏ Look at the drug container to make sure you have the right drug and the right dose.

❏ Never crush or open tablets or capsules that have a special coating. Doing so may change the drug's effectiveness by changing the way your body absorbs the drug. Ask your doctor or pharmacist if it's safe for you to crush or open a drug.

❏ Pour the prescribed number of tablets or capsules into the bottle cap. If too many pour out, drop the extra tablets or capsules back into the container without touching them. Doing so may contaminate the drug remaining in the bottle. Now pour the drug from the cap into your hand.

❏ Place the tablets or capsules as far back on your tongue as you can. You may do this with one tablet or capsule at a time or all of them at once.

❏ Tip your head slightly *forward* to prevent choking or coughing; take a drink of water or juice, and swallow.

❏ Take coated tablets with plenty of water or juice.

❏ If you have trouble swallowing a tablet or capsule, moisten your mouth with some water or juice before you take the tablet. If permissible, it may also help to crush an uncoated tablet, open a soft capsule, or split a tablet.

❏ Protect tablets and capsules from light, humidity, and air. If the drug changes color or has an unusual odor, discard it. Also discard all drugs according to the manufacturer's expiration date.

Taking liquid drugs

❏ First, wash your hands. Then get the medication and a medicine cup. Look at the container to make sure you have the right drug and to check the recommended dosage. If the drug is in a suspension, shake it vigorously before proceeding.

❏ Uncap the bottle and place the cap upside down on a clean surface to prevent contaminating the inside of the cap.

❏ Many over-the-counter liquid drugs come with a dose cap for customer convenience. These cups aren't interchangeable among different drugs, and one cupful doesn't equal one dose. Keep the dose cup with the drug it came with, and always read the label carefully and completely.

❏ Locate the marking for the recommended dose on the medicine cup. Keeping your thumbnail on the mark, hold the cup at eye level and pour in the correct amount of drug. Place the cup safely on a flat surface. Check the dose you have measured by looking at the top of the liquid from eye level. Swallow the drug.

❏ Wipe the bottle's lip with a damp paper towel, taking care not to touch the inside of the bottle. Replace the bottle cap.

❏ Wash the medicine cup with soap and hot water. Store the drug as directed on the label.

❏ When pouring liquid OTC drugs, keep the label next to your palm. This way, if any liquid spills or drips, it won't ruin the label.

❏ If you pour out too much liquid, discard the excess. Don't return it to the bottle.

❏ If a liquid drug has an unpleasant taste, consider sucking on ice to numb your tastebuds before taking the drug. You may also wish to chill an oily liquid before taking it.

❏ To relieve a bitter taste after swallowing the drug, suck on a piece of sugarless hard candy or chew a piece of gum. Gargling or rinsing your mouth with water or mouthwash may also help.

❏ Keep all drugs out of the reach of children.

❏ Don't hesitate to ask your doctor or pharmacist about drugs and any directions you don't understand.

Giving an oral drug to a child

❐ Approach your child in a matter-of-fact but friendly manner. Act as though you expect his cooperation, and praise him when he cooperates.

❐ Never guess at the amount of medication your child should receive. Children aren't small adults, and half an adult dose may be too much. Also, don't measure a dose of liquid medication using a teaspoon or tablespoon from your kitchen— the measurement won't be accurate. Instead, buy a measured-dose vial or oral syringe at the drugstore or supermarket.

❐ Many over-the-counter liquid medications come with a dose cap for customer convenience. These cups aren't interchangeable among different drugs, and one cupful doesn't equal one dose. Keep the dose cup with the medication it came with, and always read the label carefully and completely.

❐ Don't confuse the abbreviations for teaspoon (tsp) and tablespoon (tbs).

❐ Give an older child choices, if possible, to give him a sense of control. For example, offer him a choice of beverage to take with (or after) the medication (unless the label recommends not to give the medication with certain beverages or foods).

❐ Explain the relationship between illness and treatment to an older child. He may be more cooperative if he realizes that the medication will help him get better.

❐ Place a tablet or capsule near the back of your child's tongue and give him plenty of water or flavored drink to help swallow it. Then make sure he swallows it.

❐ Encourage your child to tip his head *forward* when swallowing a tablet or capsule. Throwing his head back increases the risk of inhaling the medication and choking.

❐ Give medication to an infant in a manner similar to feeding. Giving medication through a bottle's nipple, for example, takes advantage of the infant's natural sucking reflex. To make sure the infant gets the full dose, don't mix the medication with formula—he may not eat it all. What's more, he may refuse to take the formula afterward. *(continued)*

❐ You can also give infants medication through a medicine dropper. Place the dropper between the gum and cheek and toward the back of the mouth to prevent gagging. Squeeze gently. Don't squirt medication directly into the throat—it may cause choking.

❐ If you mix medication in food or fluids, use as little food or fluid as possible. Otherwise, the child may not be able to finish it all and won't get the correct dose.

❐ Be honest and careful. Never try to trick a child into taking medication. Doing so may make him resist you the next time he has to take it.

❐ Never tell a child that medication is candy. He may try to take more than the recommended dose.

❐ Don't promise that the medication will taste good if you've never tasted it or if you know that it doesn't taste good.

❐ Don't force your child to swallow his medication or try to hold his nose or mouth shut to promote swallowing. Doing so may cause choking.

❐ Don't try to give medication to a crying child; he could choke on it.

❐ Make sure you understand what side effects can occur and what constitutes an allergic reaction.

❐ Never threaten, insult, or embarrass your child if he doesn't cooperate. These actions can lead to resistance.

❐ If you can't get your child to take the medication, consult your pharmacist. The medication may come in another form that your child can tolerate.

❐ Keep all medication away from a place where your child could accidentally take it. Always use the child-resistant cap.

❐ Ask your poison control center to send you poison prevention stickers to apply to all medication containers. Teach children that the sticker means, "Stay away! Only a grownup can give this to me." Post the poison control center's number near your telephone.

❐ Note the time you gave the medication so you know when it's safe to give another dose, if needed.

Using eyedrops

❐ Begin by washing your hands thoroughly.

❐ Hold the medication bottle up to the light and examine it. If the solution is discolored or contains sediment, don't use it. Instead, take it back to the pharmacy and have it checked.

❐ If the medication looks okay, warm it to room temperature by holding the bottle between your hands for 2 minutes.

❐ Moisten a cottonball or a tissue with water and clean any secretions from around your eyes. Use a fresh cottonball or tissue for each eye. Be sure to wipe outward in one motion, starting from the area nearest your nose. Use a new tissue or cottonball for each wipe.

❐ Stand or sit before a mirror, or lie on your back, whichever is most comfortable.

❐ Tilt your head back slightly and toward the eye you're placing the drops in. Gently pull down your lower eyelid to expose your conjunctival sac (the inside of your lower eyelid).

❐ Position the dropper over the conjunctival sac and steady your hand holding the dropper by resting two fingers against your cheek or nose.

❐ Look up at the ceiling. Then squeeze the recommended number of drops into the sac. Take care not to touch the dropper to your eye, eyelashes, or fingers. Wipe away excess medication with a clean tissue.

❐ Release the lower lid. Try to keep your eye open without blinking for at least 30 seconds. Apply gentle pressure to the corner of your eye at the bridge of your nose for 1 minute. This will prevent the medication from being absorbed through your tear duct.

❐ Repeat the procedure in the other eye.

❐ Recap the bottle and store it away from light and heat.

Using eardrops

❒ Wash your hands with warm, soapy water and dry thoroughly.

❒ Warm the eardrops for comfort by holding the bottle in your hands for at least 2 minutes. Never place eardrops in the microwave or in hot water to warm the solution. Shake the bottle, as directed, and open it.

❒ Fill the dropper; then place the open bottle and dropper within easy reach.

❒ Lie on your side to expose the ear you're treating.

❒ An adult can straighten his ear canal by gently pulling the top of the ear up and back. For a child, gently pull down and back on the earlobe.

❒ Position the dropper above the ear, taking care not to touch it to the ear. Squeeze the dropper's bulb to release one drop at a time.

❒ Wait until you feel (or the child feels) the drop go in the ear. Then release another drop. Repeat these steps until you have given the recommended number of drops. To keep the drops from running out of the ear, remain on your side or keep the child on his side for about 10 minutes.

❒ Or, to keep the medication from running out of your ear, you may place a cotton-ball with a dab of petroleum jelly *at the very entrance to the ear canal.* Never place anything into the ear canal. Remove the cottonball after 1 hour.

❒ Wipe the dropper with a clean tissue, recap the bottle, and store it away from light and extreme heat, or as directed on the label.

❒ Call your doctor if the drops cause dizziness, ringing in the ear, hearing loss, severe discomfort, motion sickness, or foul-smelling drainage. Also call the doctor if symptoms are persistent despite self-treatment.

Using a vaginal medication

❑ Plan to insert your vaginal medication after bathing and just before bedtime to make sure it will stay in your vagina for the appropriate amount of time.

❑ Collect the equipment you'll need, including the medication, an applicator, water-soluble lubricating jelly, a towel, and a sanitary pad.

❑ Empty your bladder, wash your hands, and place the towel on the bed. Sit on the towel, and open the medication wrapper or container.

❑ Place the vaginal suppository or tablet in the applicator, or fill the applicator with medicated cream, ointment, or jelly. Some products have a prefilled applicator.

❑ To make insertion easier, lubricate the suppository or applicator tip with water or water-soluble lubricating jelly. Don't use petroleum jelly; it may interfere with absorption.

❑ Lie down on the bed with your knees flexed and legs spread apart.

❑ Spread apart your labia with one hand and insert the applicator tip into your vagina with the other hand.

❑ Advance the applicator about 2 inches, angling it slightly toward your tailbone.

❑ Push the plunger to insert the medication. The medication may feel cold.

❑ Remove the applicator and discard it if it's disposable. If it's reusable, wash it thoroughly with soap and water, dry it with a paper towel, and return it to its container.

❑ Remain lying down for about 30 minutes so that the medication won't leak out of your vagina. Wear a sanitary pad to avoid staining your clothes or bed linens.

OTC drug resources

Consumer Healthcare Products Association
1150 Connecticut Avenue, NW
Washington, DC 20036-4193
Tel: (202) 429-9260
Fax: (202) 223-6835
www.chpa-info.org

Cosmetic, Toiletry, and Fragrance Association
1101 17th Street, NW, Suite 300
Washington, DC 20036-4702
Tel: (202) 331-1770
Fax: (202) 331-1969
www.ctfa.org

Council on Family Health
1155 Connecticut Avenue, NW, Suite 400
Washington, DC 20036
Tel: (202) 429-6600
www.cfhinfo.org

Federal Consumer Information Center
Tel: (800) 688-9889
www.pueblo.gsa.gov

Federal Trade Commission
CRC-240
Washington, DC 20580
Tel: (877) 382-4357
www.ftc.gov

Food and Drug Law Institute
1000 Vermont Avenue, NW, Suite 200
Washington, DC 20005-4903
Tel: (202) 371-1420
Fax: (202) 371-0649
www.fdli.org

National Consumers League
1701 K Street, NW, Suite 1201
Washington, DC 20006
Tel: (202) 835-3323
Fax: (202) 835-0747
www.natlconsumersleague.org

National Institutes of Health
U.S. Department of Health and Human Services
Bethesda, MD 20892
Tel: (301) 496-4000
www.nih.gov

Office of Dietary Supplements
National Institutes of Health
31 Center Drive, Room 1B29
Bethesda, MD 20892-2086
Tel: (301) 435-2920
Fax: (301) 480-1845
http://dietary-supplements.info.nih.gov

U. S. Food and Drug Administration
5600 Fishers Lane
Rockville, MD 20857-0001
Tel: (888) 463-6332
www.fda.gov

Acknowledgments

We would like to thank the following companies for granting us permission to include their drugs in the full-color photoguide.

American Home Products Corporation

Advil® 200-mg Tablets, Caplets, Gel Caplets, Liqui-Gels®

Advil® Cold & Sinus Caplets, Tablets

Advil® Migraine 200-mg Liquid Filled Capsules

Childrens Advil® 50-mg Chewable Tablets: fruit and grape

Junior Strength Advil® 100-mg Coated Tablets, Chewable Tablets: fruit and grape

Aspirin-free Anacin® Extra Strength 500-mg Tablets

Axid® AR 75-mg Tablets

Caltrate® 600 Tablets

Caltrate® 600 + D Tablets

Caltrate® 600 Plus Chewable Tablets: assorted fruit flavors

Centrum® Silver® Tablets

Centrum® Tablets

Primatene® Tablets

Robitussin® Cold/Cold & Congestion Non-drowsy Formula Caplets and Softgels

Robitussin® Cold Multi-Symptom Cold & Flu Non-drowsy Formula Caplets and Softgels

Robitussin® Cold Severe Congestion Non-drowsy Formula Softgels

Robitussin® Cold Sinus & Congestion Caplets

Bayer Corporation Consumer Care Division

Aleve® 220-mg Tablets, Caplets, Gelcaps

Alka-Seltzer® Gas Relief Maximum Strength Liquid Softgels

Alka-Seltzer® Original, Lemon-lime, Cherry Effervescent Tablets

Alka-Seltzer Plus® Cold & Cough Liqui-Gels

Alka-Seltzer Plus® Cold & Flu Non-drowsy Liqui-Gels

Alka-Seltzer Plus® Cold & Sinus Non-drowsy Liqui-Gels

Alka-Seltzer Plus® Cold Liqui-Gels

Alka-Seltzer Plus® Night-Time Cold Liqui-Gels

Aspirin Regimen Bayer® Adult Low Strength 81-mg Enteric Coated Tablets

Aspirin Regimen Bayer® Adult Low Strength 81-mg with Calcium Caplets

Aspirin Regimen Bayer® Children's 81-mg Chewable Tablets: cherry and orange

Aspirin Regimen Bayer® Regular Strength 325-mg Enteric Coated Caplets

Extra Strength Bayer® Aspirin 500-mg Caplets, Gelcaps

Extra Strength Bayer® Aspirin Arthritis Pain Regimen 500-mg Caplets

Extra Strength Bayer® Plus
500-mg Caplets
Extra Strength Bayer® PM
Aspirin Plus Sleep Aid
Caplets
Genuine Bayer® Aspirin 325-mg
Tablets, Caplets, Gelcaps
Phillips'® Liqui-Gels®

Bristol-Myers Products
Extra Strength Excedrin®
Tablets, Caplets, Geltabs
Aspirin Free Excedrin® Extra
Strength Caplets, Geltabs
Aspirin Free Excedrin PM®
Tablets, Caplets, Geltabs
Excedrin® Migraine Tablets,
Caplets, Geltabs
Theragran-M® Advanced
Tablets

GlaxoSmithKline Consumer Healthcare, L.P.
Contac® 12 Hour Cold Non-
Drowsy Caplets
Contac® Day & Night
Allergy/Sinus Caplets
Contac® Day & Night Cold/Flu
Caplets
Contac® Severe Cold & Flu
Maximum Strength Caplets
Contac® Severe Cold & Flu
Non-drowsy Formula Caplets
Ecotrin® Adult Low Strength
81-mg Tablets
Ecotrin® Maximum Strength
Arthritis Relief 500-mg
Tablets
Ecotrin® Regular Strength
325-mg Tablets
Nicorette® 2-mg Gum original,
mint, orange
Nicorette® 4-mg Gum original,
mint, orange

Os-cal® 500 Tablets
Os-cal® 500+D Tablets
Tagamet HB 200® Tablets
Tums® Regular Strength
Peppermint Tablets

Johnson & Johnson–Merck Consumer Pharmaceuticals Co.
Mylanta® Gas Maximum
Strength Chewable Tablets:
mint
Mylanta® Gelcaps
Mylanta® Ultra Tabs Tablets:
cherry and mint
Pepcid AC® Tablets, Chewable
Tablets, Gelcaps

McNeil Consumer Brands, Inc. and McNeil-PPC, Inc.
Imodium® A-D Caplets
Imodium® Advanced Chewable
Tablets: mint
Lactaid® Extra Strength Caplets
Lactaid® Original Strength
Caplets
Lactaid® Ultra Caplets,
Chewable Tablets: vanilla
Children's Motrin® 50-mg
Chewable Tablets: orange
Junior Strength Motrin®
100-mg Caplets, Chewable
Tablets: orange
Motrin® Cold and Flu Caplets
Motrin® IB 200-mg Tablets,
Caplets, Gelcaps
Motrin® Migraine 200-mg
Caplets
Motrin® Sinus/Headache Non-
drowsy formula Caplets
Children's Tylenol® Allergy-D
Chewable Tablets: bubble
gum

Children's Tylenol® Cold
Chewable Tablets: grape

Children's Tylenol® Cold Plus
Cough Chewable Tablets:
cherry

Children's Tylenol® Sinus
Chewable Tablets: fruit burst

Junior Strength Tylenol®
160-mg Chewable Tablets:
fruit and grape

Tylenol® Allergy Sinus
Maximum Strength Multi-
Symptom Gelcaps

Tylenol® Arthritis Extended
Relief 650-mg Caplets

Tylenol® Cold Multi-Symptom
Complete Formula Caplets

Tylenol® Extra Strength 500-mg
Caplets, Gelcaps, Geltabs,
Tablets

Tylenol® Flu Maximum
Strength NightTime Gelcaps

Tylenol® PM Extra Strength
Caplets, Gelcaps, Geltabs

Tylenol® Regular Strength
325-mg Tablets

Tylenol® Sinus Non-drowsy
Maximum Strength Caplets,
Gelcaps, Geltabs

Novartis Consumer Health, Inc.

Ex-lax® Chocolated Regular
Strength Pieces

Ex-lax® Gentle Strength
Laxative Plus Stool Softener
Caplets

Ex-lax® Maximum Strength
Laxative Pills

Ex-lax® Regular Strength
Laxative Pills

Gas-X® Extra Strength 125-mg
Chewable Tablets: cherry and
peppermint

Gas-X® Regular Strength
80-mg Chewable Tablets:
cherry and peppermint

Maalox® Anti-Gas Extra
Strength Tablets: peppermint

Maalox® Quick Dissolve
Maximum Strength Chewable
Tablets: assorted flavors

Maalox® Quick Dissolve
Regular Strength Chewable
Tablets: assorted flavors

Tavist® Allergy Tablets

Tavist® Sinus Non-drowsy
Caplets

TheraFlu® Maximum Strength
Non-Drowsy Flu, Cold &
Cough Caplets

Triaminic® Softchews® Cold &
Allergy: orange

Triaminic® Softchews® Cold &
Cough: cherry

Triaminic® Softchews® Cough
& Sore Throat: grape

Schering Corporation and Schering-Plough Healthcare Products, Inc.

Chlor-Trimeton® Allergy
4-Hour Tablets

Chlor-Trimeton® Allergy
8-Hour Tablets

Chlor-Trimeton® Allergy
12-Hour Tablets

Chlor-Trimeton® Allergy-D
4-Hour Tablets

Chlor-Trimeton® Allergy-D
12-Hour Tablets

Correctol® Tablets, Caplets,
Softgels

The Proctor & Gamble Co.
Pepto-Bismol® Caplets,
   Chewable Tablets
Vicks® DayQuil® LiquiCaps®
Vicks® NyQuil® LiquiCaps®

Warner-Lambert Consumer Healthcare
Benadryl® Allergy Kapseals®
Benadryl® Allergy Ultratab®
   Tablets
Benadryl® Allergy/Cold Tablets
Benadryl® Allergy/Congestion
   Tablets
Benadryl® Allergy & Sinus
   Fastmelt Dissolving Tablets:
   cherry
Benadryl® Allergy/Sinus
   Headache Caplets, Gelcaps
Benadryl® Dye-Free Allergy
   Liqui-gels® Softgels
Rolaids® Antacid Tablets:
   peppermint, spearmint, cherry
Rolaids® Extra Strength Tablets:
   fruit
Children's Sudafed® Nasal
   Decongestant Chewables:
   orange
Sudafed® 12-hour Caplets
   120 mg
Sudafed® 24-hour Tablets
   240 mg
Sudafed® Maximum Strength
   Cold & Allergy Tablets
Sudafed® Maximum Strength
   Nasal Decongestant 30-mg
   Tablets
Sudafed® Maximum Strength
   Non-Drying Sinus Liquid
   Caps
Sudafed® Maximum Strength
   Severe Cold Formula Caplets,
   Tablets

Sudafed® Multi-Symptom
   Cold & Cough Liquid Caps
Sudafed® Multi-Symptom
   Cold & Sinus Liquid Caps
Sudafed® Sinus Headache
   Caplets
Zantac 75® Tablets

Index

---

t refers to a table; **boldface** refers to full-color photographs

t refers to a table; **boldface** refers to full-color photographs